RESPIRATORY
CARE

H A N D B O O K

RESPIRATORY CARE
HANDBOOK

Springhouse Corporation
Springhouse, Pennsylvania

STAFF FOR THIS VOLUME

CLINICAL STAFF

Clinical Director
Barbara McVan, RN

Clinical Editors
Helen Hahler D'Angelo, RN, MSN; Mary Chapman Gyetvan, RN, BSEd; Judith A. Schilling McCann, RN, BSN

PUBLICATION STAFF

Executive Director, Editorial
Stanley Loeb

Executive Director, Creative Services
Jean Robinson

Editorial Director
Matthew Cahill

Design
John Hubbard (art director), Stephanie Peters (associate art director), Mary Stangl

Editing
Regina Ford, Diane Labus, David Moreau

Copy Editing
David Prout (supervisor), Nick Anastasio, Keith de Pinho, Elizabeth B. Kiselev, Doris Weinstock, Debra Young

Art Production
Robert Perry (manager), Mark Marcin, Loretta Caruso, Anna Brindisi, Donald Knauss, Robert Wieder, Christina McKinley

Typography
David Kosten (manager), Diane Paluba (assistant manager), Nancy Wirs, Brenda Mayer, Joyce Rossi Biletz, Robin Rantz, Brent Rinedoller, Valerie L. Rosenberger

Manufacturing
Deborah Meiris (manager), T.A. Landis

Project Coordination
Aline S. Miller (supervisor), Laurie J. Sander

Library of Congress Cataloging-in-Publication Data
Respiratory care handbook.
    p.   cm.
  Includes bibliographies and index.
  1. Respiratory therapy—Handbooks, manuals, etc. 2. Respiratory disease nursing—Handbooks, manuals, etc. I. Springhouse Corporation.
  [DNLM: 1. Respiratory Therapy—handbooks. 2. Respiratory Tract Diseases—therapy—handbooks. WF 39 R434]
RC735.I5R475 1989 616.2'0046—dc19 88-22435
ISBN 0-87434-163-9

CONTENTS

ADVISORY BOARD, CONTRIBUTORS, AND CONSULTANTS

ADVISORY BOARD

CONTRIBUTORS

Joan M. Bauman, RN, BSN, CCRN, Critical Care Clinical Instructor, Holy Cross Hospital, Silver Spring, Md.

Patrice A. Castle, BS, PT, Owner, Prime Physical Therapy Group, Inc., Bala Cynwyd, Pa.

Karen Hahn, RN, MSN, Assistant Professor, Marquette University College of Nursing, Milwaukee

Amy Perrin Ross, RN, MSN, CNRN, Neuroscience Clinical Nurse Specialist, Loyola University Medical Center, Maywood, Ill.

Margaret M. Stevens, RN, BSN, C-NP, Neurosurgery Nurse Practitioner, University of Maryland Hospital/Maryland Institute of Emergency Medical Services Systems, Baltimore

Janet D'Agostino Taylor, RN, MSN, Pulmonary Rehabilitation Clinical Specialist, St. Elizabeth's Hospital, Boston

Kathy M. Witta, RN, MSN, CCRN, Critical Care Clinical Nurse Specialist, Intermediate Medical Care Unit, The Hospital of the University of Pennsylvania, Philadelphia

SPECIAL PROJECT CONSULTANT AND CONTRIBUTOR

Patricia L. Carroll, RN, RRT, BS, Independent Nurse Consultant, Fellow of the Litchfield (Conn.) Institute

CONSULTANTS

Patrice A. Castle, BS, PT, Owner, Prime Physical Therapy Group, Inc., Bala Cynwyd, Pa.

Janet D'Agostino Taylor, RN, MSN, Pulmonary Rehabilitation Clinical Specialist, St. Elizabeth's Hospital, Boston

Cindy Dillon, RN, BSN, MS, Pediatric Pulmonary Clinical Nurse Specialist, St. Christopher's Hospital—Cystic Fibrosis Center, Philadelphia

Marie O'Toole, RN, BSN, MSN, Assistant Professor, Jefferson University—Allied Health Services, Philadelphia

Gloria Sonnesso, RN, MSN, CCRN, Pulmonary Clinical Nurse Specialist, Hahnemann University Hospital, Philadelphia

Kathy M. Witta, RN, MSN, CCRN, Critical Care Clinical Nurse Specialist, Intermediate Medical Care Unit, The Hospital of the University of Pennsylvania, Philadelphia

FOREWORD

Today, with growing numbers of acutely ill patients to care for and increasingly complex treatments to master, you'll be challenged to provide competent respiratory care. To respond to this challenge confidently, you'll need a sound understanding of respiratory anatomy and physiology, assessment techniques, diagnostic tests, and treatments. You'll also need to understand the causes, pathophysiology, and symptoms of respiratory disorders.

RESPIRATORY CARE HANDBOOK gives you the practical, comprehensive knowledge you need to deliver competent respiratory care. Despite its comprehensive nature, the handbook is designed for fast reference. It's conveniently divided into 15 chapters. Each chapter contains an introduction that briefly presents the central concepts of that chapter, illustrations and charts that explain or supplement important information from the text, and selected references.

The handbook's first chapter lays a solid foundation by reviewing the respiratory system's anatomy and physiology. Chapter 2 follows with a step-by-step guide to respiratory assessment, including points specific to pediatric and geriatric patients.

Chapter 3 covers diagnostic procedures and monitoring techniques used in detecting and treating respiratory disorders. It covers a full range of procedures, including such common ones as sputum culture and pulmonary function tests and such specialized ones as thoracic computed tomography and pulmonary artery catheterization.

Chapters 4 to 8 address the pathophysiology and treatment of many pulmonary conditions, including restrictive and obstructive disorders, pulmonary vascular conditions, inhalation disorders, and the respiratory complications of neurological disturbances. In Chapter 9, you'll find a thorough discussion of acute respiratory failure and adult respiratory distress syndrome.

In Chapters 10 to 14, you'll learn about current respiratory therapy, including chest physiotherapy, oxygen and aerosol therapies, airway management procedures, ventilatory support procedures, and thoracic surgery and chest tubes. In Chapter 15, you'll find a complete discussion of respiratory drug therapy, including such drug classes as adrenergics, xanthine derivatives, antituberculars, anti-infectives, anti-inflammatories, mucolytics, anticholinergics, and neuromuscular blockers.

Helpful appendices follow the main text. These include an outline of basic life support, equations, a sample pulmonary rehabilitation program, commonly used abbreviations, and drugs that are toxic to the pulmonary system. Finally, you'll find a thorough index to help you locate information quickly and accurately.

No matter what your specialty, RESPIRATORY CARE HANDBOOK offers you a wealth of seasoned advice.

Suzanne C. Lareau, RN, MS
Pulmonary Clinical Nurse Specialist
Jerry L. Pettis Memorial Veterans
Administration Hospital
Loma Linda, Calif.

1 RESPIRATORY ANATOMY AND PHYSIOLOGY

Introduction

Technologic advances in respiratory care have increased the life span of patients with severe acute and chronic respiratory diseases. Also, advances in treating other physical disorders have increased the number of patients who survive critical illness but who are left with severe respiratory impairment.

Today's expanded responsibilities for respiratory care require proficiency in many skills—from patient assessment to evaluation. The function, physiology, and pathophysiology of the respiratory system must be fully understood to meet these responsibilities. The more you know about this system, the more confident you will be when caring for patients in respiratory distress.

The respiratory system is central to the functioning of most body systems. When it performs effectively, it supports other body systems, contributing to their organ function. Likewise, an impaired respiratory system can cause failure in other body systems, resulting in life-threatening organ failure.

Although the respiratory system contributes to the functioning of other body systems, it also depends on some of them. For example, the respiratory system needs the circulatory and nervous systems to exchange carbon dioxide and oxygen in the lungs. When people breathe, their lungs draw in oxygen from the air, distribute it to the blood, and then remove carbon dioxide from the blood for expulsion into the air.

Besides performing this vital gas exchange, the respiratory system helps maintain the body's acid-base balance to ensure a stable hydrogen-ion concentration. Its other functions include warming the lungs' inhaled air, filtering the air through the nasal hairs, and permitting speech by distributing air to the vocal cords.

When another body system experiences a physiologic deficit, the respiratory system usually compensates. In diabetic ketoacidosis, for example, the respiratory system tries to maintain acid-base balance by working harder to eliminate carbon dioxide.

Some respiratory structures have important nonrespiratory functions. For example, the lungs:
• act as a reservoir for blood from the heart
• provide a minor excretion route for specific drugs and metabolites (for example, anesthetic vapors and gases)
• help inactivate the potent vasoconstrictor serotonin by taking it up in endothelial cells
• protect the heart, brain, and kidneys from emboli by filtering particles from venous blood before they enter the systemic circulation
• help regulate water balance
• synthesize, release, activate, inactivate, and store chemical substances (such as prostaglandins, angiotensin I, bradykinin, norepinephrine, acetylcholine, histamine, and surfactant).

Respiratory anatomy

The respiratory system exchanges carbon dioxide, produced by cellular metabolism, for atmospheric oxygen. Divided into upper and lower tracts, it includes the organs responsible for external respiration. (See *The Respiratory System*.)

Upper respiratory tract

The upper respiratory tract consists of the nose, mouth, nasopharynx, oropharynx, laryngopharynx, and larynx.

Nose and mouth

The two portals for air are the nose and the mouth. During inspiration, air enters the body through the nostrils (nares), where small hairs (vibrissae) filter out dust and large particles. Divided at the midline by a septum, each nasal passage is formed anteriorly by cartilaginous walls and posteriorly by light, spongy bony structures known as conchae or turbinates.

Covered with a ciliated mucus layer, the conchae warm and humidify air before passing it through the nasopharynx. These tiny projections form eddies in the flowing air, forcing it to rebound in several different directions during its passage through the nose. This action traps finer particles, which the cilia then propel to the pharynx to be swallowed. If the air passage around the conchae is bypassed—for example, when a patient is on a ventilator—air must be humidified and heated outside the body. The conchae also divide nasal passages into the superior, middle, and inferior meatuses. The four paranasal sinuses, which provide speech resonance, drain through the meatuses near the conchae.

The maxillary and frontal sinuses are large mucus-covered, air-filled cavities; the sphenoidal and ethmoidal sinuses—also mucus-coated—consist of several small spaces in the nasal cavity's bony posterior portion.

Nasopharynx

Air flows from the nasal cavity through the conchae, which remain constantly open, into the muscular nasopharynx. The pharyngeal tonsils and the eustachian tube openings are nestled in the lateral walls of the nasopharynx above the soft palate. (The eustachian tubes regulate middle ear pressure.)

Oropharynx and laryngopharynx

The mouth's posterior wall, the oropharynx, joins the nasopharynx to the laryngopharynx. Extending to the esophagus, the laryngopharynx is the lowest pharyngeal region.

Larynx

The larynx, which contains the vocal cords, connects the pharynx with the trachea by means of cartilaginous and muscular walls. Two of its nine cartilages—the large, shield-shaped thyroid cartilage (Adam's apple) and the cricoid cartilage just below it—can be palpated in the neck.

The epiglottis, a leaf-shaped, flexible cartilage, hangs over the larynx. Its most important function is to prevent food or liquid from entering the airways. The epiglottis snaps shut during swallowing, routing food to the esophagus. It opens to allow air to enter the trachea and lungs.

The larynx aids in coughing, an important protective mechanism. When dust, dirt, or other irritants stimulate laryngeal sensory receptors, the abdominal and thoracic muscles contract, pushing against the diaphragm and increasing pressure within the tracheobronchial tree. The vocal cords open suddenly in a cough, forcing air and foreign particles out of the lungs.

Lower respiratory tract

The lower respiratory tract is subdivided into the conducting airways (trachea, primary bronchi, lobar and segmental bronchi) and the acinus (respiratory bronchioles, alveolar ducts, and alveoli), which is the area of gas exchange. Mucous membrane lines the

The Respiratory System

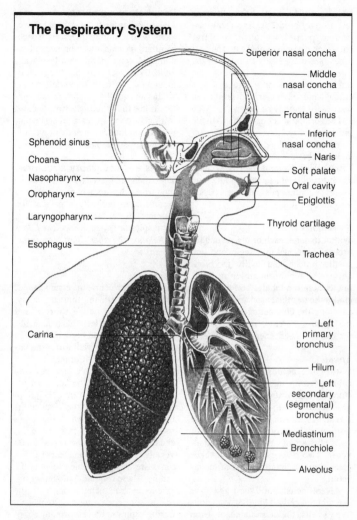

- Superior nasal concha
- Middle nasal concha
- Frontal sinus
- Inferior nasal concha
- Naris
- Soft palate
- Oral cavity
- Epiglottis
- Thyroid cartilage
- Trachea
- Left primary bronchus
- Hilum
- Left secondary (segmental) bronchus
- Mediastinum
- Bronchiole
- Alveolus

- Sphenoid sinus
- Choana
- Nasopharynx
- Oropharynx
- Laryngopharynx
- Esophagus
- Carina

respiratory tract, and constant movement of mucus by ciliary action cleanses the tract and carries foreign matter upward for swallowing or expectoration.

Trachea
The tubular trachea, half in the neck and half in the thorax, extends about 5″ (12 cm) from the only complete tracheal ring, the cricoid cartilage, to the carina at the level of the sixth or seventh thoracic vertebra. C-shaped cartilaginous rings reinforce and protect the trachea, preventing its collapse.

Bronchi
The trachea branches into two primary (mainstem) bronchi at the carina. The right primary bronchus, a more direct passageway from the trachea, is wider

and about 1″ (2.5 cm) shorter than the left primary bronchus. As a result, aspirated particles entering the trachea—or a malpositioned endotracheal tube—are more likely to fall into the right bronchus than the left. Like the trachea, the bronchi are lined with a ciliated mucous layer and reinforced with cartilaginous rings.

The primary bronchi then divide into secondary (lobar) branches. Accompanied by blood vessels, nerves, and lymphatics, they enter the lungs at the hilum. Each of the five secondary bronchi (right upper, middle, and lower, and left upper and lower) passes into its own lung lobe.

Bronchioles

Within its lobe, each of the secondary bronchi branches into segmental and smaller bronchi and finally into bronchioles. Each bronchiole, in turn, branches into a lobule. The lobule includes the terminal bronchioles, which conclude the conducting airways, and the acinus, the chief respiratory unit for gas exchange. (See *The Lobule*.)

Alveoli

Within the acinus, terminal bronchioles branch into respiratory bronchioles, which structurally resemble bronchioles but also feed directly into alveoli at sites along their walls. These respiratory bronchioles end in alveolar sacs, clusters of capillary-swathed alveoli. Two-way gas diffusion takes place through the thin walls of the alveoli.

Alveoli consist of Type I and Type II epithelial cells. Thin, flat squamous Type I cells, the most abundant, form the alveolar walls through which gas exchange occurs. Type II cells aid gas exchange by producing surfactant, a lipid-type substance that coats the alveolus, preventing total alveolar collapse, and facilitates gas exchange by lowering surface tension.

Respiratory membrane

The alveolar cells described above, along with a minute interstitial space, capillary basement membrane, and endothelial cells in the capillary wall, collectively make up the "respiratory membrane," which separates the alveolus and capillary. The entire structure is less than 1 μ thick. Any increase in thickness or decrease in surfactant production reduces the rate of gas diffusion across the membrane.

Lungs and accessory structures

The lungs and accessory structures, the pleura, the thoracic cavity, and the mediastinum (actually a part of the thoracic cavity), are essential parts of the respiratory system. (See *The Lungs in Relation to Other Chest Structures,* page 6.)

Lungs

Straddling the heart, the cone-shaped, spongy lungs fill the thoracic cavity, the right lung being shorter and broader than the left. Each lung has an apex, base, three borders, and two surfaces. The chest wall forms the lateral boundary for both lungs.

Each lung's concave base rests on the diaphragm, and the apex extends slightly above the first rib. The hilum lies above and behind the heart and is the opening through which the lung's root structures pass: primary bronchus, pulmonary and bronchial blood vessels, lymphatics, and nerves. The lungs are freely movable except at the hilum, where root and pulmonary ligaments anchor them. Along with the diaphragm, each lung base moves up during expiration and down during inspiration.

Fissures partially divide each lung into lobes—three lobes for the larger right lung, two for the left. The left lung's medial anterior surface wraps around and under the heart, forming a tongue-like structure known as the lingula pulmonis sinistri. The diaphragm, the floor of the thoracic cavity, separates the inferior surfaces of

The Lobule

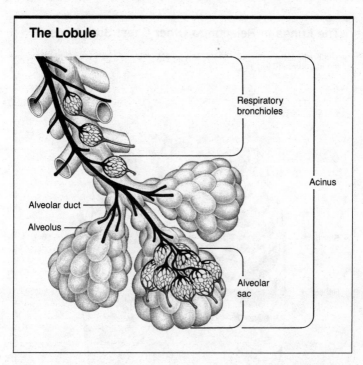

Respiratory bronchioles

Acinus

Alveolar duct

Alveolus

Alveolar sac

both lower lobes from the abdominal viscera.

Pleura

Composed of a visceral layer and a parietal layer, the pleura totally encloses the lung. The visceral pleura, a tough, elastic-like membrane, hugs the contours of the lung surface, including the fissures between lobes. It separates each lung from mediastinal structures, such as the heart and its great vessels, the trachea, the esophagus, and the bronchi. A similar membrane, the parietal pleura, lines the chest wall's inner surface and the diaphragm's upper surface, then doubles back around the mediastinum. The parietal and visceral pleurae meet at the hilum to form a narrow fold known as the pulmonary ligament. Both the visceral and parietal pleurae contain connective and epithelial tissues and a single layer of secreting epithelium.

An airtight region between the membranes, the pleural space or pleural cavity is only a potential space. It can be seen only when air or water collects in it, such as in pneumothorax or pleural effusion. Normally, a thin film of serous fluid fills this space, lubricating the pleural surfaces to slide smoothly against each other. It also creates a vacuum between the layers, which compels the lungs to move synchronously with the chest wall during breathing.

Thoracic cavity

The area within the chest wall, the thoracic cavity, is bounded below by the diaphragm; above by the scalene

The Lungs in Relation to Other Chest Structures

The lungs occupy most of the thoracic cavity. Note the heart projected over the sternum and left lung.

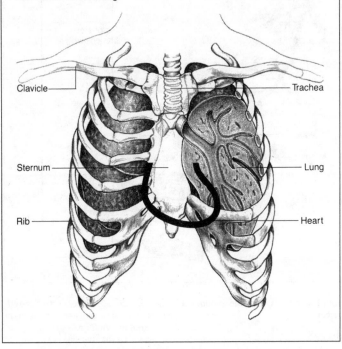

muscles and the fascia of the neck; and circumferentially by the ribs, intercostal muscles, vertebrae, sternum, and ligaments. Some of the body's vital organs and structures are housed in the thoracic cavity. The thoracic cage, the bones, and the muscles surrounding the thoracic cavity protect the thoracic organs and support the chest wall, allowing it to move during respiration.

Mediastinum
A thick extension of thoracic fascia envelops the mediastinal space between the lungs. Extending from the sternum to the vertebral column, the mediastinum houses the heart and pericardium; thoracic aorta; pulmonary artery and veins, vena cavae, and azygos veins; thymus, lymph nodes, and vessels; trachea, esophagus, and thoracic duct; and vagus, cardiac, and phrenic nerves.

Pulmonary circulation
The respiratory system's primary purpose, of course, is to exchange carbon dioxide and oxygen. To achieve this exchange, the airways of the tracheobronchial tree are shadowed by a similar network of blood vessels. Oxygen-depleted blood being routed to the lungs for replenishment is pumped from the right ventricle to the pulmonary trunk. This trunk branches

laterally into the right and left pulmonary arteries, which further divide into smaller arteries and closely follow the bronchial airways throughout the lungs. Eventually, the pulmonary arteries branch into arterioles and venules that form capillary beds around and protrude into the alveoli, the site of gas exchange. After oxygen diffusion, oxygenated blood travels to the left atrium via the pulmonary veins to be pumped throughout the systemic circulation.

The tissues of the lung and pleura receive blood from the bronchial arteries, which arise from the aorta and its branches. The bronchial arteries are a part of the systemic circulation and play no part in the oxygenation of blood.

An extensive network of lymph vessels drains the pulmonary pleura in the dense connective tissue around the bronchi, respiratory bronchioles, pulmonary arteries, and veins. Circulating freely, lymph flows into collecting trunks, which empty into the bronchopulmonary lymph nodes at the hilum.

Respiratory physiology

Breathing involves two actions: inspiration, an active process, and expiration, a relatively passive one. Breathing is regulated by both mechanical and chemical factors, and is influenced by lung expansibility (compliance) and by the size of airways and the resistance to flow that they impart. (See *Mechanics of Normal, Quiet Breathing*.)

Neurologic control of breathing

Neurologically regulated, with the help of chemoreceptors and certain physiologic factors, breathing is mainly automatic and usually involuntary. Working together, these various control mechanisms regulate ventilation to provide continuous airflow in and

---

Mechanics of Normal, Quiet Breathing

Inspiration
● Central nervous system (CNS) transmits impulses to the diaphragm via the phrenic nerve, stimulating diaphragm contraction.
● Diaphragm descends as it contracts, vertically enlarging thorax; external intercostal muscles also contract (especially during deep or forced inspiration), raising and rotating ribs and sternum and horizontally enlarging thorax.
● Thoracic expansion lowers intrapleural pressure; pleural cohesion causes lungs to expand with thorax; lung expansion lowers intrapulmonic (bronchoalveolar) pressure below atmospheric pressure.
● Intrapulmonic/atmospheric pressure gradient pulls air into lungs until the two pressures equalize.

Expiration
● CNS impulses to diaphragm cease; diaphragm slowly relaxes and moves up in the thorax; lungs and thorax recoil to resting size and position.
● This recoil (usually passive, but aided during deep or forced expiration by CNS-stimulated contraction of internal intercostal muscles) reduces thorax to resting size.
● Compression of lungs and thorax causes intrapulmonic pressure to rise above atmospheric pressure.
● Intrapulmonic/atmospheric pressure gradient forces air out of lungs until the two pressures equalize.

---

out of the lungs; however, the amount of air that actually reaches the lungs with oxygen and then departs carrying carbon dioxide depends on lung volume and capacity, resistance to airflow, and compliance. (See *Measuring Lung Volumes*, page 8.)

Measuring Lung Volumes

Certain lung volumes can be measured using a spirometer, and others can be calculated from the results. Typically, you'll measure tidal volume and vital capacity.

• *Tidal volume (TV):* the amount of air that enters or leaves the lungs during normal, quiet breathing. Average inspiratory and expiratory tidal volumes each equal 500 ml.

• *Inspiratory reserve volume (IRV):* the amount of air that can be inhaled after normal inhalation. Average is 3,000 ml.

• *Expiratory reserve volume (ERV):* the amount of air that can be exhaled after normal exhalation. Average expiratory reserve volume is 1,200 ml.

Certain lung volumes can't be measured with a spirometer:

• *Residual volume (RV):* the amount of air remaining in the lungs after the deepest possible expiration. Unresponsive to voluntary effort, it can be removed only by collapse of the lungs. Average residual volume is 1,200 ml. Adding various lung volumes allows evaluation of several lung capacities:

• *Vital capacity (VC):* the amount of air exhaled by the deepest possible expiration after the deepest possible inspiration. As the sum of tidal, inspiratory reserve, and expiratory reserve volumes, it's usually about 4,700 ml.

• *Functional residual capacity (FRC):* the amount of air remaining in the lungs after normal expiration. As the sum of the expiratory reserve and residual volumes, it ensures a steady supply of air in the lungs, so that gas exchange can occur continuously, even between breaths.

• *Inspiratory capacity (IC):* the maximum amount of air inhaled after normal expiration. It's the sum of the tidal and inspiratory reserve volumes.

• *Total lung capacity (TLC):* the amount of air in the lungs after the fullest possible inspiration. The sum of vital capacity and residual volume, it's usually about 5,900 ml.

• *Minute volume or minute ventilation (VE):* the product of the tidal volume multiplied by the number of respirations per minute. For example, a person with a tidal volume of 500 ml, breathing 12 times per minute, has a minute volume of 6,000 ml.

• *Maximal breathing capacity:* the amount of air moved in and out of the lung in 1 minute of forced breathing. This can be calculated by having a person breathe as rapidly and deeply as possible for 15 seconds, and then multiplying that number by 4 to arrive at a figure for a minute's respiration. The resulting figure may reach 100 liters/minute during strenuous exercise.

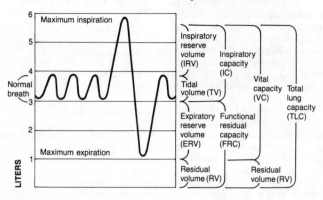

Neurologic regulators

The regulators for the mechanical aspects of breathing reside in the medulla oblongata and the pons. Called respiratory centers, they are really groups of scattered neurons that function as a unit to regulate breathing. The primary location in the medulla is called the medullary respiratory center. Here, neurons associated with inspiration apparently interact with neurons associated with expiration to regulate respiratory rate and depth. They also react to impulses from other areas, particularly the pons. In the pons, two neuron groups, or centers, interact with the medullary respiratory center to smooth the transitions from inspiration to expiration and back, thereby regulating respiratory rhythm. The apneustic center of the pons stimulates inspiratory neurons in the medulla to precipitate inspiration. In turn, these inspiratory neurons stimulate the pneumotaxic center of the pons to precipitate expiration. They do this in two ways: by inhibiting the apneustic center and by stimulating the expiratory neurons in the medulla. Thus, as a pacemaker, the pons regulates rhythm, while the medulla regulates rate and depth. (See *Innervation of Respiratory Structures,* page 10.)

Conscious control of breathing through nerve impulses from the motor areas of the cerebral cortex can override the involuntary respiratory centers. This permits voluntary breath control for such activities as speaking, singing, and swimming. This conscious control is only temporary, however, and the respiratory centers, in turn, will override cortical impulses to meet ventilatory needs.

Central and peripheral chemoreceptors

Responding to changes in blood CO_2, O_2, and pH, the central and peripheral chemoreceptors monitor the body's ventilatory status and signal the respiratory centers to adjust respiratory rate and depth. The central chemoreceptors, located in the anterior medulla, are particularly sensitive to alterations in PCO_2 and acid-base balance. For example, physical exertion raises the level of carbon dioxide in the blood; the gas diffuses easily from cerebral capillaries into the cerebrospinal fluid bathing the central nervous system, where it reacts with water to form carbonic acid and yield hydrogen ions. Chemoreceptors detect this rising acidity and stimulate the respiratory centers to increase respiratory rate and depth. As expiration of carbon dioxide lowers carbonic acid levels, the chemoreceptors stimulate the respiratory centers to reduce respiratory rate and depth. Conversely, if blood levels of carbon dioxide fall below normal, the central chemoreceptors initiate a cessation of breathing (apnea) until ongoing cellular metabolism produces sufficient carbon dioxide to stimulate the respiratory centers again.

Peripheral chemoreceptors, located in the aortic and carotid bodies, primarily monitor the blood-oxygen level. When the blood level of oxygen falls, the oxygen content of interstitial fluid around the peripheral chemoreceptors also falls, and the receptors stimulate the respiratory centers to increase respiratory rate and/or depth to introduce additional oxygen.

Physiologic factors

Along with the important chemical and neurologic factors, several physiologic factors significantly affect breathing: lung inflation, changes in blood pressure and temperature, airway irritation, and sensory stimulation. (See *Pulmonary Innervation,* page 11.)

Lung inflation. Lung inflation stimulates stretch receptors in the alveolar ducts, which send a stream of impulses along the vagus nerves to the central nervous system. These afferent impulses inhibit the inspiratory center, which then stops sending expansion impulses to the

Innervation of Respiratory Structures

Stimulation from external sources and from higher brain centers acts on respiratory centers in the pons and medulla. These centers in turn send impulses to the various parts of the respiratory apparatus to alter respiration
patterns.

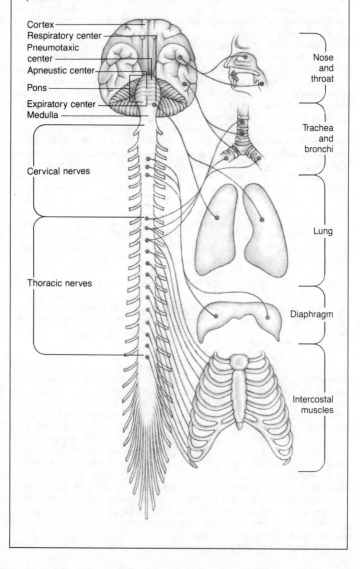

diaphragm and external intercostal muscles. Consequently, these muscles stop expanding, and passive expiration follows. This reflex, the *Hering-Breuer reflex*, is an important regulator of normal respiration; however, a secondary mechanism independent of the vagus nerves is also operative and becomes apparent when the normal pathway is blocked. For example, cutting the vagus nerves prolongs and deepens inspiration, but eventually the inspiratory center stops sending expansion messages and allows expiration to occur.

Blood pressure changes. Sudden, sharp changes stimulate pressoreceptors in the aortic and carotid sinuses. With a sudden rise in blood pressure, the receptors send impulses along vagus and glossopharyngeal nerves to the respiratory centers. These impulses depress respiratory activity and temporarily make respirations lower and shallower. With a sudden blood pressure drop, as occurs with severe hemorrhage, pressoreceptor impulses slow down. The respiratory center activity quickens correspondingly, increasing respiratory rate and depth.

Temperature changes. Changes in the temperature of the blood passing through the respiratory centers may also trigger changes in respiration. A temperature increase from fever or exertion quickens the respiratory rate, and a temperature drop, as in hypothermia, decreases the respiratory rate.

Airway irritation. Foreign particles stimulate the protective "irritant" receptors in the mucous membrane that lines the respiratory tract. In the nose, a sneeze results to expel the irritant. In the larynx or trachea, such an invasion induces a cough.

Sensory stimulation. Stimulation of various receptors may cause a temporary reflex reaction. Sudden heat or cold or alarming sounds or sights may provoke a gasp, accelerated respiratory rate, or momentary apnea.

Pulmonary Innervation

Vagal and sympathetic efferents and vagal afferents innervate the lungs, forming networks around the bronchial and arterial trees. Stimulation via the vagal efferents causes bronchoconstriction, and via the sympathetic efferents, vasoconstriction.

The three main vagal afferents have varied responses. *Irritant* receptors lie just under the surface of the airways and seem to respond to irritant gases, smoke, dust, and histamine by causing coughing and bronchoconstriction. *J (juxtacapillary)* receptors are believed to lie in the alveolar walls and to respond to exercise, emboli, edema, and irritant gases by causing hyperventilation. *Stretch* receptors lie in the smooth muscle of the smaller airways and respond to lung distention by signaling the central nervous system to halt inspiration (Hering-Breuer reflex).

Physical forces

Effective gas exchange is opposed by three forces of resistance that can restrict respiration and add to the work of breathing: elastic resistance, nonelastic (viscous) resistance, and airflow resistance.

Elastic resistance

The lung's natural tendency to contract because of the elasticity of its tissue is known as elastic resistance. This elasticity derives partly from elastic fibers throughout the lung, which stretch during inspiration and spring back during expiration. It derives primarily, however, from the surface tension of the fluid lining the alveoli, which constantly promotes alveolar collapse. Two forces counteract lung elasticity: chest-wall rigidity combined with pleural fluid tension, and secretion of surfactant in the alveoli to reduce alveolar surface tension.

During inspiration, the cohesive force of the fluid between the visceral and parietal pleurae combined with negative intrapleural pressure causes the lung to expand with the chest wall and, during expiration, halts lung deflation at the chest wall's point of maximum contraction. The lung and chest wall function smoothly as a counterbalanced unit, as long as the pleurae remain intact. When the pleurae are interrupted, such as by external puncture or by rupture of a bleb, this pleural force of attraction is broken and lung collapse results, as in pneumothorax.

In the alveoli, epithelial cells secrete surfactant, a lipoprotein, which coats the fluid lining the alveoli and prevents fluid contact with alveolar air. This creates a surface tension 2 to 14 times less than the fluid-air tension and reduces alveolar tendency to collapse. Thus, any disease process that interferes with surfactant production promotes lung collapse.

Nonelastic (viscous) resistance
Nonelastic resistance results from the force exerted on the thorax by the diaphragm and the abdominal contents, which inhibits the thorax from expanding downward. Though not usually sufficient to compromise inspiration, such resistance may become a problem with obesity, abdominal distention, ascites, and late-term pregnancy.

Airflow resistance
Airflow resistance derives from a change in airway radius or in airflow pattern. Airway radius, a critical factor, decreases as large bronchi branch out through the lung. It also decreases when accumulated secretions narrow the bronchi or when condensation narrows ventilator tubing. A 50% reduction in airway radius causes a sixteenfold increase in resistance to gas flow. For the patient on a ventilator, airway length is also a factor. The ventilator tubing becomes an extension of the tracheobronchial tree, and this change in airway length directly affects airway resistance: doubling the length doubles the resistance.

Airflow pattern—whether laminar, turbulent, or transitional (see *Airflow Patterns*)—also affects resistance. Laminar flow offers minimal resistance to gas flow. The smooth angles in the small airways of the bronchial tree produce this desirable flow pattern. Turbulent flow creates added friction and raises resistance to flow. While considered normal in the trachea and larger bronchi, turbulent flow can occur in the smaller airways as a result of bronchoconstriction or excessive secretions. For the patient on a ventilator, condensation in the tubing can also change the flow pattern. Keep in mind that high gas flow rates also induce turbulence and thus require higher pressures to deliver a normal tidal volume. A mix of patterns, called transitional flow, occurs around obstructions and at transitional points in the larger airways, such as branches.

Compliance

$$E = \frac{1}{C}$$

The reciprocal of elasticity, compliance is the lung's ability to expand, to yield to intra-alveolar pressure during inspiration. Compliance has two affecting factors: lung expansibility and chest-wall expansibility, including the thorax and diaphragm. Chest-wall compliance isn't routinely measured, because it's affected by skeletal muscle contraction and valid measurement demands total muscle relaxation. Lung compliance, however, doesn't depend on physical relaxation for valid measurement. Lung compliance may be static or dynamic. The most common measurement, static compliance, is made under static conditions. It's a product of the tidal volume divided by the pressure required to maintain that volume; this determines the change in volume for every centimeter of water pressure increase. Normal static compliance is 100 ml/cm H_2O. Dynamic compliance is measured under nonstatic conditions, usually during inspiration. Normal dynamic compliance is 50 ml/cm H_2O.

Understanding diffusion

Gas moves from an area of greater pressure to one of lesser pressure. Ventilation is the mechanical movement of air into and out of the lungs. The action of the chest wall, pleurae, and lungs produces changes in intrapulmonic and intrapleural pressure that are necessary to accomplish ventilation. (See *Understanding Shunt and Dead Space,* page 14.) The next step in gas exchange, external respiration, is the actual diffusion of oxygen into and carbon dioxide out of the blood. This occurs because the partial pressures of those gases on each side of the respiratory membrane create steep pressure gradients that promote gas transfer in opposite directions. (See *Gas Diffusion and the Law of Partial Pressures,* page 15.)

Rapid gas exchange

Normally, gas exchange takes place in half the time allowed for it. Exposure of blood to the respiratory membrane lasts about 0.8 second at rest. Almost full oxygen saturation of the blood occurs in half that time, and carbon dioxide exchange occurs 20 times faster than oxygen exchange. So, if a specific lung area receives an adequate volume of blood flow, flow rate will not compromise gas exchange.

The speed at which gas exchange occurs and the specific pressure needed to affect the exchange depend on the degree to which a gas is soluble in blood. Because carbon dioxide is much more soluble than oxygen, it diffuses more rapidly than oxygen and requires a much lower pressure gradient to do so, even when resistance to diffusion increases. With added resistance from a thickened respiratory membrane, as occurs with pulmonary fibrosis, carbon dioxide may still diffuse outward with its partial pressure in systemic blood remaining normal, while oxygen diffusion and PO_2 decrease.

Airflow Patterns

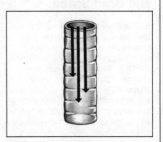

Laminar flow
This linear pattern, found mostly in the small peripheral bronchial passages, offers minimal resistance.

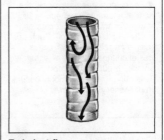

Turbulent flow
This eddying pattern increases resistance. It is normal in the trachea and large central bronchi, where flow rates are high.

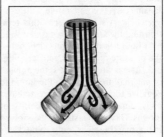

Transitional flow
This mixed pattern occurs in low-flow regions—for example, where larger airways join or branch.

Understanding Shunt and Dead Space

- *Shunt:* areas of the lung that are perfused but not ventilated. This abnormality commonly occurs in adult respiratory distress syndrome (ARDS). Shunt affects gas exchange more often than dead space.
- *Dead-space air:* air filling respiratory airways that conduct air to the alveoli but play no part in gas exchange. These airways include the nose, mouth, pharynx, larynx, trachea, and bronchial tree, but not the alveoli. Average dead-space air is 150 ml for an adult male and 110 ml for an adult female.
- *Physiologic dead-space air:* the sum of anatomic dead-space air and air in any nonfunctioning or partly functioning alveoli. Such defective alveoli, no longer active in gas exchange, may be adequately ventilated but lack a blood supply. This abnormality commonly occurs in pulmonary embolism.

Oxygen transport

Once diffusion occurs, internal respiration takes place. Arterial blood transports oxygen to the tissues in two ways: physically, dissolved in plasma; and chemically, bound to hemoglobin. Plasma carries comparatively little oxygen. Henry's law governs this relationship: the amount of a gas dissolved in a liquid is directly proportional to the pressure of the gas against the liquid. As gas pressure rises, the amount of gas that dissolves into the liquid to equalize that pressure differential also rises, depending on the solubility of the gas. Oxygen resists being dissolved in plasma; therefore, only about 3% is transported in this manner.

Hemoglobin carries about 97% of the oxygen in the blood, depending on the PO_2 level. (See *Oxyhemoglobin Dissociation Curve*, page 16.) High PO_2, as in pulmonary capillaries, causes oxygen to bind to the proteins' iron (heme or Fe^{++}) molecules to form oxyhemoglobin (HbO_2). Low PO_2, as at the cellular level, reverses the bond, so oxygen is released. Barriers to this process include certain chemicals, such as nitrites and carbon monoxide. Nitrites convert hemoglobin to a ferric state (Fe^{+++}), called methemoglobin, thereby preventing it from combining with oxygen. Carbon monoxide, which is more strongly attracted to hemoglobin than oxygen, easily displaces oxygen in the bonding process.

Hemoglobin bound to oxygen to its fullest extent (normally about 1.34 ml of oxygen per gram of hemoglobin) is considered 100% saturated. Less complete combinations are expressed in lower percentages. Saturation near 100% turns hemoglobin bright red, as in normal arterial blood. Desaturated (reduced) hemoglobin is purple and imparts the bluish tone of cyanosis to the skin.

Cyanosis, however, is unreliable as an indicator of hypoxemia (decreased blood oxygen), because it doesn't show up until at least 5 g of hemoglobin is desaturated—a situation more serious clinically for the anemic patient with total hemoglobin of only 8 g than for the polycythemic patient with a total hemoglobin of 20 g.

When oxygen-laden arterial blood reaches body tissues, internal respiration or gas exchange between systemic capillaries and interstitial fluid takes place along pressure gradients. Oxygen moves into the interstitial fluid to nourish the cells, and carbon dioxide leaves the fluid to travel in the blood. Blood then moves across the capillaries from the arterial to the venous system to begin its journey to the lungs, where the CO_2 waste is exchanged for oxygen.

Carbon dioxide transport

The blood carries carbon dioxide to the lungs in three ways: (1) dissolved in plasma; (2) coupled with hemoglobin as carbaminohemoglobin; and (3)

Gas Diffusion and the Law of Partial Pressures

The concept of diffusion draws on Dalton's law of partial pressures. This law states that in a mixture of gases, the pressure (tension) exerted by each gas is independent of the other gases present and directly corresponds to the percentage it represents of the total mixture.

Here's how Dalton's law works. Atmospheric air inspired at sea level exerts a pressure of 760 mm Hg against all parts of the body. Oxygen represents 21% of air, and therefore exerts a partial pressure (PO_2) of 158 mm Hg, or 21% of 760 mm Hg. Carbon dioxide, a trace element of atmospheric air, has a partial pressure (PCO_2) of 0.3 mm Hg. Nitrogen, making up 78% of air, has a partial pressure of 596 mm Hg. Lastly, water vapor has a partial pressure (PH_2O) of 5.7 mm Hg.

During inspiration, the upper respiratory tract warms and humidifies atmospheric air, increasing the partial pressure of water vapor to @37°C

47 mm Hg. Partial pressures of the other gases decline because total pressure must remain at 760 mm Hg. Before entering the alveoli, inspired air mixes with gas that was not exhaled on the previous expiration. Because this gas contains more carbon dioxide and less oxygen than inspired air, partial pressures must change again.

Gas that finally enters the alveoli for diffusion across the respiratory membrane registers still further partial pressure changes but remains high in oxygen pressure and low in carbon dioxide pressure. It's met by deoxygenated blood from the right ventricle with low oxygen and high carbon dioxide pressure. The differential in partial pressures of oxygen and carbon dioxide causes the two gases to cross the respiratory membrane toward the lower side of their respective pressure gradients. Oxygen diffuses into the blood and carbon dioxide diffuses outward, equalizing the gas pressures on both sides of the respiratory membrane.

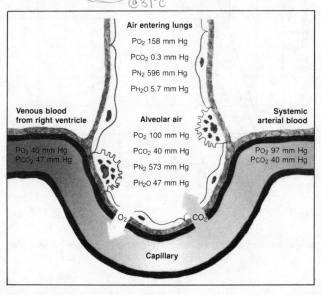

Air entering lungs

PO_2 158 mm Hg

PCO_2 0.3 mm Hg

PN_2 596 mm Hg

PH_2O 5.7 mm Hg

Venous blood from right ventricle

Alveolar air

PO_2 100 mm Hg

PCO_2 40 mm Hg

PN_2 573 mm Hg

PH_2O 47 mm Hg

Systemic arterial blood

PO_2 40 mm Hg
PCO_2 47 mm Hg

PO_2 97 mm Hg
PCO_2 40 mm Hg

O_2 CO_2

Capillary

Oxyhemoglobin Dissociation Curve

The oxyhemoglobin dissociation curve shows hemoglobin saturation (affinity for oxygen) at any Po_2 and thus the efficiency of oxygen transport and delivery. Note that the curve flattens out at a Po_2 of about 75 mm Hg; at this level, most of the hemoglobin is saturated, and an increase in Po_2 won't greatly improve saturation. Note, too, that when Po_2 falls below 60 mm Hg, rapid and extensive desaturation can occur, resulting in hypoxia.

Factors that alter hemoglobin affinity and shift the curve include pH, Pco_2, and temperature. A rise in pH, or a drop in Pco_2 or temperature, induces hemoglobin to bond with oxygen, producing higher saturation at a given Po_2 and shifting the curve to the left. But these same factors inhibit oxygen release at the cellular level. Conversely, a drop in pH, or a rise in Pco_2 or temperature, induces hemoglobin to release oxygen, producing lower saturations at a given Po_2 and shifting the curve to the right. But these factors also inhibit hemoglobin bonding in the lungs.

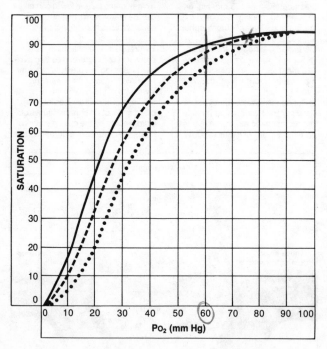

Key:

Normal $\big\}$ Middle Curve

$\uparrow$ pH
$\downarrow$ Temp $\big\}$ Left Curve
$\downarrow$ Pco_2

$\downarrow$ pH
$\uparrow$ Temp $\big\}$ Right Curve
$\uparrow$ Pco_2

combined with water as carbonic acid and its component ions. (See *Carbon Dioxide Transport*.) Only 7% is carried in blood plasma, and the reaction requires many seconds to complete. Some of this 7% has a measurable partial pressure; the rest reacts very slowly with water to form carbonic acid (H_2CO_3), which may further break down into hydrogen ions (H^+) and bicarbonate ions (HCO_3^-); both processes are reversible.

About 23% of the carbon dioxide reacts somewhat faster with hemoglobin in the red blood cells and forms the compound carbaminohemoglobin.

About 70% of the carbon dioxide converts to carbonic acid in the red blood cells, a process that occurs in a fraction of a second because of the presence of the catalyzing enzyme, carbonic anhydrase. Equally fast, the carbonic acid breaks down into hydrogen ions and bicarbonate ions; the hydrogen ions remain cell-bound, neutralized by the hemoglobin, while the bicarbonate ions trade places with chloride ions in the surrounding plasma. Red blood cells expel excess bicarbonate yet remain electrically neutral in this process, called chloride shift.

When venous blood enters the lung for gas exchange, all reversible chemical processes reverse, reforming carbon dioxide. The gas diffuses into the alveoli and is expired.

The degree to which oxygen in the alveoli trades places with carbon dioxide in the blood depends largely on the amount of oxygen the lungs can draw in and the amount of blood available in the lungs to absorb it. This ratio of ventilation to perfusion determines the effectiveness of gas exchange.

Ventilation/perfusion ratio (respiratory quotient)

Effective gas exchange depends on an adequate volume of oxygen reaching the alveoli and on sufficient blood flow (perfusion) through pulmonary capillaries. The relationship between the

Carbon Dioxide Transport

The tissues release carbon dioxide into the bloodstream, where it travels to the lungs in three forms: as a gas dissolved in plasma, combined with hemoglobin, and combined with water as carbonic acid.

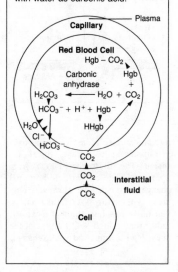

two shows the ventilation/perfusion ($\dot{V}/\dot{Q}$) ratio or, as it is also known, the respiratory quotient.

Ideally, the respiratory quotient would be 1. Gravity's effects, however, markedly reduce both ventilation and perfusion. In the upper lung, perfusion is affected more than ventilation; the $\dot{V}/\dot{Q}$ ratio may rise to 2.4. The situation reverses in the lower lung, with perfusion slightly exceeding ventilation. (See *Normal Ventilation and Perfusion*, page 18.)

Because the quality of the $\dot{V}/\dot{Q}$ match affects the quality of gas exchange, the result is an unequal exchange pattern throughout the lung. Because of reduced blood flow, the PO_2 at the apex is more than 40 mm Hg lower than the PO_2 at the base, al-

Normal Ventilation and Perfusion

This diagram shows matched perfusion and ventilation. Deoxygenated blood in the pulmonary artery enters the respiratory unit, then emerges oxygenated into the pulmonary vein.

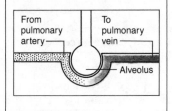

though exercise increases apical oxygen uptake as it increases apical perfusion. The difference in PCO_2 from apex to base, as reflected by pH change, is much less. However, only areas with a low $\dot{V}/\dot{Q}$ ratio (that is, ventilation is less than perfusion), rather than a high $\dot{V}/\dot{Q}$ ratio as at the apex, lead to impaired gas exchange.

Respiratory pathophysiology

Understanding respiratory anatomy and physiology is fundamental to identifying respiratory pathophysiology and understanding its implications and the ramifications of treatment. All are increasingly important today, given the nurse's expanding role in health assessment. The ability to interpret clinical findings for specific respiratory disorders rests on an understanding of the overall mechanisms of respiratory dysfunction.

Ineffective gas exchange

Ineffective gas exchange between the alveoli and the pulmonary capillaries is a major problem in respiratory dis-

orders and can affect all body systems. (See *Effects of Chronic Ineffective Gas Exchange,* pages 20 and 21.) For gas exchange to be effective, ventilation and perfusion must match as closely possible. Ventilation/perfusion (V/Q) mismatch accounts for most of the defective gas exchange in respiratory disorders. Such mismatching may result from a V/Q dysfunction or a change in lung mechanics.

Ventilation/perfusion dysfunction

When ineffective exchange results from a physiologic abnormality, the effect may be reduced ventilation to a unit (shunt), reduced perfusion to a unit (dead-space ventilation), or both (silent unit). (See *Effects of Inadequate Ventilation and Perfusion.*) Note that shunting refers to unoxygenated blood being returned to the left heart. An abnormal shunt may occur because an actual physical defect, such as congenital heart disease, allows unoxygenated blood to bypass fully functioning alveoli, or because a collapsed alveolus prevents oxygen from reaching an adequately perfused area of the lung. However, keep in mind that a physical shunt occurs in the normal lung. The pulmonary veins collect oxygen-depleted blood from the bronchial artery, which perfuses the bronchi, and form the thebesian veins, which drain the heart muscle. Shunting of this poorly oxygenated blood into arterial blood depresses arterial PO_2, but not significantly for the normal person. The person with heart disease, however, may also have a physical defect between the right and left sides of the heart, which diverts greater amounts of unoxygenated blood directly into arterial blood flow and seriously depresses arterial PO_2. Most abnormal shunting, though, results from alveolar collapse.

Changes in lung mechanics

Ineffective gas exchange also can occur because changes in lung mechanics demand higher internal pressures to produce adequate breath volumes. Thus, the work of breathing is increased and the effectiveness of diffusion is reduced. Changes in mechanics fall into two classes: changes in compliance and changes in resistance.

Changes in compliance. Changes in expansibility can occur in either the lung or the chest wall. Lung compliance decreases in interstitial and alveolar pulmonary diseases—such as pulmonary edema, pulmonary fibrosis, sarcoidosis, and adult respiratory distress syndrome (ARDS)—because characteristic cellular changes make inspiration more difficult.

Chest-wall compliance is affected by thoracic deformity, muscle spasm, and abdominal distention. Compliance may decrease in ankylosing spondylitis, kyphosis, marked obesity, extreme pectus excavatum, scoliosis, and disorders causing muscle spasticity.

Changes in resistance. Changes in the pressure needed to produce airflow may occur in the lung tissue itself, as with sarcoidosis and other interstitial lung diseases; in the chest wall, as with pleurisy and other pleural disorders; or in the airways. Airway resistance alone, however, accounts for 80% of all respiratory system resistance. Airway resistance typically mounts with such obstructive diseases as asthma, chronic bronchitis, and emphysema. Consequently, the work of breathing increases, particularly during expiration, to compensate for narrowed airways and diminished gas exchange.

Results of ineffective gas exchange

When gas exchange is ineffective, one end result is hypoxia (tissue-oxygen deficiency), although this deficiency may be evident only on exertion when oxygen demand intensifies. This deficiency may occur at any point from ventilation to transport to cell metabolism, but the end result is oxygen deficiency at the cellular level. Such a decrease in cellular oxygen concentration means the cell must resort to an-

Effects of Inadequate Ventilation and Perfusion

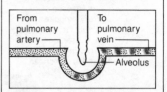

Inadequate ventilation (shunt)
In the low $\dot{V}/\dot{Q}$ unit shown above, alveolar collapse causes hypoxemia. It usually results from acute diseases, such as atelectasis, pneumonia, and adult respiratory distress syndrome.

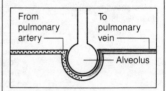

Inadequate perfusion (space ventilation)
When the $\dot{V}/\dot{Q}$ ratio is high, as in the unit pictured above, the alveolus receives inadequate blood flow. Note the narrowed capillary, indicating poor perfusion. This usually results from a perfusion defect, such as pulmonary embolism.

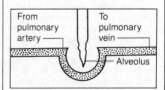

Inadequate ventilation and perfusion (silent unit)
The silent unit, as shown above, has poor perfusion and ventilation. By diverting blood flow to better-ventilated lung areas, the silent unit helps compensate for a $\dot{V}/\dot{Q}$ imbalance. This can stem from multiple causes, such as pulmonary embolism and chronic alveolar collapse.

Effects of Chronic Ineffective Gas Exchange

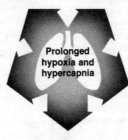

Renal system
• Release of erythropoietin
• Increased retention of bicarbonate ion, sodium, and water
• Fluid overload

Neurologic system
• Dulling of medullary respiratory center
• Respiration stimulated by aortic and carotid bodies

Musculoskeletal system
• Pulmonary osteoarthropathy (arthralgia, digital clubbing, subperiosteal proliferation of long bones)
• Increased myoglobin in muscles

Prolonged hypoxia and hypercapnia

Cardiovascular system
• Pulmonary capillary vasoconstriction
• Increased pulmonary vascular resistance
• Pulmonary hypertension
• Shunting of oxygenated blood
• Cor pulmonale

Hematopoietic system
• Polycythemia
• Increased risk of embolism and thrombosis

Prolonged hypoxia and hypercapnia, as seen in patients with chronic respiratory disorders, eventually take their toll on other vital systems.

Neurologic system
With progressive hypercapnia, the regulatory mechanisms of respiration may adjust to tolerate higher PCO_2 levels. But severe hypercapnia dulls the medullary respiratory center, forcing peripheral chemoreceptors in the aortic and carotid bodies to direct respiration. Because these receptors respond to low PO_2, and any treatment involving high concentrations of oxygen will suppress this hypoxic drive and thus suppress respiration, oxygen therapy must be strictly controlled in accordance with blood gas analysis.

Cardiovascular system
Respiratory neuromuscular disorder or lung or pulmonary vascular disease can produce cor pulmonale,

acute for chronic enlargement of the right ventricle. Usually, cor pulmonale is chronic, secondary to chronic obstructive pulmonary disease, such as emphysema. In acute form, cor pulmonale may develop from massive pulmonary embolism, with or without heart failure, or from acute pulmonary infection or other conditions that sharply increase hypoxemia. Cor pulmonale may result from widespread destruction of lung tissue or pulmonary capillaries that reduces the pulmonary vascular bed, from increased pulmonary vascular resistance, from shunting of unoxygenated blood, or from pulmonary vasoconstriction and pulmonary artery hypertension because of decreased PO_2. Pulmonary hypertension, the most common cause, may occur sporadically at first under conditions of increased pulmonary blood flow, as with exertion or fever. Eventually constant, it leads to right ventricular muscle hypertrophy, followed by right-heart failure, reduced cardiac output, and cardiovascular collapse.

Musculoskeletal system

A compensatory increase in muscle content of the oxygen-binding heme protein myoglobin improves oxygen transport to contracting muscles when Po_2 is low. In addition, an increase in pulmonary vasculature in response to chronic hypoxia may be the cause of pulmonary osteoarthropathy, also called secondary hypertrophic osteoarthropathy. This conditon—which shows up as bone and tissue changes in the extremities (arthralgia, clubbing, proliferation of subperiosteal tissues in long bones)—may accompany bronchial carcinoma, bronchiectasis, or pulmonary abscess.

Renal system

Sustained hypercapnia causes renal retention of bicarbonate ions, sodium, and water to dilute the effects of excess hydrogen ions, a compensatory action that can lead to fluid overload. Sustained hypoxia stimulates the kidneys to release erythropoietic factor into the blood. This factor causes a plasma transport protein to yield erythropoietin, the compound that spurs red blood cell production and raises hematocrit.

Hematopoietic system

Chronic hypoxemia often causes polycythemia, a compensatory attempt to increase the blood's oxygen-carrying capacity by increasing the number of red blood cells. However, such an increase thickens the blood, which makes embolism and thrombosis more likely, and increases the heart's work load—dangers that outweigh the advantage of improved oxygen capacity, especially for the patient with cor pulmonale.

aerobic metabolism to supply its energy needs, a situation that leads to lactic acidosis.

The mechanisms of hypoxia vary because oxygen delivery to the cells depends on the blood's oxygen-carrying capacity, cardiac output, and peripheral blood flow. For example, insufficient hemoglobin, as in anemia, reduces the blood's ability to transport adequate oxygen. Low blood volume, as from severe hemorrhage or an embolus or other vascular impedance, also reduces the amount of blood available to carry oxygen to the cells.

Another result of ineffective gas exchange is hypoxemia, which refers to a decrease in the oxygen concentration of the blood and is often used incorrectly as a synonym for hypoxia. Hypocapnia, another result of ineffective gas exchange, is a decrease in the carbon dioxide concentration of the blood. Conversely, hypercapnia is an increase in blood retention of carbon dioxide.

Ineffective gas exchange not only leads to poor tissue oxygenation, but also promotes retention of carbon dioxide and threatens homeostasis by tipping the systemic acid-base balance. The body has three normal regulatory mechanisms for dulling this toxic effect before it can tax other body systems.

Compensatory mechanisms

Normally, the body's acid-base balance hovers at 7.4 or remains within a very narrow pH range of 7.35 to 7.45. This is crucial, because an acute drop to 7.1 (acidosis) or a rise to 7.5 (alkalosis) may be life-threatening. Anything that tips the balance to the acid side, by producing hydrogen ions, lowers the pH; conversely, anything that tips the balance toward the basic side, by producing bicarbonate ions, decreases acidity and raises the pH. Body fluids fluctuate constantly, their composition altered by acids, carbon dioxide, and water from the cellular metabolism of carbohydrates, proteins, and fats. Carbon dioxide and water unite to form carbonic acid, which dissociates into hydrogen ions and bicar-

$$CO_2 + H_2O \rightleftharpoons \quad \rightleftharpoons H^+ + HCO_3^-$$

bonate ions. Three regulatory mechanisms neutralize or eliminate an excess of either hydrogen or bicarbonate ions and maintain the body's normal pH: acid-base buffers, the respiratory system itself, and the renal system.

Buffer systems. Pairs of weak acids and related bases operate in seconds to reduce the danger of stronger incoming acids and bases. By combining with a strong acid, which would dissociate to yield many hydrogen ions and thus sharply lower the pH, these buffers create a weaker acid that dissociates into fewer hydrogen ions and has a gentler effect on pH. They react similarly to neutralize a strong base, thereby keeping pH fluctuations to a minimum. Chief buffers of body fluids are bicarbonates, phosphates, and proteins, such as hemoglobin. The bicarbonate buffers, however, are mainly responsible for monitoring blood and interstitial fluid. Among the buffer systems, the bicarbonates alone have a limitless outlet in the respiratory system to reduce acidity and renew themselves by increased expiration of carbon dioxide.

Respiratory system. The second acid-base regulator is the respiratory system, which normally can restore homeostasis within minutes. Because the amount of carbon dioxide in plasma determines the amount of carbonic acid and hydrogen ions produced, any rise in PCO_2 means a rise in acidity; any drop in PCO_2 means a rise in alkalinity. Working together to detect and correct pH changes, the medullary respiratory centers and the lungs strive to keep PCO_2 at 40 mm Hg, a level that makes it possible for the lungs to excrete carbon dioxide at the same rate the cells produce it. They succeed by altering the respiratory rate and depth to eliminate more or less carbon dioxide, and therefore acid, as necessary to control pH. Respiratory alkalosis or acidosis results, however, when the respiratory disorder itself causes prolonged hyperventilation or hypoven-

tilation beyond the limits needed to adjust pH or otherwise prevents effective carbon dioxide exchange.

Renal system. The body's third and long-term regulator is the renal system. Within several hours or over several days, the kidneys adjust pH by excreting nonvolatile (fixed) acids— those which the lungs can't excrete— and by either excreting hydrogen ions and reabsorbing bicarbonate ions to correct excess acidity or reversing this action to correct alkalosis. In cases of metabolic acidosis or metabolic alkalosis that stem from altered metabolic rather than respiratory patterns, renal and respiratory compensatory mechanisms work together. The kidneys adjust the levels of appropriate ions, while the lungs change respiratory rate and depth to reduce or conserve carbon dioxide.

Thus, coping mechanisms exist to offset the effects of inefficient gas exchange. Compensation for acid-base imbalance involves a systemic shift in the opposite direction that moves pH back within normal limits. A primary respiratory imbalance produces an opposing compensatory metabolic response; the reverse also holds true. For example, respiratory acidosis provokes conservation of bicarbonate ions and excretion of hydrogen ions (compensatory metabolic alkalosis).

Multiple systemic dysfunction requiring outside intervention occurs when a disorder keeps compensatory systems from operating effectively. For example, the patient with chronic obstructive pulmonary disease (COPD) who develops diabetic ketoacidosis can't compensate by increasing expiration of carbon dioxide. Remember, too, that the COPD patient will show an elevated bicarbonate level as his kidneys compensate for carbon dioxide retention to maintain a normal pH; correcting the elevated bicarbonate level only aggravates acidosis. Thus, in treating systemic dysfunction, it's crucial to treat the primary problem, not the compensatory response.

Anatomic and physiologic variations in children

A child's developing respiratory system makes him more susceptible than an adult to certain respiratory diseases. For instance, upper respiratory tract infections commonly occur in children because a child's respiratory tract is immature, and the mucous membranes often can't produce enough mucus to warm and humidify inhaled air. Also, a child's developing immune system can't fight bacteria and viruses as well as an adult's can.

Kiesselbach's triangle, the cricoid cartilage, and the sinuses are key structures in a child's upper respiratory tract. Kiesselbach's triangle—also present in adults—is a fine network of small blood vessels near the tip of the nose. In children, it's the most common site of nosebleeds. The cricoid cartilage, located just below the epiglottis, is the narrowest cartilage ring in the developing larynx; thus, swelling or small amounts of mucus easily can occlude the narrow lumen. At birth, the ethmoidal and maxillary sinuses are present, the sphenoidal sinuses are very small, and the frontal sinuses are absent. The sphenoidal sinuses develop fully after puberty; the frontal, at age 7 or 8.

Because the lower respiratory tract is small in infants and children, breath sounds are louder and more bronchial, expiration is longer, and vesicular sounds are harsher. Breath sounds are transmitted throughout the chest and are difficult to localize. The infant's thorax is round, with equal antero-posterior transverse diameters. The lateral diameter increases rapidly with growth, resulting in characteristic adult proportions by age 6. (The thin chest wall and lack of muscle allow palpation of the floating ribs in young children.) The chest walls of newborns and infants consist mostly of cartilage. Therefore, any kind of obstruction to airflow results in prominent retractions. In children, the right mainstem bronchus is more prominently vertical than is the adult's. Aspiration on the right side is more common than left-sided aspiration. Also, a child's airway diameter is markedly less than the adult's. Thus, minimal swelling with inflammation, such as occurs in croup, can cause serious airway obstruction.

Infants are obligate nose breathers, which is one reason colds are more serious for them. A child's breathing should be primarily abdominal until age 6 or 7 (longer if the patient has done breathing exercises for singing or athletics). Abdominal breathing beyond this age may indicate pain or splinting of the chest walls, as in pleuritis; respiratory movements before this age suggest pain or splinting of the abdomen, as in peritonitis.

A child's respiratory rate may double in response to exercise, illness, or emotion. Normally, the rate for newborns is 30 to 80 breaths/minute; for toddlers, 20 to 40; and for children of school age and older, 15 to 25. Children usually reach the adult rate (12 to 20) at about age 15.

Selected References

Guyton, A.C. *Textbook of Medical Physiology,* 7th ed. Philadelphia: W.B. Saunders Co., 1986.

Respiratory Disorders. Nurse's Clinical Library. Springhouse, Pa.: Springhouse Corp., 1984.

Respiratory Problems. NurseReview Series. Springhouse, Pa.: Springhouse Corp., 1986.

Shapiro, B.A., et al. *Clinical Applications of Respiratory Care,* 3rd ed. Chicago: Year Book Medical Pubs., Inc., 1985.

Wade, J.F. *Comprehensive Respiratory Care: Physiology and Technique,* 3rd ed. St. Louis: C.V. Mosby Co., 1982.

2 RESPIRATORY ASSESSMENT

Introduction

Respiratory assessment is essential on hospital admission, at regular intervals during illness, and during routine health evaluation and screening. Perform respiratory assessment daily for ambulatory patients and more frequently for acutely ill patients; for those particularly susceptible to disease (pediatric and geriatric patients, for example); or for those whose activities are limited by medication, surgery, or debilitating diseases. Using correct assessment techniques, you can detect changes in a patient's respiratory system early and intervene quickly, perhaps preventing serious complications.

History

Begin gathering data by asking the patient open-ended questions. If possible, ask these questions systematically, to avoid overlooking important information. The interview may have to be conducted in several short sessions, depending on the severity of the patient's condition.

Biographical data
Determine the patient's age, sex, marital status, occupation, education, religion, and ethnic background. These factors provide clues to potential risks and to the patient's interpretation of his condition. Old age, for example, suggests physiologic changes, such as decreased vital capacity. Or the patient's occupation may alert you to problems related to hazardous materials.

Chief complaint
Assessing your patient's chief complaint helps you rapidly identify problems associated with respiratory distress. Ask him to tell you the "story" of his chief complaint, using questions like these: *When did you first notice that you didn't feel well? What's happened since then to bring you to the hospital?*

History of present illness
The most common chief complaints for respiratory disorders are cough (with or without sputum production or hemoptysis), dyspnea, and chest pain. You may want to ask the questions listed below to explore fully the history of your patient's present illness.

Cough
Does your cough usually occur at a specific time of day? How does it sound—dry, hacking, barking, congested? Family members may be asked about the frequency of a cough, because a chronic cough may not even be noticed by the patient. Try to determine whether the patient's cough is related to cigarette smoking or irritants. (The most common causes of coughing are smoking and chronic bronchitis.)

Are you taking any medication or receiving treatment to clear the cough? How frequently do you take the medication or receive treatment? Have you recently been exposed to anyone with a similar cough? Was this person's cough caused by a cold or flu?

Sputum production
How much sputum are you coughing up per day? Remember, the tracheobronchial tree can produce up to 3 oz (90 ml) of sputum per day.

At what time of day do you cough up the most sputum? Many smokers cough when they get up in the morning; nonsmokers usually don't. Coughing from an irritant occurs most often during exposure to it—for example, at work.

Is sputum production increasing? This may result from external stimuli or from such internal causes as chronic bronchial infection or a lung abscess. Excess production of sputum that separates into layers may indicate bronchiectasis.

Does the sputum contain mucus or look frothy? What color is it? Has the color changed? Does it smell bad? Foul-smelling sputum may result from an anaerobic infection, such as an abscess. Blood-tinged or rust-colored sputum may result from trauma caused by coughing or from underlying pathology, such as bronchitis, pulmonary infarction or infection, tuberculosis, and tumors. A color change from white to yellow or green indicates infection.

Dyspnea
Are you always short of breath or do you have attacks of breathlessness? Onset of dyspnea may be slow or abrupt, and the degree varies among patients. For example, a patient with asthma may experience acute dyspnea intermittently.

What relieves the attacks—positioning, relaxation, medication? Do the attacks cause your lips and nail beds to turn blue? Does body position, time of

day, or a certain activity affect your breathing? Paroxysmal nocturnal dyspnea and orthopnea are commonly associated with chronic lung disease, but they may be related to cardiac dysfunction.

How many stairs can you climb or blocks can you walk before you begin to feel short of breath? Do activities such as taking a shower or shopping make you feel this way? Dyspnea from activity suggests poor ventilation or perfusion, or inefficient breathing mechanisms.

Do you experience associated signs and symptoms, such as cough, diaphoresis, or chest discomfort? Does the breathlessness seem to be stable, or is it getting worse? Is it accompanied by external sounds, such as wheezing or stridor? Wheezing results from small-airway obstruction (for example, from an aspirated foreign body, from a tumor, from asthma, or from congestive heart failure). Stridor results from tracheal compression or laryngeal edema.

Chest pain
Is the pain localized? Describe the nature of the pain. Is it sharp, stabbing, crushing, or achy? Is it constant, or do you experience attacks? Have you ever had a chest injury? Does a specific activity (such as movement of the upper body or exercise) produce pain? Chest pain may be associated with cardiovascular disorders, but respiratory disorders usually cause musculoskeletal chest pain. (The lungs have no pain-sensitive nerves. However, the parietal pleura and the tracheobronchial tree are sensitive to pain.)

Is the pain accompanied by other signs and symptoms, such as coughing, sneezing, or shortness of breath? Does the pain occur when you breathe deeply? This distinction is important in determining whether your patient's pain is pleuritic.

Does splinting relieve the pain?

Past medical history

Information obtained through a medical history helps explain existing symptoms and also identifies patients at risk for developing respiratory difficulty. Focus on the following body systems, procedures, and conditions when reviewing your patient's history:

• *Respiratory system*. Ask whether your patient has ever had pneumonia, pleurisy, asthma, bronchitis, emphysema, or tuberculosis. Also ask him how often he gets colds.

• *Cardiovascular system*. Ask if your patient has ever had high blood pressure, a heart attack, congestive heart failure, or pulmonary edema. A history of such a disorder is particularly significant because of the close relationship between the cardiovascular system and the respiratory system.

• *Chest surgery*. Find out if the patient has had lung surgery, a mastectomy, or other chest surgery. Remember that physical examination findings differ for patients who have undergone such procedures as thoracoplasty or pneumonectomy.

• *Invasive medical procedures*. Ask the patient if he has undergone any chest or lung-related procedures, such as bronchoscopy or thoracentesis.

• *Chest deformities*. Note that congenital or trauma-related deformities may distort cardiac and pulmonary structures.

• *Laboratory tests*. Ask your patient for the dates and results of his last chest X-ray, pulmonary function test, electrocardiogram, arterial blood gas analysis, sputum culture, and skin test for tuberculosis.

• *Allergies*. Ask whether the patient reacts to common allergens, such as medications, food, pets, dust, or pollen. Also ask if he has any allergic signs and symptoms, such as coughing, sneezing, sinusitis, or dyspnea. Chronic allergies may predispose him to other respiratory disorders. Has he ever been treated for an allergy?

• *Medications*. Ask the patient if he takes any prescription or over-the-counter drugs for cough control, expectoration, nasal congestion, chest pain, or dyspnea. Also note any other medications the patient is taking, including over-the-counter medications.

• *Vaccinations*. Ask the patient if he has ever been vaccinated against pneumonia or flu.

Family history

When reviewing your patient's family history, ask if any family member has ever had asthma, cystic fibrosis, or emphysema, all of which may be genetically transmitted. Other important disorders to ask about include lung cancer and infectious diseases, such as tuberculosis. Also inquire about chronic allergies, cardiovascular disorders (such as hypertension, myocardial infarction, and congestive heart failure), and respiratory disturbances (such as frequent colds or episodes of flu, pneumonia, asthma, or emphysema). Disorders involving other body systems may be associated with pulmonary dysfunction, so ask about a family history of such conditions as kyphosis, scoliosis, obesity, and neuromuscular dysfunction.

Psychosocial history

Focus your questions about the patient's psychosocial history on the following aspects of his life:

• *Home conditions*. Persons living near a constant source of air pollution, such as a chemical factory, may develop respiratory disorders. Exposure to cigarette smoke in the home may aggravate respiratory symptoms, and crowded living conditions facilitate the transmission of communicable respiratory diseases.

• *Work*. Exposure on the job to cigarette smoke or to other substances that may be irritating to the respiratory system may be significant.

• *Pets*. Exposure to animals may precipitate allergic or asthmatic attacks.

• *Hobbies*. Seemingly innocent pastimes, such as building model airplanes or refinishing old furniture, may expose the patient to harsh chemical irritants.

• *Travel*. Persons traveling to unusual places or emigrating from countries where health care is poor are at increased risk of acquiring an infectious respiratory disorder.

• *Stress*. Some respiratory conditions, such as asthma and infection, can be aggravated by stress.

• *Smoking*. Ask the patient if he smokes cigarettes, cigars, pipe tobacco, marijuana, or any other type of cigarette, such as clove cigarettes. If he smokes cigarettes, find out how many packs he smokes each day and how long he's been smoking at this rate. Note the number of pack years. (See *Determining Pack Years*.) If the patient doesn't smoke now, ask if he used to smoke and how much. Learning about a patient's smoking habits is vital to completing a comprehensive respiratory history. Smoking can be associated with numerous and varied pathologies, such as lung cancer, chronic bronchitis, and emphysema.

• *Diet and alcohol intake*. Ask the patient about alcohol use and about his diet, because his nutritional status may influence his risk of respiratory infection.

• *Daily routine*. Respiratory signs and symptoms can interfere with such activities as climbing stairs or traveling to work. It may be appropriate to talk with family members about the patient's daily routine, because the patient may not realize the adaptations he has made for shortness of breath.

Review of systems

Complete your patient's health history by asking about the following signs and symptoms commonly associated with respiratory disorders:

• *General*. Fever, chills, and fatigue may occur in association with respiratory symptoms.

Determining Pack Years

If your patient smokes cigarettes, he's at higher risk for such respiratory diseases as lung cancer, emphysema, and bronchitis. By calculating pack years, you can assess his risk. Use the following formula:

number of packs smoked per day
×
number of years the
patient has smoked

For example, a patient who has smoked 2 packs of cigarettes per day for 42 years has incurred 84 pack years.

• *Skin*. Nocturnal diaphoresis may be associated with tuberculosis. Flushing can be associated with increased PCO_2.

• *Blood*. Anemia decreases the blood's oxygen-carrying capacity; polycythemia may occur in response to chronic hypoxemia.

• *Nose*. Nasal discharge, sinus pain or infection, or postnasal drip may result from seasonal allergies or from chronic sinus problems.

• *Mouth and throat*. Halitosis may result from a pulmonary infection, such as an abscess or bronchiectasis.

• *Cardiovascular system*. Ankle edema, paroxysmal nocturnal dyspnea, orthopnea, or chest pain that worsens with exercise, eating, or stress may reflect a cardiovascular disorder rather than a respiratory one.

• *Gastrointestinal system*. Weight loss suggests possible deterioration from disease, such as from lung cancer.

• *Nervous system*. Confusion, inability to concentrate, syncope, and restlessness may be associated with cerebral hypoxia. A headache upon awakening can indicate increased PCO_2.

• *Musculoskeletal system*. Chronic hypoxia may cause fatigue and weakness.

• *Psychological status.* Some respiratory signs (for example, wheezing and hyperventilation) may reflect emotional problems.

Physical examination

Environment and equipment
Before assessing your patient, be sure the examining area is quiet so you can auscultate his lungs accurately. Make sure the lighting is adequate to detect skin color variations. (If possible, use natural light, because fluorescent light doesn't show true skin color.)

You'll need a nasal speculum, a tongue depressor, a penlight, a cotton-tipped applicator, and a stethoscope. You may also wish to use a marking pen and a centimeter stick to mark points of reference on the patient's body.

Preparation and positioning
Tell the patient to undress to the waist and to put on a loose-fitting examining gown. (If the patient is a woman wearing a bra, ask her to remove it.) Be sure the patient is adequately draped for privacy and warmth.

Place the patient in a comfortable position that allows you access to his posterior and anterior chest. If he experiences shortness of breath, elevate his head. If the patient's condition permits, have him sit on the edge of a bed or examining table or in a chair, leaning slightly forward, with his arms folded across his chest. If this isn't possible, place him in the semi-Fowler's position for the anterior chest examination. Then ask him to lean forward slightly, using the side rails or mattress for support, so you can examine his posterior chest. If the patient can't lean forward for posterior chest examination, place him in a lateral position.

Remember that when you position the patient laterally in bed to examine his posterior chest, the mattress and the displacement of the patient's organs distort sounds and lung expansion. To offset these effects, examine the uppermost side of your patient's chest first; then roll him on his other side and repeat the examination, for comparison.

When you assess the patient's thorax, keep in mind the three portions to be examined—posterior, anterior, and lateral. You can examine any of these areas first and perform the lateral examination during the posterior or anterior assessment. The most important point is to proceed systematically, always comparing one side of the patient's thorax with the other side. (In this way, the patient serves as his own control.) Remember to examine the apices during the posterior and the anterior examinations.

Overview of respiratory status
Before starting detailed pulmonary assessment, quickly observe the patient for the following signs and symptoms of severe hypoxia or other acute respiratory difficulty:
• low level of consciousness
• shortness of breath when speaking
• rapid, deep, shallow, or depressed respirations
• use of accessory muscles when breathing
• intercostal and sternal retractions
• cyanosis
• external sounds (such as crowing, wheezing, or stridor)
• diaphoresis
• nasal flaring
• extreme apprehension or agitation.

A patient exhibiting most or all of these signs and symptoms requires immediate intervention and notification of the doctor.

Baseline data
The patient's vital signs—temperature, blood pressure, pulse, and respirations—provide baseline data for

your respiratory assessment. Deviations from normal may signal changes in respiratory status.

• Fever commonly indicates respiratory infection, which impairs diffusion of gases from the lungs to the bloodstream. Tissue metabolic rates rise with temperature, causing increased oxygen demand. The combination of impaired diffusion from the infection and a fever above 100.6° F. (38.1° C.) stresses the body's ability to meet respiratory needs.

Make sure you obtain an accurate temperature reading. You may, for instance, obtain a spuriously low oral temperature if your patient can't keep his lips closed, if he's receiving humidified oxygen, or if he's tachypneic (respirations greater than 20 breaths/minute). Under any of these circumstances, take a rectal temperature reading.

• Blood pressure, normally ranging from 90/60 to 140/90 mm Hg, may be normal, elevated, or depressed in a patient with respiratory problems. Changes depend on the patient's previous physical status and on his ability to compensate for existing respiratory difficulty. With acute respiratory distress, blood pressure initially remains normal or rises slightly, as a compensatory mechanism. During decompensation, blood pressure falls.

• With hypoxia (insufficient oxygen for tissue needs), pulse rate increases above the normal of 60 to 90 beats/minute in response to sympathetic stimulation. (Other possible reasons for an elevated pulse include exertion, anxiety, and smoking.) An irregular pulse may reflect such cardiac dysrhythmias as atrial fibrillation (commonly seen in patients with chronic respiratory problems) and premature atrial contractions (a common response to hypoxia). Premature ventricular contractions (a regular pulse rate interrupted by pauses or extra beats) also may occur. If you detect an irregular, thready, or weak pulse, assume that tissue and pulmonary perfusion has diminished.

• Respiration changes in response to hypoxia. Initially, the body compensates by increasing respiratory rate and depth. But when the body tires, respiratory rate and depth decrease. Respiratory failure may follow. (See *Common Respiratory Patterns*, pages 30 and 31, for information on differences in respiratory rates, rhythms, and depths.)

These baseline data guide the rest of your assessment. Take vital signs frequently, and be sure to document them properly.

Hyperventilation and *hypoventilation* describe the amount of carbon dioxide in arterial blood in conjunction with an abnormal rate and depth of respiration. *Hyperventilation* refers to a faster than normal respiratory rate, deeper breathing, and a lower than normal PCO_2 level. *Hypoventilation* refers to a slower than normal respiratory rate, shallower breathing, and a higher than normal PCO_2 level.

Skin color and condition

Begin your detailed respiratory examination by inspecting your patient's skin color. Look for central cyanosis in highly vascular areas: the lips, the nail beds, the tip of the nose, the ear helices, and the underside of the tongue. For a patient with dark brown or black skin, inspect those areas where cyanotic changes would be apparent: the nose, the cheeks, and the mucosa inside the lips. Facial skin may be pale gray in a cyanotic dark-skinned patient.

Central cyanosis, which affects all body organs, results from prolonged hypoxia. Its presence helps you gauge the severity of a patient's illness. (Remember, though, that severely anemic patients with respiratory difficulty don't appear cyanotic, and polycythemic patients may appear cyanotic and not be hypoxic because of the extra

Common Respiratory Patterns

To determine the rate, rhythm, and depth of your patient's respirations, observe him at rest. Make sure he's unaware that you're counting his respirations. A person conscious of his respirations may alter his natural pattern.

Always count respirations for at least 1 minute. If you count for only a fraction of a minute and then multiply, your count may be off by as much as 4 respirations per minute.

Your patient's respiratory rhythm should be even, except for an occasional deep breath.

Use this chart as a guide for noting differences in respiratory rates, rhythms, and depths.

Type	Characteristics
Eupnea	Normal respiration rate and rhythm. For adults and teenagers, 12 to 20 breaths/minute; ages 2 to 12, 20 to 30 breaths/minute; newborns, 30 to 50 breaths/minute. Also, occasional deep breaths at a rate of 2 or 3 breaths/minute.
Tachypnea	Increased respirations, as seen in fever. Respirations increase about 4 breaths/minute for every degree Fahrenheit above normal.
Bradypnea	Slower but regular respirations. Can occur when the brain's respiratory control center is affected by opiate narcotics, tumor, alcohol, a metabolic disorder, or respiratory decompensation. Normal during sleep.
Apnea	Absence of breathing, may be periodic.
Hyperpnea	Deeper respirations, rate normal.
Cheyne-Stokes	Respirations gradually become faster and deeper than normal, then slower, over a 30- to 170-second period. Periods of apnea for 20 to 60 seconds alternate.
Biot's	Faster and deeper respirations than normal, with abrupt pauses in between. Each breath has same depth. May occur with spinal meningitis or other CNS conditions.

Common Respiratory Patterns *(continued)*	
Type	**Characteristics**
Kussmaul's 	Faster and deeper respirations without pauses. In adults, over 20 breaths/minute. Breathing usually sounds labored, with deep breaths that resemble sighs. Can occur from renal failure or metabolic acidosis.
Apneustic 	Prolonged gasping inspiration, followed by extremely short, inefficient expiration. Can occur from lesions in the brain's respiratory center.

hemoglobin that cannot be saturated.) Be sure you know how to distinguish central cyanosis from peripheral cyanosis, which is caused by local vasoconstriction and is only apparent in the nail beds and sometimes the lips.

For all patients, examine the skin for dryness—a possible sign of dehydration—or for diaphoresis, which may be associated with fever and infection. Bright cherry-red mucous membranes may result from carbon monoxide poisoning. Flushed skin can indicate increased PCO_2. While inspecting the skin, observe the fingers for clubbing, a sign of chronic respiratory dysfunction as well as certain cardiovascular and, rarely, gastrointestinal disorders. (See *Assessing for Clubbed Fingers,* page 32.)

Upper respiratory tract

Inspect your patient's facial structures, observing for symmetry, deformities, and inflammation. Check his nasal septum for deviation and perforations. Using a nasal speculum, examine his nostrils for discharge, for the condition and color of their mucosa (it should be slightly redder than oral mucosa), for swelling and bleeding, and for any obstructions.

Next, palpate his nose to detect any swelling, pain, or fractures. Palpate the maxillary sinuses for tenderness and swelling by pressing on the patient's cheeks over the maxillary areas. Palpate his frontal sinuses by placing your thumbs just below the patient's eyebrows and pressing upward. While observing and palpating these facial structures, listen for external sounds of moisture or mucus and for stridor or wheezing.

If the patient wears dentures, ask him to remove them. Then, using a tongue depressor, a cotton-tipped applicator, and a penlight, examine his oropharynx for color changes, inflammation, white patches, ulcerations, bleeding, exudate, and lesions. Be sure to check his soft palate, anterior and posterior pillars of fauces, uvula, tonsils, posterior pharynx, teeth, gums, tongue, mouth floor, mucous membranes, and lips. Remember that a dark-skinned patient has dark patches on his mucous membranes.

Using a tongue depressor, bring the patient's pharynx into view and ask him to say "eh." Observe for symmetrical rise and fall of the soft palate. Next, touch both sides of his posterior pharynx with the applicator to check his gag reflex. (This test is particularly helpful when you're assessing an older patient with decreased sensitivity to

Assessing for Clubbed Fingers

To quickly assess the fingers for clubbing, have the patient place the first phalanges of the forefingers together. Normally, the bases of the nails are concave and create a small, diamond-shaped space when the first phalanges are opposed (as shown in the illustration at top). When clubbed fingers are opposed, the now-convex bases of the nails can touch without leaving a space (as shown in the illustration at bottom).

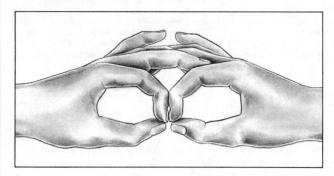

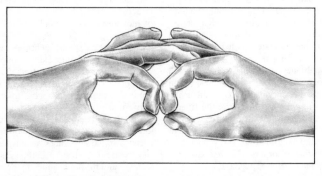

touch, or one who has suffered a cerebrovascular accident (CVA); it helps you determine the patient's ability to swallow oral secretions and food.) To determine the patient's ability to clear his respiratory tract of accumulated secretions, ask him to cough. If your patient is debilitated by CVA or other cerebral trauma or by drug or alcohol ingestion, elicit a cough by gently touching his posterior oropharynx with a cotton-tipped applicator.

Inspect the patient's trachea for midline position, and observe again for any use of accessory neck muscles in breathing. If you can't see his trachea, palpate for it at the midline position, using the fingertips of one hand. Starting at the middle base of the patient's lower jaw, gently slide your fingertips down the center of his neck. After locating his larynx, you should be able to feel his trachea in the area of the sternal notch. Any deviation of the trachea to either side indicates deformity and calls for further investigation. Also, observe and palpate the patient's neck over the trachea for swelling, bruises, tenderness, and masses that might obstruct breathing.

Posterior chest inspection

Instruct the patient to sit and lean forward, with his shoulders rounded and his arms crossed on his chest. (Always note the patient's tolerance of position changes.) After checking his posterior chest for wounds, lesions, masses, or scars, observe the rate, rhythm, and depth of his respirations. The normal respiratory rate for an adult is 12 to 20 breaths/minute. Respirations should be regular and inaudible, with the sides of the chest expanding equally. Normal respirations consist of inspiration, a slight pause, and a slightly longer expiration. Prolonged expiratory time suggests impedance of air outflow.

Next, observe the patient's chest for impaired movement. Normally, the chest moves upward and outward symmetrically on inspiration. Impaired movement may result from pain, exertion from poor positioning, or obstruction from abdominal distention. Paradoxical movement of the chest wall may result from fractured ribs or flail chest.

Note the slope of the patient's ribs. Check for retraction of intercostal spaces during inspiration and for abnormal bulging of intercostal spaces during expiration. Then observe for spinal deformities, such as lordosis, kyphosis, and scoliosis.

Posterior chest palpation

Palpate the patient's posterior chest to assess his thorax, to identify thoracic structures, and to check expansion and vocal or tactile fremitus. (See *Palpation Sequences*, page 34.) Begin by feeling for muscle mass with your fingers and palms (use a grasping action of the fingers to assess position and consistency). Normally, it feels firm, smooth, and symmetrical. As you palpate muscle mass, also check skin temperature and turgor. Be sure to note the presence of crepitus (especially around a wound site). Then palpate the thoracic spine, noting tenderness, swelling, or deformities, such as lordosis, kyphosis, and scoliosis.

Next, using your metacarpophalangeal joints and fingerpads, gently palpate the patient's intercostal spaces and ribs for abnormal retractions, bulging, and tenderness. Normally, the intercostal spaces delineate a downward sloping of the ribs. In a patient with an increased anteroposterior diameter caused by obstructive lung disease, you'll feel ribs that are abnormally horizontal.

Now palpate the thoracic landmarks to identify underlying lobe structures. (See *Thoracic Landmarks*, page 35.) To help you identify the division between the patient's upper and lower lobes, instruct him to raise his arms above his head; then palpate the borders of his scapulae. The inner edges of the scapulae should line up with the divisions between the upper and lower lobes. (See *Lung Lobe Positions*, pages 36 and 37.)

The inferior border of the lower lobes is usually located at the 10th thoracic spinous process and may descend, on full inspiration, to the 12th thoracic spinous process. To locate the lower lung borders in a patient lying laterally, palpate the visible free-floating ribs or costal margins; then count four intercostal spaces upward for the general location of the lower lung fields.

Palpate for symmetrical expansion of the patient's thorax (respiratory excursion) by placing your palms—fingers together and thumbs abducted toward the spine—flat on the bilateral sections of his lower posterior chest wall. Position your thumbs at the 10th rib level, and grasp the lateral rib cage with your hands. As the patient inhales, his posterior chest should move upward and outward, and your thumbs should move apart; when he exhales,

Palpation Sequences

Follow the sequences illustrated here to palpate the posterior and anterior chest.

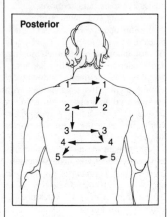

Posterior

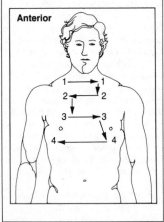

Anterior

your thumbs should return to midline and touch each other again. Repeat this technique on his upper posterior chest.

Palpate for vocal or tactile fremitus by using the top portion of each palm and following the palpation sequence illustrated in *Palpation Sequences*. To check for vocal fremitus, ask your pa-

tient to repeat "99" as you proceed. Palpable vibrations will be transmitted from his bronchopulmonary system, along the solid surfaces of his chest wall, to your palms and fingers.

Note the symmetry of the vibrations and the areas of enhanced, diminished, or absent fremitus. (Remember, fremitus should be most pronounced in the patient's upper chest where the trachea branches into the right and the left mainstem bronchi, and less noticeable in the lower regions of the thorax.)

You can estimate the level of your patient's diaphragm on both sides of his posterior chest by placing the ulnar side of your extended hand parallel to the anticipated diaphragm level. Instruct the patient to repeat "99" as you move your hand downward. The level where you no longer feel fremitus corresponds approximately to the diaphragm level.

Posterior chest percussion

To learn the density and location of such anatomic structures as the patient's lungs and diaphragm, you must identify five percussion sounds: flat, dull, resonant, hyperresonant, and tympanic. (See *Percussion Sounds*, page 38.) Start by percussing across the top of each shoulder. The area overlying the lung apices—approximately 2" (5 cm)—should be resonant. Then percuss downward toward the patient's diaphragm, at 2" intervals, comparing right and left sides as you proceed. (See *Percussion and Auscultation Sequences*, page 39.) Remember to avoid his scapulae and other bony areas. The thoracic area (except over the scapulae) should produce resonance when you percuss. At the level of the diaphragm, resonance should change to dullness. A dull sound over the lungs indicates fluid or solid tissue. Hyperresonance or tympany over a patient's lung suggests pneumothorax or large emphysematous blebs. A marked

Thoracic Landmarks

Posterior view

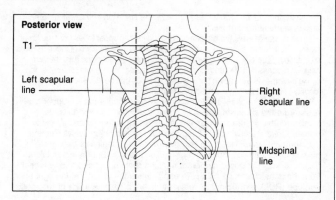

- T1
- Left scapular line
- Right scapular line
- Midspinal line

Anterior view

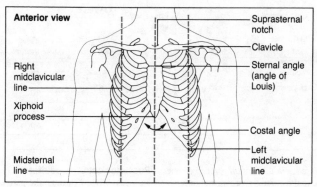

- Suprasternal notch
- Clavicle
- Sternal angle (angle of Louis)
- Right midclavicular line
- Xiphoid process
- Costal angle
- Midsternal line
- Left midclavicular line

Lateral view

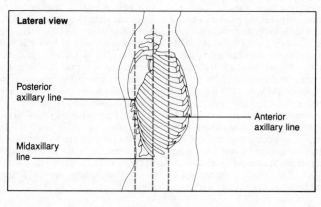

- Posterior axillary line
- Anterior axillary line
- Midaxillary line

Lung Lobe Positions

To locate lung lobes, you'll need to know the common chest wall landmarks shown in these illustrations.

In the posterior view, the oblique fissures divide the upper lobes from the lower lobes of both lungs. Externally, you can approximate the location of these fissures by imagining bilateral lines drawn laterally and inferiorly from the third thoracic spinous process to the inferior border of the scapula. You should remember that unlike the other views shown here, where all lobes can be identified, you can identify only two lobes in each lung in the posterior view.

In the left lateral view, the left oblique fissure divides the left upper lobe (LUL) from the left lower lobe (LLL). Externally, you can approximate the location of this fissure by imagining a line drawn anteriorly and inferiorly from the third thoracic spinous process to the sixth rib, midclavicular line.

In the right lateral view, you can determine the location of the right oblique fissure as you did for the left oblique fissure. But the right oblique fissure divides the upper *portion* of the lung (both upper and middle lobes) from the right lower lobe (RLL). To approximate the division of the right upper lobe (RUL) and the right middle lobe (RML), imagine a line drawn medi-

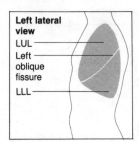

Left lateral view
LUL
Left oblique fissure
LLL

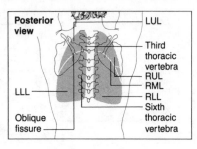

Posterior view
LUL
Third thoracic vertebra
RUL
RML
RLL
Sixth thoracic vertebra
LLL
Oblique fissure

difference in diaphragm level from one side to the other is an abnormal finding.

Next, measure diaphragmatic excursion. Instruct the patient to take a deep breath and hold it while you percuss downward until dullness identifies the lower border of the lung field. Mark this point. Now ask the patient to exhale and again hold his breath, as you percuss upward to the area of dullness. Mark this point, too. Repeat this entire procedure on the opposite side of the patient's chest. Now measure the distances between the two marks on each side. Normal diaphragmatic excursion measures about 1¼″ to 2¼″ (3 to 6 cm). (A person's diaphragm is usually slightly higher on his right side.)

Posterior chest auscultation

To assess airflow through the patient's respiratory system, auscultate his lungs and identify normal and abnormal (adventitious) breath sounds. (See *Normal and Abnormal Breath Sounds,* pages 40 and 41.) Lung auscultation helps detect abnormal fluid or mucus as well as obstructed passages. You can also determine the condition of the alveoli and surrounding pleura.

Before auscultating the posterior chest, remove clothing and bed linen from the body area to be examined. If the patient has a lot of hair on his posterior chest, wet and mat it with a damp washcloth to prevent it from

In the anterior view, you can locate the apices and the inferior borders of both lungs using external landmarks on the chest. The apices lie ¾″ to 1½″ (2 to 4 cm) above the inner portion of the clavicle. The inferior borders run from the sixth rib, midclavicular line, to the eighth rib, midaxillary line.

The horizonal fissure divides the right upper lobe from the right middle lobe. Externally, you can approximate the location of this fissure by imagining a line drawn anteriorly and superiorly from the fifth rib, midaxillary line, to the fourth rib, midclavicular line.

The right and left oblique fissures divide the lower lobe from the upper and middle lobes. Externally, you can approximate the location of these fissures by imagining bilateral lines drawn medially and inferiorly from the fifth rib, midaxillary line, to the sixth rib, midclavicular line.

Locating chest wall landmarks and the imaginary lines noted above will help you perform a complete thoracic assessment of your patient.

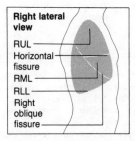

Right lateral view
RUL
Horizontal fissure
RML
RLL
Right oblique fissure

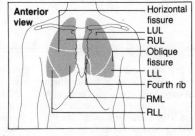

Anterior view
Horizontal fissure
LUL
RUL
Oblique fissure
LLL
Fourth rib
RML
RLL

causing rubbing sounds that can be confused with crackles.

When auscultating the patient's chest, instruct him to take full, slow breaths through his mouth. (Nose breathing changes the pitch of the lung sounds.) Listen for one full inspiration and expiration before moving the stethoscope. Remember, a patient may try to accommodate you by breathing quickly and deeply with every movement of the stethoscope—which can cause hyperventilation. If your patient becomes light-headed or dizzy, stop auscultating and allow him to breathe normally for a few minutes.

Using the diaphragm of the stethoscope, begin auscultating above the patient's scapulae. Move to the area between the scapulae and the vertebral column. Then move laterally beneath the scapulae, to the right and left lower lobes. Move the stethoscope's diaphragm methodically, and compare the sounds you hear on both sides of the chest before moving to the next area.

Normally, you'll hear vesicular breath sounds—soft, low-pitched sounds lasting longer during inspiration—at the lung bases. Bronchovesicular breath sounds—medium-pitched sounds that are equal in duration on inspiration and expiration—can be heard between the scapulae. Decreased or absent breath sounds may result from bronchial obstruction, muscle weakness, obesity, or pleural disease.

Percussion Sounds

Sound	Pitch	Intensity	Quality	Indication
Flatness	High	Soft	Extreme dullness	*Normal:* sternum; *abnormal:* atelectatic lung
Dullness	Medium	Medium	Thudlike	*Normal:* liver area, cardiac area, diaphragm; *abnormal:* pleural effusion
Resonance	Low	Moderate to loud	Hollow	*Normal:* lung
Hyper-resonance	Lower than res-onance	Very loud	Booming	*Abnormal:* emphysematous lung or pneumothorax
Tympany	High	Loud	Musical, drumlike	*Normal:* stomach area; *abnormal:* air-distended abdomen

If you hear an adventitious breath sound, note its location and at which point during the respiratory process it occurs—during inspiration, for example. Then continue auscultating the patient's posterior chest.

After auscultating, instruct the patient to cough and breathe deeply. Let him rest, and listen again to the area where you heard the adventitious sound or sounds. Note any changes. Sometimes crackles and rhonchi can be cleared by coughing; wheezes and friction rubs can't be cleared this way.

If you've detected any respiratory abnormality during palpation, percussion, or auscultation, assess your patient's voice sounds for vocal resonance. The significance of vocal resonance is based on the principle that sound carries best through a solid, not as well through fluid, and poorly through air. Normally, you should hear vocal resonance as muffled, unclear sounds, loudest medially and less intense at the lung periphery. Voice sounds that become louder and more distinct signal bronchophony, an abnormal finding except over the trachea and posteriorly over the upper right lobe. To elicit bronchophony, ask your patient to say "99" or "one, two, three" while you auscultate his thorax in the systematic way described above.

Whispered pectoriloquy reveals the presence of an exaggerated bronchophony. Ask your patient to whisper a simple phrase like "one, two, three." Hearing the words clearly through the stethoscope is an abnormal finding.

Egophony is another form of abnormal vocal resonance. Ask your patient to say "ee-ee-ee." Transmission of the sound through the stethoscope as "ay-ay-ay" is an abnormal finding, possibly indicating compressed lung tissue, as in a pleural effusion.

You may hear increased vocal resonance, whispered pectoriloquy, and egophony in any patient with consolidated lungs.

Anterior chest inspection

To inspect your patient's anterior chest, place him in semi-Fowler's position.

Percussion and Auscultation Sequences

Follow the sequences illustrated here to percuss and auscultate the patient's lungs. Remember to compare sound variations from one side to the other as you proceed, and to avoid bony areas. Document any abnormal sounds and describe them carefully, including their location.

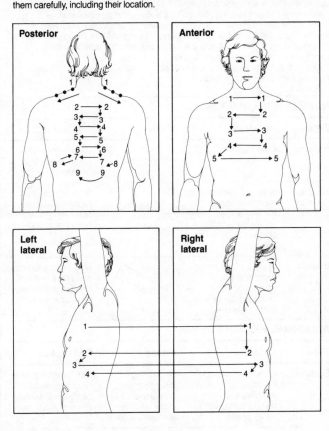

Begin by inspecting for draining, open wounds, bruises, abrasions, scars, cuts, and punctures, as well as for rib deformities, fractures, lesions, or masses. Then inspect the rate, rhythm, and depth of respirations. Remember that men, infants, and children are normally diaphragmatic (abdominal) breathers, as are athletes, singers, and persons who practice yoga. Women are usually intercostal (chest) breathers.

Your patient's face should look relaxed when he breathes. Abnormal findings include nasal flaring, pursed-lip breathing, use of neck or abdominal muscles on expiration, and inter-

Normal and Abnormal Breath Sounds

Breath sounds are produced by air moving through the tracheobronchoal-veolar system. Normal breath sounds are labeled *bronchial, bronchovesicu-lar*, and *vesicular*. They're described according to location, ratio of inspira-tion to expiration, intensity, and pitch.

Abnormal (adventitious) breath sounds occur when air passes either through narrowed airways or through moisture, or when the membranes lin-ing the chest cavity and the lungs become inflamed. These sounds include *crackles, rhonchi, wheezes*, and *pleural friction rub*. You may hear them su-perimposed over normal breath sounds.

Use this chart as a guide to assess both normal and abnormal breath sounds. Document your findings.

NORMAL BREATH SOUNDS

Type	Location	Ratio	Description
Bronchial	Over trachea	I / 2:3 \ E	Loud, high pitched, and hollow, harsh, or coarse
Broncho-vesicular	Anteriorly, near the mainstem bronchi in the first and second intercostal spaces; posteriorly, between the scapulae	I / 1:1 \ E	Soft, breezy, and pitched about two notes lower than bronchial sounds
Vesicular	In most of the lungs' peripheral parts (cannot be heard over the presternum or the scapulae)	I / 3:1 \ E	Soft, swishy, breezy, and about two notes lower than bronchov-esicular sounds

ABNORMAL BREATH SOUNDS

Type	Location	Cause	Description
Crackles	Anywhere; heard in lung bases first with pulmonary edema, usually during inspi-ratory phase	Air passing through mois-ture, especially in the small air-ways and alveoli	Light crackling, pop-ping, nonmusical; can be further clas-sified by pitch: high, medium, or low
Rhonchi	In larger airways, usually during expir-atory phase	Fluid or secre-tions in the large airways or nar-rowing of large airways	Coarse rattling, usu-ally louder and lower pitched than crackles; can be described as sonorous, bubbling, moaning, musical, sibilant, and rumbly

Normal and Abnormal Breath Sounds *(continued)*

ABNORMAL BREATH SOUNDS

Type	Location	Ratio	Description
Wheezes	Anywhere; occur during expiration	Narrowed airways	Creaking, groaning; always high-pitched, musical squeaks
Pleural friction rub	Anterolateral lung field, on both inspiration and expiration (with the patient in an upright position)	Inflamed parietal and visceral pleural linings rubbing together	Superficial squeaking or grating

costal or sternal retractions. Inspect for impaired chest wall movement. Observe for thoracic deformities, such as pectus excavatum (funnel chest) and pectus carinatum (pigeon chest). (See *Chest Deformities*, page 42.) Check the patient for barrel chest by noting the ratio between the anteroposterior diameter of his chest and its lateral diameter; the normal ratio ranges from 1:2 to 5:7.

Anterior chest palpation

Begin palpating your patient's anterior chest using your fingers and palms. Feel for areas of tenderness, muscle mass, and skin turgor and elasticity. Note any crepitus during your palpation, especially around wound sites, subclavian catheters, and chest tubes.

Palpate his sternum and costal cartilages for tenderness and deformities, and then, using your metacarpophalangeal joints and finger pads, palpate his intercostal spaces and ribs for abnormal retractions, bulging, and tenderness. Remember to proceed to the lateral aspects of the thorax.

Next, palpate the thoracic landmarks used to identify underlying structures.

To assess for symmetrical respiratory expansion, place your thumbs along each costal margin, pointing toward the xiphoid process, with your hands along the lateral rib cage. Ask the patient to inhale deeply, and observe for symmetrical thoracic expansion.

Now palpate for vocal or tactile fremitus, remembering to examine the lateral surfaces and to compare symmetrical areas of the patient's lungs. (See *Palpation Sequences*, page 34.) (If your patient is a woman, you may have to displace her breasts to examine her anterior chest.) Remember that fremitus will usually be decreased or absent over the patient's pericardium.

Anterior chest percussion

Percussing the patient's anterior chest allows you to determine the location and density of his heart, lungs, liver, and diaphragm. Begin by percussing the lung apices (the supraclavicular areas), comparing right and left sides. Then percuss downwards in $1\frac{1}{4}''$ to $2''$ (3- to 5-cm) intervals. You should hear resonant tones until you reach the third or fourth intercostal space (ICS), to the left of the sternum, where you'll hear a dull sound produced by the heart. This sound should continue as you percuss down toward the fifth ICS

Chest Deformities

FUNNEL CHEST
Physical characteristics
- Sinking or funnel-shaped depression of lower sternum
- Diminished anteroposterior chest diameter

Signs and associated conditions
- Postural disorders, such as forward displacement of neck and shoulders
- Upper thoracic kyphosis
- Protuberant abdomen
- Functional heart murmur

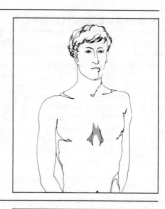

PIGEON CHEST
Physical characteristics
- Projection of sternum beyond abdomen's frontal plane. Evident in two variations: projection greatest at xiphoid process and projection greatest at or near center of sternum

Signs and associated conditions
- Functional cardiovascular or respiratory disorders

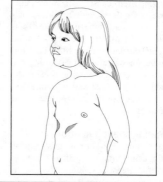

BARREL CHEST
Physical characteristics
- Enlarged anteroposterior and transverse chest dimensions; chest appears barrel-shaped
- Prominent accessory muscles

Signs and associated conditions
- Chronic respiratory disorders
- Increasing shortness of breath
- Chronic cough
- Wheezing

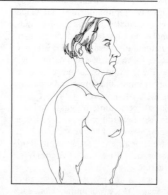

and laterally toward the midclavicular line. At the sixth ICS, at the left midclavicular line, you'll hear resonance again. As you percuss down toward the rib cage, you'll hear tympany over the stomach. On the right side, you should hear resonance, indicating normal lung tissue. Near the fifth to seventh ICS you'll hear dullness, marking the superior border of the liver.

To percuss his lateral chest, instruct the patient to raise his arms over his head. If he is short of breath, have him lean forward with his arms on the overbed table. Percuss laterally, comparing right and left sides as you proceed. These areas should also be resonant.

Anterior chest auscultation

In the same way you auscultated the patient's posterior chest, auscultate his anterior and lateral chest, comparing sounds on both sides before moving to the next area.

Begin auscultating the anterior chest at the trachea, where you should hear bronchial (or tubular) breath sounds.

Next, listen for bronchovesicular breath sounds where the mainstem bronchi branch from the trachea (near the second intercostal space, ¾" to 1¼" [2 to 3 cm] to either side of the sternum). Bronchial and bronchovesicular sounds are abnormal when heard over peripheral lung areas.

Now, using the standard chest landmarks, listen over the patient's peripheral lung fields for vesicular sounds. Be sure to auscultate his lateral chest walls, comparing right and left sides as you proceed. On the left side, heart sounds diminish breath sounds; on the right side, the liver diminishes them.

If you hear adventitious breath sounds, describe them and note their location and timing. After you've listened to several respirations in the area of the adventitious sound, instruct the patient to cough and breathe deeply.

Then, using the technique described on pages 36 to 38 for the posterior chest, auscultate the area producing the abnormal sound and, if necessary, auscultate for bronchophony, whispered pectoriloquy, and egophony.

Pediatric assessment

Pediatric history data

Ask the parents how often the child has had upper respiratory tract infections. Remember that a history of more than six ear, nose, or throat infections a year necessitates further evaluation of the child, because colds in preschool children are often a sign of streptococcal infection. Find out if the child has had other respiratory signs and symptoms, such as dyspnea, wheezing, rhinorrhea, or a stuffy nose. Ask if these appear to be related to the child's activities or to seasonal changes.

Also, ask if the child has had a cough that interrupts his sleep or causes vomiting. If so, does it produce sputum? Is the sputum blood-tinged? Has the child had a pertussis vaccine? Ask if anyone in the family has ever had cystic fibrosis or other major respiratory diseases, such as asthma.

Examination considerations

Positioning a child for a respiratory examination depends, of course, on his age, condition, and disposition. The sitting position offers you easiest access to his thorax, and usually a parent can help by holding the child in his lap. You and the parent can also form a mock examining table by sitting opposite each other, placing your knees together, and allowing the child to sit on the parent's lap.

If the child is quiet, auscultate his lungs first. If you hear fluid, place the stethoscope's diaphragm over his nose to determine if the fluid is in the nose or upper respiratory tract. This is important in children, because the sound of fluid in the nose can be transmitted through the short distance between the nose and the lungs.

To examine the child's nostrils for patency, occlude one, put the stethoscope's diaphragm over the other, and listen and watch for condensation on the diaphragm. With infants and young children, perform this procedure after auscultating the lungs, because crying (which the procedure may provoke) can cause an unnatural respiration rate and interfere with breath sound auscultation. Also, crying usually elicits mouth breathing, which can make determining the nostrils' patency difficult. To quiet a crying baby and relax his breathing, hand him a plastic windmill and ask him to blow on it, or have him pretend to blow out a candle.

The procedure you should use for inspecting the child's mouth and throat also depends on his age and disposition. Position the infant on his back, and ask the parent to hold him still. If the patient is a young child, have the parent hold the child on his lap, restraining the child's head with one arm and his arms with the other. Or the parent can raise and hold the child's arms over his head, immobilizing the head between the arms. A child age 6 or older will probably sit on the examining table without restraint. (To ease his anxiety, you might allow him to handle the equipment.)

Use a flashlight and tongue depressor to examine the child's mouth and throat. You can also use the tongue depressor to elicit the gag reflex in infants. Remember, however, that you should never test this reflex or examine the pharynx in a child suspected of having epiglottitis, because these procedures can cause complete laryngeal obstruction, which could be fatal.

While examining the posterior thorax of the older child, be sure to check for scoliosis. If you observe an abnormality, refer him for treatment. Also, remember that Harrison's groove (a horizontal ridge at the diaphragm level, accompanied by some flaring of

the ribs below the groove, as by rickets or congenital syphilis) is considered normal in infants and young, thin children—if other pathologic signs aren't present.

Childhood respiratory disorders

You may see laryngotracheobronchitis (croup)—the most common cause of respiratory distress in children over age 3—in a child with a history of upper respiratory tract infections, a barking cough ("seal bark"), fever, stridor, and diminished breath sounds with rhonchi. Signs and symptoms of this usually benign disease are similar to those for epiglottitis. Usually, a chest X-ray determines the cause of respiratory distress in children.

Epiglottitis, a bacterial infection preceded by a minor respiratory illness, sometimes may be present in a child with sudden respiratory distress and high fever, hoarseness, and anoxia. Remember: excitement or stress that causes the child to cry can produce immediate airway obstruction. Epiglottitis is more common in children between ages 3 and 8; croup, which has similar signs and symptoms, is more common in children between ages 2 and 5.

In assessing the toddler, evaluate wheezing carefully. In this age-group, wheezing often results from an accumulation of secretions that narrows the airway (as in bronchiolitis) and not necessarily from bronchospasm (as in asthma).

Intracostal, subcostal, and suprasternal retractions and expiratory grunts are always serious signs in children. Refer an infant or child with any of these signs for treatment immediately. He may have pneumonia, respiratory distress syndrome, or left-sided heart failure. An infant with untreated pneumonia can die within hours.

When a child's signs and symptoms include retractions, nasal flaring, cyanosis, restlessness, and apprehension—primarily on inspiration—the trachea or mainstem bronchi may be obstructed. If these signs and symptoms occur on expiration, his bronchioles may be obstructed, as seen with asthma or bronchitis. Regardless of the specific cause, these signs and symptoms indicate serious respiratory distress. Foreign body aspiration may also result in childhood respiratory distress.

Geriatric assessment

Health history concerns
During the health history interview, remember that the elderly patient may be confused or his mental function may be slow, especially if he has hypoventilation and hypoperfusion from respiratory disease. Also, keep in mind that because an elderly patient has reduced sensations, he may describe his chest pain as heavy or dull, whereas a younger patient would describe the same pain as sharp. When recording a retired patient's psychosocial history, be sure you ask about his former occupation, because it may have involved exposure to harmful substances.

Examination findings
As you inspect an elderly patient's thorax, be especially alert for degenerative skeletal changes, such as kyphosis. Palpating for diaphragmatic excursion may be more difficult in the elderly patient because of loose skin covering his chest. Therefore, when you position your hands, slide them toward his spine, raising loose skinfolds between your thumbs and the spine.

When you percuss an elderly person's chest, remember that loss of elasticity stretches the alveoli and bronchioles, producing hyperresonance. Pulmonary function also decreases. During auscultation, carefully observe how well your patient tolerates the examination. He may tire easily because of low tolerance to oxygen debt. Also, taking deep breaths during auscultation may produce light-headedness or syncope faster than in a younger patient. You may hear diminished sounds at the lung bases because some of his airways are closed.

Risk of illness
Elderly persons are subject to the same respiratory disorders and diseases as younger adults. In cold, damp weather, however, they're at an increased risk for chronic respiratory disease, colds, and flu. Also, these patients run a greater risk of developing pneumonia because their weakened chest musculature reduces their ability to clear secretions.

Selected References
Bates, B., and Hoeckelman, R.A. *A Guide to Physical Examination and History Taking,* 4th ed. Philadelphia: J.B. Lippincott Co., 1987.

Glass, L., and Jenkins, C. "The Ups and Downs of Serum pH," *Nursing83* 13(9):34-41, September 1983.

Health Assessment Handbook. Springhouse, Pa.: Springhouse Corp., 1985.

Malasanos, L., et al. *Health Assessment,* 3rd ed. St. Louis: C.V. Mosby Co., 1985.

Respiratory Disorders. Nurse's Clinical Library. Springhouse, Pa.: Springhouse Corp., 1984.

Respiratory Problems. NurseReview Series. Springhouse, Pa.: Springhouse Corp., 1986.

Sana, J., and Judge, R. *Physical Assessment Skills for Nursing Practice,* 2nd ed. Boston: Little, Brown & Co., 1982.

Westra, B. "Assessment Under Pressure: When Your Patient says, 'I Can't Breathe,'" *Nursing84* 14(5):34-39, May 1984.

3 DIAGNOSTIC TESTS AND MONITORING PROCEDURES

Introduction

The pulmonary and circulatory systems provide the body with a continuous supply of oxygen and remove carbon dioxide quickly and efficiently. The pulmonary system controls gas exchange between the atmosphere and blood; the circulatory system transports gases between the lungs and cells. A dysfunction in either system disrupts homeostasis and causes anoxia or even cell death.

The procedures and tests described in this chapter help identify and assess such dysfunction. Typically, clinical evaluation of a patient with suspected pulmonary dysfunction begins with a thorough patient history and a physical examination. A chest X-ray usually follows initial assessment and, depending on its results, a sputum specimen may be collected to determine if dysfunction results from cancer, bacteria, or parasites. Arterial blood gas determinations evaluate the patient's ability to exchange a sufficient amount of carbon dioxide for oxygen.

Pulmonary function tests may then identify obstructive or restrictive ventilatory defects. Such tests measure lung capacity volume and flow and help screen patients preoperatively to evaluate their surgical risk.

Endoscopic examination permits direct observation of the larger airways. This may serve both diagnostic and therapeutic purposes. For example, endoscopy allows removal of foreign bodies (with a rigid bronchoscope), secretions, and blood.

Finally, radiographic and scanning tests serve various purposes, from screening for asymptomatic cancer to determining perfusion and ventilation abnormalities. These tests can visualize the entire pulmonary system or provide a three-dimensional view of a specific area.

Pulmonary function tests

These dynamic tests examine how the pulmonary system works. The most common pulmonary function tests (PFTs) are spirometric measurements of volume (the amount of exhaled air) and flow rates (the speed of exhalation). (See *Reading a Spirogram*.) Generally, volumes decrease in restrictive disease; flow rates decline in obstructive disease.

These tests can also determine the degree of respiratory impairment. They're increasingly used as screening tests in patients without overt pulmonary symptoms, such as preoperative patients and asymptomatic smokers.

Other PFTs require specialized equipment and are usually used in patients with identified pulmonary disease. These tests measure CO_2 response, peak flow, and uniformity of ventilation and estimate volumes that can't be measured directly. (See *Specialized Pulmonary Function Tests*, page 49.)

Reading a Spirogram

The following diagram represents normal lung volumes. Rising lines represent inspiration; falling lines represent exhalation.

To read a spirogram, you'll need to understand the following terms.
• *Volumes* measure the amount of air.
• *Capacities* consist of two or more volumes.
• *Tidal volume (TV)* reflects the volume of air breathed in and out during a normal breath.
• *Inspiratory reserve volume (IRV)* reflects the volume of air inhaled with a normal inhalation.
• *Expiratory reserve volume (ERV)* reflects the volume of air exhaled with a normal exhalation.
• *Residual volume (RV)* reflects the volume of air in the lungs at all times that can't be exhaled. It must be measured indirectly.
• *Inspiratory capacity (IC)* reflects the total amount of air that can be inhaled after normal exhalation (IRV + TV).
• *Forced vital capacity (FVC)* reflects the total amount of air that can be exhaled after maximal inhalation (IRV + TV + ERV).
• *Functional residual capacity (FRC)* reflects the total amount of air that remains in the lungs after normal exhalation (RV + ERV). It must be measured indirectly.
• *Total lung capacity (TLC)* reflects the total amount of air in the lungs at peak inspiration (IRV + TV + ERV + RV).

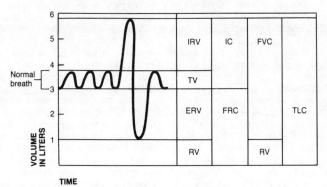

Adapted with permission from R.F Wilson, ed., *Critical Care Manual: Principles and Techniques of Critical Care*, Vol. 1. Kalamazoo, Mich.: Upjohn Co., 1976.

Test results may be plotted on a curve (see *Restrictive and Obstructive Lung Disease*, page 50), with normal breathing shown by the tidal volume (TV). Maximal exhalation after a maximal inhalation is called forced vital capacity (FVC); this curve's used as the basis for most measurements. Forced expiratory volume in the first second of exhalation (FEV_1) reflects how much air the patient can exhale at the beginning of an exhalation. The FEV_1/FVC ratio—the most common gross measurement of obstructive disease—indicates how much of the total exhaled volume the patient exhaled in the first second of exhalation. In short, it indicates how fast the patient exhales.

Two flow parameters are measured from the routine spirogram: FEV 25% to 75% (forced expiratory flow in the middle 50% of exhaled volume) and mid-maximum expiratory flow rate (MMEFR). These indicate flow more sensitively than the FEV_1/FVC ratio. With some spirometers, measurments must be calculated from the graph itself. (The newer automated spirometers display the numbers.)

Purpose
• To determine the cause of dyspnea
• To assess the effectiveness of therapy
• To distinguish obstructive from restrictive disorders
• To estimate the degree of pulmonary dysfunction
• To establish baseline pulmonary function for future comparison
• To provide objective evidence of subjective symptoms
• To provide documentation of disability for compensation
• To detect early signs of respiratory impairment in asymptomatic patients

Procedure
Explain to the patient that the test evaluates his lung function. Instruct him not to eat a heavy meal within a few hours before the test. Tell him where the test will be performed and by whom. (The test will take place in a pulmonary laboratory, a doctor's office, or at the bedside with a portable spirometer.)

Emphasize that test accuracy depends on his cooperation and effort. Let him know he will have to wear a nose clip. Assure him that although the test may be tiring, it will be painless; reassure him that he'll be allowed to rest as necessary.

If ordered, withhold bronchodilators. (If the test is being done to evaluate the treatment regimen, continue all medications.) Steroids are rarely withheld because their effects wear off so slowly.

Just before the test, have the patient void and loosen any restrictive clothing. If he wears dentures, tell him to leave them in place because this will help keep his mouth sealed around the mouthpiece.

During the test, the patient will sit next to the spirometer. A noseclip will be placed on his nose and positioned so that he can breathe only through his mouth. (This prevents air leakage from his nose, which would decrease the measurements.) He'll then put the mouthpiece, which attaches to a hose connected to the machine, in his mouth. Then he'll be instructed to breathe normally through the mouthpiece until he's comfortable, and the examiner has tested for and corrected any leaks.

Next, the patient will be told to breathe in as deeply as he can and to hold his breath momentarily. Then he should blow into the machine as forcefully, rapidly, and completely as he can until he's told to stop. Even if he feels that he's exhaled all the air he can, he should continue exhaling until instructed to stop.

He'll then breathe normally through the machine, then repeat the procedure until two measurements come within 5% to 10% of each other, confirming that he gave maximal effort and that the volumes and flows are accurate. (*Note:* This proves especially critical in patients undergoing disability testing because it's almost impossible to reproduce two falsely low curves within 10% accuracy.)

If ordered, the test will be repeated after the patient has inhaled a bronchodilator to determine if he has reversible obstructive airway disease or to objectively document the efficacy of such medication. Be sure the medication has enough time to take effect before the test is repeated; also, be sure to communicate that the patient received a bronchodilator so that he doesn't receive another dose too soon. (If a pre- and post-bronchodilator test

Specialized Pulmonary Function Tests

Test	Description
Peak flow	Measures peak flow as patient exhales as hard as possible into peak flow meter. Peak flow is shown by an indicator on the unit. Test is commonly used to allow patients to evaluate their response to bronchodilator therapy. It can also help the patient to objectively evaluate severity or progression of an asthma attack and determine if he should go to a hospital emergency room.
CO_2 response	Determined by measuring patient's respiratory rate and tidal volume in response to breathing of various CO_2 concentrations. Reduced CO_2 response may indicate chronically elevated arterial CO_2 level with a resultant blunted chemoreceptor response or other cause of chemoreceptor depression (as in narcotic overdose).
Thoracic gas volume	Measures total volume of gas in chest via body plethysmography. Increased gas volume occurs in obstructive disease with air trapping; decreased volume may indicate restrictive disease or atelectasis.
Flow volume loop	Spirometric tracing that graphically represents both inhalation and exhalation. Tracings allow measurement of large airway obstruction (usually more evident on inspiratory curve). It also allows more precise measurement of small airway flow.
Nitrogen washout test	Determines ventilatory uniformity. Patient breathes 100% oxygen to wash nitrogen out of lungs. One measurement of nitrogen in exhaled air will give an indication of uniformity of ventilation. Another measurement of exhaled volumes and fraction of nitrogen in exhaled air allows functional residual capacity (FRC) calculation.
Helium dilution	Patient breathes helium from closed system until helium in system and in lungs equilibrates. Allows calculation of FRC by analyzing new helium concentration.

is done, bronchodilators are routinely withheld before testing.)

Precautions
PFTs are contraindicated in patients with acute coronary insufficiency, angina, recent myocardial infarction, cerebrovascular accident, or intolerance for Valsalva's maneuver.

Post-test care
Check to see if the patient received a bronchodilator during testing, and ad-just the medication schedule appropriately. Resume previously ordered activities and diet. Be sure test results are documented, especially if the patient is scheduled for surgery.

Normal values
Normal values are predicted for each patient based on his age, height, and gender. Results are usually expressed

Restrictive and Obstructive Lung Disease

The shape of the spirogram tracing as well as the numerical values help determine if the patient has obstructive or restrictive disease. As these graphs of forced vital capacity (FVC) maneuvers show, the volume decreases but flow remains normal in restrictive disease. Notice that the curve—although smaller—resembles a normal curve in shape. With obstructive disease, flow decreases and the curve takes longer to flatten out at the bottom. The dropoff is not as steep because the patient exhales more slowly through obstructed airways.

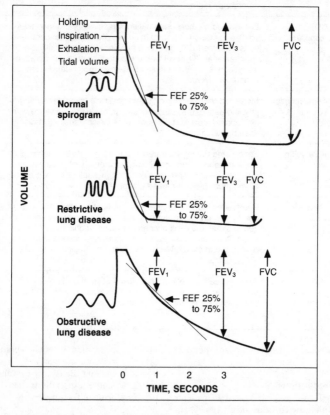

Adapted with permission from N.B. Slonim and L.H. Hamilton, *Respiratory Physiology*, 3rd ed. St. Louis: C.V. Mosby Co., 1976.

as a percentage of the predicted value. A nomogram listing normal values can be obtained from manufacturers of mechanical spirometers; these values are programmed into electronic spirometers. A predicted value of 85% or more is considered normal.

Implications of abnormal results

Forced vital capacity (FVC) can be evaluated by looking at the exhalation curve shape and the numerical values. Curve shape proves important because the numerical value may approach normal in the patient with obstructive disease—he may be able to exhale the appropriate amount of air if he's given enough time. (Look for a curve with a diminished drop-off or exhalation that extends more than 5 seconds.) An increased FVC may occur in well-conditioned patients, in singers who have relatively large lung capacities, and in patients with chronic lung disease and overinflated lungs. A decreased FVC indicates a restrictive disorder or obstructive disease so severe that the patient traps air and can't exhale completely. A decreased FEV_1 usually indicates obstructive disease. However, because FEV_1 reflects volume, it also decreases in restrictive disease.

The FEV_1/FVC ratio reflects flow and decreases in obstructive disease. With severe obstruction, the ratio drops below 40%; with moderate obstruction, it ranges between 40% and 60%; and with mild obstruction, it ranges from 60% to 70%. A ratio between 70% and 80% warrants follow-up (a ratio above 80% is considered normal). This is how FEV_1 can be used to determine obstructive disease—not just the volume itself. A ratio above 95% is usually insignificant unless you suspect the patient isn't inhaling deeply enough or exhaling completely. If the patient is deliberately trying to do poorly, the FEV_1/FVC ratio may be extremely high because he's exhaling a smaller total volume.

Two flow parameters are measured from the routine spirogram: the forced expiratory flow in the middle 50% of exhaled volume (FEV 25%-75%) and MMEFR. These are more sensitive indicators of flow than the FEV_1/FVC ratio; a decrease can indicate obstruction in smaller airways. In asymptomatic smokers, for example, decreased flow parameters may accompany a normal FEV_1/FVC ratio, indicating early small-airway disease. These measurements prove especially helpful in screening asymptomatic patients. As with FEV_1/FVC, elevated values are usually insignificant.

Decreased tidal volume (TV) values indicate restrictive disease; increased values occur in nonrespiratory problems, such as fever, diabetic ketoacidosis, neurologic abnormalities, and salicylate intoxication. However, TV usually isn't measured in standard spirometry.

Interfering factors

• Lack of patient cooperation (patients must be awake, coherent, and able to follow instructions)
• Inability to keep a tight seal on the mouthpiece
• Severe shortness of breath that precludes FVC maneuver

Arterial blood gas analysis

Arterial blood gas (ABG) analysis evaluates gas exchange in the lungs by measuring the partial pressures of oxygen (PaO_2) and carbon dioxide ($PaCO_2$) and the pH of an arterial blood sample. PaO_2 indicates how much oxygen the lungs deliver to the blood; $PaCO_2$ indicates how efficiently the lungs eliminate carbon dioxide. The pH reflects the blood's acid-base level or the hydrogen ion (H^+) concentration. An acidic pH indicates H^+ excess; an alkaline pH, H^+ deficit. Oxygen content

(O_2CT), oxygen saturation (O_2Sat), and bicarbonate (HCO_3^-) values also aid diagnosis. A blood sample for ABG analysis may be drawn by percutaneous arterial puncture or from an arterial line.

Purpose
• To evaluate the efficiency of pulmonary gas exchange
• To assess integrity of the ventilatory control system
• To determine the blood's acid-base level
• To monitor respiratory therapy

Procedure
Explain to the patient that this test evaluates how well his lungs deliver oxygen to blood and eliminate carbon dioxide. Inform him that he needn't restrict food or fluids. Tell him the test requires a blood sample. Also, tell him who will perform the arterial puncture and when, and which site (radial, brachial, or femoral artery) has been selected for the puncture.

Instruct the patient to breathe normally during the test, and warn him that he may experience brief cramping or throbbing pain at the puncture site. Perform an arterial puncture, and document the procedure.

Precautions
• If the patient has recently had intermittent positive-pressure breathing (IPPB) treatment, wait at least 20 minutes before drawing arterial blood.
• If the patient is receiving oxygen therapy, find out whether the order for ABG measurements specifies that these be obtained on room air or on oxygen therapy. If the order indicates room air, discontinue oxygen therapy for 15 to 20 minutes before drawing the sample and monitor the patient carefully while he's without oxygen. Replace the oxygen if the patient shows signs of respiratory distress, and call the doctor to clarify the order.

• Wait approximately 30 minutes after suctioning or making any ventilator change before drawing blood for ABG measurement.
• Before sending the sample to the laboratory, include the following information on the requisition slip:
—Indicate whether the patient was breathing room air or receiving oxygen therapy when the sample was drawn. If he was receiving oxygen therapy, note the flow rate or the FIO_2 from a Venturi mask.
—If the patient's on a ventilator, note the FIO_2, tidal volume, and rate.
—Record the patient's rectal temperature and respiratory rate.

Post-test care
Apply pressure to the puncture site. Monitor the patient's vital signs and be alert for signs and symptoms of circulatory impairment, such as swelling, discoloration, pain, numbness, or tingling in the affected arm or leg. Watch for bleeding from the puncture site and for hematoma formation.

Normal values
Normal ABG values fall within the following ranges:
PaO₂: 75 to 100 mm Hg (decreases with age)
PaCO₂: 35 to 45 mm Hg
pH: 7.35 to 7.42
O₂CT: 15% to 23%
O₂ Sat: 94% to 100%
HCO₃⁻: 22 to 26 mEq/liter.

Implications of abnormal results
Below-normal PaO_2, O_2CT, and O_2Sat values, in combination with a high $PaCO_2$ value, indicate alveolar hypoventilation and may result simply from rebreathing air in a poorly ventilated room. More serious underlying causes include respiratory muscle weakness or paralysis (as in Guillain-Barré syndrome), respiratory center inhibition (from head injury, brain tumor, or drug abuse, for example), and airway obstruction (possibly from mucus plugs,

obstructive lung disease, or a tumor). Similarly, these low values may result from bronchiolar obstruction caused by asthma or emphysema, from an abnormal ventilation-perfusion ratio resulting from partially blocked alveoli or pulmonary capillaries, or from damaged or fluid-filled alveoli because of disease, hemorrhage, or near-drowning.

When inspired air contains insufficient oxygen, then PaO_2, O_2CT, and O_2Sat values also decrease; however, the $PaCO_2$ value may remain normal. Such findings commonly accompany pneumothorax, impaired diffusion between alveoli and blood (from interstitial fibrosis, for example), an arteriovenous shunt that permits blood to bypass the lungs, and early stages of adult respiratory distress syndrome (ARDS) and asthma.

A below-normal O_2CT value—with normal PaO_2, O_2Sat, and, possibly, $PaCO_2$ values—may result from severe anemia, decreased blood volume, and reduced hemoglobin oxygen-carrying capacity, such as in sickle cell anemia.

Besides identifying blood oxygen disorders, ABG measurements provide valuable information about acid-base disorders, as shown in the accompanying chart. (See *Respiratory Acidosis or Alkalosis?*, page 54.)

Interfering factors
• Exposing the sample to air affects PaO_2 and $PaCO_2$ levels and interferes with accurate interpretation of results.
• Failure to heparinize the syringe, place the sample correctly in an iced bag, or immediately send the sample to the laboratory adversely affects the test results.
• Venous blood in the sample may lower the PaO_2 value and elevate the $PaCO_2$ value.
• IPPB treatment less than 20 minutes before arterial puncture alters ABG values.
• Bicarbonate, ethacrynic acid, hydrocortisone, metolazone, prednisone, and thiazides may elevate $PaCO_2$ levels. Acetazolamide, methicillin, nitrofurantoin, and tetracycline may decrease $PaCO_2$ levels.

Pleural fluid analysis

The pleura, a two-layer membrane covering the lungs and lining the thoracic cavity, maintains a small amount of lubricating fluid between its layers to minimize friction during respiration. Increased fluid in this space—the result of such diseases as cancer, tuberculosis, or blood or lymphatic disorders—can cause respiratory difficulty.

In pleural fluid aspiration (thoracentesis), the doctor punctures the patient's thoracic wall to obtain a specimen of pleural fluid for analysis or to relieve pulmonary compression and resultant respiratory distress. The specimen is examined for color, consistency, glucose and protein content, cellular composition, and the enzymes lactic dehydrogenase (LDH) and amylase; it's also examined cytologically for cancer cells and cultured for pathogens. To lessen the risk of puncturing the lung, liver, or spleen, thoracentesis may be preceded by physical examination and chest radiography or ultrasound study to locate the fluid.

Purpose
To provide a fluid specimen to determine the cause and nature of pleural effusion

Procedure
Explain to the patient that the test assesses the space around the lungs for fluid. Inform him that he needn't restrict food or fluids. Tell him who will perform the test and where.

Inform the patient that chest radiography or ultrasound study may precede the test to help locate the fluid. Check the patient's history for hypersensitivity

Respiratory Acidosis or Alkalosis?

RESPIRATORY ACIDOSIS

Alveolar hypoventilation causes respiratory retention of CO_2, leading to carbonic acid excess and a decreased pH. Arterial P_{CO_2} above 45 mm Hg and pH below 7.35.

Predisposing factors
- Airway obstruction
- Chest-wall injury
- Neuromuscular disease
- Drug overdose (CNS depression)
- ARDS (late stages)
- Pneumothorax
- Pneumonia
- Pulmonary edema

Signs and symptoms
- Tachycardia
- Dyspnea
- Dysrhythmias
- Diaphoresis
- Lethargy
- Confusion
- $P_{CO_2} >45$, pH<7.35, but HCO_3^- 22 to 26 (normal)

Compensation
- Over time, in the presence of *increased* P_{CO_2}, the kidneys compensate by excreting hydrogen ions and reabsorbing HCO_3 to bring pH back to normal

Interventions
- Give O_2 (low concentrations in patients with chronic obstructive pulmonary disease) if the P_{O_2} is decreased.
- Give intravenous fluids.
- Give inhaled or intravenous bronchodilators.
- Start mechanical ventilation if hypoventilation can't be corrected immediately.
- Monitor ABGs and electrolytes.
- Expect to treat the underlying cause. For example, remove or dislodge obstruction of the airway.

RESPIRATORY ALKALOSIS

Alveolar hyperventilation causes excess exhalation of CO_2, leading to carbonic acid deficit and an elevated pH. Arterial P_{CO_2} below 35 mm Hg and pH above 7.45.

Predisposing factors
- Extreme anxiety
- CNS injury to respiratory center
- Fever
- Overventilation during mechanical ventilation
- Pulmonary embolism
- Congestive heart failure
- Salicylate intoxication (early)

Signs and symptoms
- Tachycardia
- Deep, rapid breathing
- Light-headedness
- Numbness and tingling or arm and leg paresthesias
- Carpopedal spasm
- Tetany
- $P_{CO_2} <35$, pH>7.45, but HCO_3^- 22 to 26 (normal)

Compensation
- Over time, in the presence of *decreased* P_{CO_2}, the kidneys compensate by retaining hydrogen ions and *not* reabsorbing HCO_3 to bring pH back to normal

Interventions
- Have the patient rebreathe into a paper bag. (Rebreathing his CO_2 increases his P_{CO_2}.)
- Administer sedatives and give calm reassuring support. (Hyperventilation is often triggered by anxiety attacks.)
- Monitor ABGs and electrolytes.
- Expect to treat the underlying cause. For example, perform gastric lavage if salicylate overdose caused the alkalosis.

to local anesthetics. Warn the patient that he may feel a stinging sensation on anesthetic injection and some pressure during fluid withdrawal. Advise him not to cough, breathe deeply, or move during the test, to minimize the risk of lung injury.

Record baseline vital signs. Shave the area around the needle insertion site, if necessary. Position the patient properly to widen intercostal spaces and to allow easier access to the pleural cavity; make sure he's well-supported and comfortable. (See *Positioning the Patient for Thoracentesis*.) Preferably, seat him at the edge of the bed, with a chair or stool supporting his feet and his head and arms resting on a padded overbed table. If he can't sit up, position him on his unaffected side, with the arm on the affected side elevated above his head. Remind him not to cough, breathe deeply, or move suddenly during the procedure.

After the patient is properly positioned, the doctor disinfects the skin, drapes the area, injects local anesthetic into the subcutaneous tissue, and inserts the thoracentesis needle above the rib to avoid lacerating intercostal vessels. When the needle reaches the fluid pocket, he attaches the 50-ml syringe and the stopcock and opens the tubing clamps to aspirate fluid into the container. During aspiration, check the patient for signs of respiratory distress, such as weakness, dyspnea, pallor, cyanosis, heart rate changes, tachypnea, diaphoresis, blood-tinged frothy mucus, and hypotension. Because the amount of pressure necessary to puncture the pleura may be uncomfortable and frightening, continually reassure the patient during the procedure.

After the needle is withdrawn, apply slight pressure and a small adhesive bandage to the puncture site.

Label the specimen(s) and record the test date and time, and the amount, color, and character of the fluid (clear, frothy, purulent, bloody) on the request slip. Note any signs of distress

Positioning the Patient for Thoracentesis

To prepare the patient for thoracentesis, place him in one of the three positions shown below: (1) sitting on the edge of the bed with arms on overbed table; (2) sitting up in bed with arms on overbed table; or (3) lying partially on the side, partially on the back with arms over the head. These positions serve to widen the intercostal spaces and permit easy access to the pleural cavity. Using pillows as shown will make the patient more comfortable.

Sitting on edge of bed

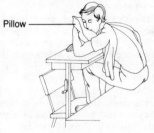

Pillow

Sitting up in bed

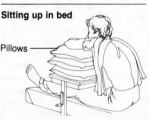

Pillows

Lying partially on side, partially on back

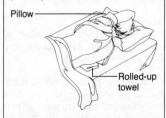

Pillow

Rolled-up towel

the patient showed during the procedure. Document the exact location where fluid was removed; this information may aid diagnosis.

Precautions

• Thoracentesis is contraindicated in patients with a history of bleeding disorders.
• Use strict aseptic technique.
• Note the patient's temperature and antibiotic therapy, if applicable, on the laboratory slip.
• Add a small amount (about 0.5 ml) of sterile heparin to the container to prevent fluid from coagulating.
• Send the specimen to the laboratory immediately.

Post-test care

Reposition the patient comfortably on the affected side or as ordered by the doctor. Tell the patient to remain on his side for at least 1 hour to seal the puncture site. Elevate the head of the bed to facilitate breathing.

Monitor vital signs every 30 minutes for 2 hours, then every 4 hours until they're stable. Tell the patient to immediately report difficulty breathing.

Watch for signs and symptoms of pneumothorax, tension pneumothorax, and fluid reaccumulation; if a large amount of fluid was withdrawn, also check for signs of pulmonary edema or cardiac distress caused by mediastinal shift. Usually, the doctor orders post-test radiography to detect these complications before clinical signs and symptoms appear.

Check the puncture site for any fluid leakage. Consider a large amount of leakage abnormal.

Normal findings

Normally, the pleural cavity maintains negative pressure and contains less than 20 ml of serous fluid.

Implications of abnormal results

Pleural effusion results from abnormal formation or reabsorption of pleural fluid. Certain characteristics classify pleural fluid as a transudate (a low-protein fluid that has leaked from normal blood vessels) or an exudate (a protein-rich fluid that has leaked from blood vessels with increased permeability). (See *Characteristics of Pulmonary Transudate and Exudate*.) Pleural fluid may contain blood (hemothorax), chyle (chylothorax), or pus and necrotic tissue (empyema). Blood-tinged fluid may indicate a traumatic tap; if so, the fluid should clear as aspiration progresses.

Transudative effusion usually results from diminished colloidal pressure, increased negative pressure within the pleural cavity, ascites, systemic and pulmonary venous hypertension, congestive heart failure, hepatic cirrhosis, and nephritis.

Exudative effusion results from disorders that increase pleural capillary permeability (possibly with changes in hydrostatic or colloid osmotic pressures), lymphatic drainage interference, infections, pulmonary infarctions, and neoplasms. Exudative effusion associated with depressed glucose levels, elevated LDH, rheumatoid arthritis cells, and negative smears, cultures, and cytologic examination may indicate pleurisy associated with rheumatoid arthritis.

The most common pathogens found in pleural fluid include *Mycobacterium tuberculosis, Staphylococcus aureus, Streptococcus pneumoniae* and other streptococci, and *Hemophilus influenzae*; with a ruptured pulmonary abscess, anaerobes, such as bacteroides, may appear. Usually, cultures are positive during early infection stages; however, antibiotic therapy may cause a negative culture despite a positive Gram stain and grossly purulent fluid. Empyema may result from complications of pneumonia, pulmonary abscess, esophageal perforation, or penetration from mediastinitis. A high neutrophil percentage suggests septic inflammation; predominating lymphocytes suggest tuberculosis or fungal or viral effusions.

Characteristics of Pulmonary Transudate and Exudate

Characteristic	Transudate	Exudate
Appearance	Clear	Cloudy, turbid
Specific gravity	<1.016	>1.016
Clot (fibrinogen)	Absent	Present
Protein	<3 g/dl	>3 g/dl
WBCs	Few lymphocytes	Many; may be purulent
RBCs	Few	Variable
Glucose	Equal to serum level	May be less than serum level
LDH	Low	High

Serosanguineous fluid may indicate pleural extension of a cancerous tumor. An elevated LDH level in a nonpurulent, nonhemolyzed, bloodless effusion may also suggest cancer. Pleural fluid glucose levels 30 to 40 mg/dl lower than blood glucose levels may indicate cancer, bacterial infection, nonseptic inflammation, or metastases. Increased amylase levels occur with pleural effusions associated with pancreatitis.

Interfering factors
• Failure to use aseptic technique may contaminate the specimen.
• Antibiotic therapy before fluid is aspirated for culturing may decrease the number of bacteria, making isolation of the infecting organisms difficult.
• Failure to send the specimen to the laboratory immediately or to add heparin to the container may alter test results.

Pleural biopsy

Pleural biopsy is the removal of pleural tissue, by needle biopsy or open biopsy, for histologic examination. Needle pleural biopsy, performed with the patient under local anesthetic, generally follows thoracentesis, which is performed when the effusion has an unknown cause (however, it can be performed separately from the aspiration).

Open pleural biopsy (a small thoracotomy), performed in the absence of pleural effusion, permits direct visualization of the pleura and the underlying lung. It's performed in the operating room, with the patient under general anesthetic.

Purpose
• To differentiate between tuberculosis and cancer, particularly in the elderly
• To diagnose viral, fungal, or parasitic disease and collagen vascular disease of the pleura

Procedure
Before needle biopsy, describe the procedure and ask the patient if he has any questions. Explain that this test permits microscopic examination of pleural tissue. Inform him that he needn't restrict food or fluids before the test. Tell him who will perform the

biopsy and where, and that the procedure takes 30 to 45 minutes. Advise him that the test requires three tissue specimens from different pleural sites, but that the needle remains in the pleura less than 1 minute. Test results should be available in 1 day.

Inform the patient that blood studies (prothrombin time, activated partial thromboplastin time, arterial blood gas analysis, and platelet count) will be performed before the biopsy and that chest X-rays will be taken before and immediately after the procedure.

Make sure the patient or an appropriate family member has signed a consent form. Check the patient's history for hypersensitivity to the local anesthetic. Tell the patient that he'll receive a local anesthetic and should experience little, if any, pain during the biopsy, although he may feel pressure.

Just before the procedure begins, record vital signs. Then place the patient in one of the following positions: sitting on the side of the bed, with his feet resting on a stool and his arms supported by the overbed table; or leaning the upper part of his body on the overbed table. Instruct him to maintain this position and remain as still as possible during the procedure. Prepare the skin over the biopsy site and drape the area. The local anesthetic is then administered.

Vim-Silverman needle biopsy

The doctor inserts the needle through the appropriate intercostal space into the biopsy site, with the outer tip distal to the pleura and the central portion pushed in deeper and held in place. The doctor inserts the outer case about $\frac{3}{8}''$ (1 cm), rotates the entire assembly 360 degrees, then withdraws the needle and tissue specimen.

Cope's needle biopsy

The doctor introduces the trocar through the appropriate intercostal space into the biopsy site. He then removes the sharp obturator and inserts a hooked stylet through the trocar. He directs the opened notch against the pleura along the intercostal space, then slowly withdraws it. Holding the outer tube stationary, he twists the inner tube to cut off the tissue specimen, then withdraws the entire assembly.

The pleural specimen is immediately placed in a properly labeled specimen bottle containing 10% neutral buffered formaldehyde solution.

Cleanse the skin around the biopsy site and apply an adhesive bandage. Document the procedure.

Precautions

• Pleural biopsy is contraindicated in patients with severe bleeding disorders.
• Send the specimen to the laboratory immediately.

Post-test care

Check vital signs every 15 minutes for 1 hour, then every hour for 4 hours or until they're stable. Make sure the chest X-ray is repeated immediately after the biopsy is completed.

Watch for signs of respiratory distress and possible complications, such as pneumothorax (immediate) and pneumonia (delayed).

As ordered, instruct the patient to use an incentive spirometer to expand his lungs and improve vital capacity.

Normal findings

The normal pleura consists primarily of mesothelial cells flattened in a uniform layer. Layers of areolar connective tissue containing blood vessels, nerves, and lymphatics lie below the mesothelial cells.

Implications of abnormal results

Histologic examination of the tissue specimen can reveal cancer, tuberculosis, or viral, fungal, parasitic, or collagen vascular disease. Primary neoplasms of the pleura, which may be localized or diffuse, are usually fibrous. Localized lesions are rarely cancerous; diffuse mesothelioma of the pleura invariably proves fatal.

Interfering factors

Failure to use the proper fixative solution or to obtain representative pleural specimens may interfere with accurate determination of test results.

Direct laryngoscopy

For this procedure, the doctor visualizes the larynx by use of a fiberoptic endoscope or laryngoscope passed through the mouth and pharynx to the larynx. Direct laryngoscopy usually follows indirect laryngoscopy, the more common procedure. (See *Indirect Laryngoscopy*.)

Permitting visualization of areas inaccessible through indirect laryngoscopy, direct laryngoscopy is indicated for children; patients with a strong gag reflex caused by anatomic abnormalities; patients with evidence of pharyngeal or laryngeal disease, such as stridor or hemoptysis; and those who have not responded to short-term symptomatic therapy. The procedure may include collection of secretions or tissue for further study and removal of foreign bodies.

Normally, the test is contraindicated for patients with epiglottitis, because trauma can quickly cause edema and airway obstruction. However, if absolutely necessary in such patients, the test may be performed in the operating room, with a surgeon ready to do an emergency tracheotomy and resuscitative equipment available.

Purpose
• To detect lesions, strictures, or foreign bodies in the larynx
• To aid diagnosis of laryngeal cancer
• To remove benign lesions or foreign bodies from the larynx
• To examine the larynx when the view provided by indirect laryngoscopy is inadequate

Indirect Laryngoscopy

Indirect laryngoscopy, normally an office procedure, allows visualization of the larynx, using a warm laryngeal mirror positioned at the back of the throat, a head mirror held in front of the mouth, and a light source.

The patient sits erect in a chair and sticks his tongue out as far as possible. The tongue is grasped with a piece of gauze and held in place with a tongue depressor. If the patient's gag reflex is sensitive, a local anesthetic may be sprayed on the pharyngeal wall. Then the larynx is observed at rest and during phonation. A simple excision of polyps may also be performed during this procedure.

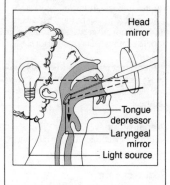

Procedure
Explain to the patient that this test determines laryngeal abnormalities. Instruct him to fast for 6 to 8 hours before the test. Tell him who will perform the procedure and that it will take place in a darkened operating room.

Inform the patient that before the procedure, he'll receive a sedative to help him relax and atropine to reduce secretions; during the procedure, he'll receive a general or local anesthetic. Also, reassure him that laryngoscopy won't obstruct the airway.

Make sure the patient or an appropriate family member has signed a consent form. Check the patient's history for hypersensitivity to the anesthetic. Obtain baseline vital signs. Administer the sedative and atropine as ordered (usually 30 minutes to 1 hour before the test). Just before the test, instruct the patient to remove dentures, contact lenses, and jewelry, and tell him to void.

To begin the procedure, place the patient in a supine position. Encourage him to relax with his arms at his sides and to breathe through his nose. A general anesthetic is administered or a local anesthetic is sprayed on his mouth and throat. With the patient's head in the proper position, the doctor introduces the laryngoscope through the patient's mouth, then examines the larynx for abnormalities; he may remove a specimen or secretions for further study. Minor surgery, such as polyp or nodule removal, may be performed at this time.

Place specimens for histology, cytology, and microbiology in their respective containers. Document the procedure.

Precautions
Send the specimens to the laboratory immediately.

Post-test care
As ordered, place the conscious patient in semi-Fowler's position; place the unconscious patient on his side with his head slightly elevated to prevent aspiration.

Check the patient's vital signs every 15 minutes until they're stable, then every 30 minutes for 4 hours, every hour for the next 4 hours, and, finally, every 4 hours for 24 hours. (This procedure may also be done as outpatient surgery; in this case, the patient will remain in the hospital only for several hours after the test.) Immediately report any adverse reaction to the anesthetic or seda-

tive (tachycardia; palpitations; hypertension; euphoria; excitation; or rapid, deep respirations).

Apply an ice collar to prevent or minimize laryngeal edema. Also, provide an emesis basin and instruct the patient to spit out saliva rather than swallow it. Observe sputum for blood, and notify the doctor immediately if excessive bleeding occurs.

Instruct the patient to refrain from clearing his throat and coughing, which may dislodge the clot at the biopsy site and cause hemorrhaging. Also, advise him to avoid smoking until vital signs stabilize and complications can be ruled out.

Immediately report any subcutaneous crepitus around the patient's face and neck—a possible indication of tracheal perforation.

Observe the patient with epiglottitis for signs of airway obstruction. Immediately report signs of respiratory difficulty, such as laryngeal stridor and dyspnea, resulting from laryngeal edema or laryngospasm. Keep emergency resuscitative equipment and a tracheotomy tray available for 24 hours.

Restrict food and fluids until the gag reflex returns (usually 2 hours). Then have the patient resume his usual diet, beginning with sips of water. Reassure him that voice loss, hoarseness, and sore throat are temporary. Provide throat lozenges or a soothing liquid gargle when his gag reflex returns.

Normal findings
A normal larynx shows no evidence of inflammation, lesions, strictures, or foreign bodies.

Implications of abnormal results
The combined results of direct laryngoscopy, biopsy, and radiography may indicate laryngeal carcinoma. Direct laryngoscopy may show benign lesions, strictures, or foreign bodies

and, with a biopsy, may distinguish laryngeal edema from radiation reaction or tumor.

Interfering factors
Failure to place the specimens in the appropriate containers and to send them to the laboratory immediately may interfere with the accurate determination of test results.

Bronchoscopy

Bronchoscopy is the direct visualization of the trachea and tracheobronchial tree through a standard metal bronchoscope or fiberoptic bronchoscope—a slender flexible tube with mirrors and a light at its distal end. A brush, biopsy forceps, or a catheter may be passed through the bronchoscope to obtain specimens for cytologic and bacteriologic examination.

A flexible fiberoptic bronchoscope is used more commonly than a rigid bronchoscope because it's smaller, allows a greater viewing range of the segmental and subsegmental bronchi, and carries less risk of trauma. However, foreign object removal, endobronchial lesion excision, and control of massive hemoptysis necessitate use of a large, rigid bronchoscope.

Complications resulting from bronchoscopy may include bleeding, infection, and pneumothorax.

Purpose
• To visually examine a possible tumor, obstruction, secretion, or foreign body in the tracheobronchial tree, as demonstrated on radiography
• To help diagnose bronchogenic carcinoma, tuberculosis, interstitial pulmonary disease, or fungal or parasitic pulmonary infection by obtaining a specimen for bacteriologic and cytologic examination
• To locate a bleeding site in the tracheobronchial tree

• To remove foreign bodies, cancerous or benign tumors, mucus plugs, or excessive secretions from the tracheobronchial tree

Procedure
Describe the procedure to the patient and explain that this test determines the nature of pulmonary dysfunction. Instruct him to fast for 6 to 12 hours before the test. Tell him who will perform the test and where; that the room will be darkened; and that the procedure takes 45 to 60 minutes. Advise him that test results are usually available in 1 day—except the tuberculosis report, which may take up to 6 weeks.

Tell the patient that chest X-ray studies and blood studies (prothrombin time, activated partial thromboplastin time, platelet count, and possibly arterial blood gas measurement) will be performed before bronchoscopy. Advise him that he may receive an I.V. sedative to help him relax. For children and for extremely apprehensive adults, a general anesthetic may be administered in the operating room. If the patient won't receive a general anesthetic, inform him that a local anesthetic will be sprayed into his nose and mouth to suppress the gag reflex. He may also receive an aerosolized anesthetic via nebulizer before the procedure. Warn him that the spray has an unpleasant taste and that he may experience some discomfort during the procedure. Reassure him that his airway won't be blocked and he will receive oxygen through the bronchoscope.

Make sure the patient or an appropriate family member has signed a consent form. Check the patient's history for hypersensitivity to anesthetic. Obtain baseline vital signs. Administer a preoperative sedative, as ordered. If the patient wears dentures, instruct him to remove them just before the test.

To begin the procedure, place the patient in a supine position on a table or bed or have him sit upright in a chair. Tell him to remain relaxed, with his arms at his sides, and to breathe through his nose. After the local anesthetic is sprayed into the patient's throat and takes effect (usually 1 or 2 minutes), the doctor introduces the bronchoscope (possibly tipped with lidocaine jelly) through the patient's mouth or nose. (See *Performing Bronchoscopy*.) When the bronchoscope's just above the vocal cords, the doctor flushes approximately 3 to 4 ml of 2% to 4% lidocaine through the scope's inner channel to the vocal cords to anesthetize deeper areas. He then inspects the anatomic structure of the trachea and bronchi, observes mucosal lining color, and notes any unusual masses or inflamed areas. Then he may use biopsy forceps to remove a tissue specimen from a suspicious area, a bronchial brush to obtain cells from a lesion surface, or suction apparatus to remove foreign bodies or mucus plugs.

Place the resulting specimens for microbiology, histology, and cytology in their respective containers. Document the procedure.

Bronchoscopy requires fluoroscopic guidance for distal lesion evaluation or for transbronchial biopsy in alveolar areas. Permanent X-ray films of pathologic findings may be obtained using bronchography. (See *Bronchography,* page 64.)

Precautions
• A patient with severe respiratory failure who can't breathe adequately by himself should be placed on a ventilator before bronchoscopy. Bronchoscopy can then be performed through the endotracheal tube.
• Send the specimens to the laboratory immediately.

Post-test care
Monitor the patient's vital signs. Notify the doctor immediately of any adverse reaction to the anesthetic or sedative.

As ordered, place the conscious patient in semi-Fowler's position; place the unconscious patient on his side, with the head of the bed slightly elevated to prevent aspiration.

Provide an emesis basin and instruct the patient to spit out saliva rather than swallow it. Observe sputum for blood, and notify the doctor immediately if excessive bleeding occurs.

For 24 hours after bronchoscopy, collect all sputum for cytologic examination—irritation produced during bronchial brushing commonly results in delayed shedding of cancer cells.

Instruct the patient who had a biopsy to refrain from clearing his throat or coughing, which may dislodge the clot at the biopsy site and cause hemorrhaging.

Immediately report any subcutaneous crepitus around the patient's face and neck—a possible indication of tracheal or bronchial perforation.

Watch for and immediately report symptoms of respiratory difficulty, such as laryngeal stridor and dyspnea resulting from laryngeal edema or laryngospasm. Observe for signs of hypoxemia (cyanosis), pneumothorax (dyspnea, cyanosis, diminished breath sounds on the affected side), bronchospasm (dyspnea, wheezing), or bleeding (hemoptysis). Keep resuscitative equipment and a tracheotomy tray available for 24 hours after the test. Restrict food and fluids until the gag reflex returns (usually in 2 hours). Then the patient may resume his usual diet, beginning with sips of clear liquid or ice chips.

Reassure the patient that hoarseness, voice loss, and sore throat after this procedure are only temporary. Provide lozenges or a soothing liquid gargle to ease discomfort when his gag reflex returns.

Normal findings
The trachea, measuring 4½" (11.3 cm), extends from the larynx to the bronchi. Lined with ciliated mucosa,

Performing Bronchoscopy

The bronchoscopic tube, inserted through the nostril into the bronchi, has four channels (see inset). Two light channels (A) provide a light source; one visualizing channel (B) to see through; and one open channel (C) to accommodate biopsy forceps, cytology brush, suctioning, lavage, anesthetic, or oxygen.

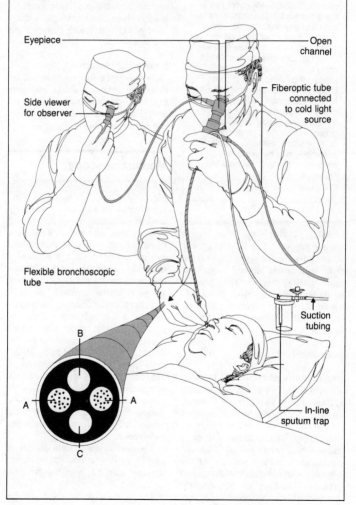

Bronchography

Bronchography is X-ray examination of the tracheobronchial tree after instillation of a radiopaque iodine contrast agent through a catheter into the lumens of the trachea and bronchi. The contrast agent coats the bronchial tree, permitting visualization of any anatomic deviations. Bronchography has been performed infrequently since the development of tomography and the flexible bronchoscope. Currently, it's used primarily for guidance during bronchoscopy or to provide permanent films of pathologic findings.

Bronchography may be performed using a local anesthetic instilled through the catheter or bronchoscope, although a general anesthetic may be necessary for children or during concurrent bronchoscopy.

it normally consists of smooth muscle containing C-shaped cartilage rings at regular intervals. The bronchi appear structurally similar to the trachea; the right bronchus is slightly larger and more vertical than the left. Smaller secondary bronchi, bronchioles, alveolar ducts, and eventually alveolar sacs and alveoli branch off from the main bronchi. Microscopic end structure walls have a single layer of squamous epithelial tissue.

Implications of abnormal results

Bronchial wall abnormalities include inflammation, swelling, protruding cartilage, ulceration, tumors, enlarged mucous gland orifices, and submucosal lymph nodes. Abnormalities of endotracheal origin include stenosis, compression, ectasia (dilation of the tubular vessel), anomalous (irregular) bronchial branching, and abnormal bifurcation from diverticulum. Abnormal substances in the bronchial lumen include blood, secretions, calculi, and foreign bodies.

Results of tissue and cell studies may indicate interstitial pulmonary disease, bronchogenic carcinoma, tuberculosis, or other pulmonary infections. Bronchogenic carcinomas include epidermoid or squamous cell carcinoma, small-cell (oat cell) carcinoma, adenocarcinoma, and large-cell (undifferentiated) carcinoma. Radiographic, bronchoscopic, and cytologic findings must be correlated with clinical signs and symptoms.

Interfering factors

Failure to place specimens in the appropriate containers and to send them to the laboratory immediately may interfere with accurate determination of test results and diagnosis.

Mediastinoscopy

Mediastinoscopy allows direct visualization of mediastinal structures—through an exploring speculum with built-in fiber light and side slit—and palpation and biopsy of paratracheal and carinal lymph nodes. A mass of tissues and organs behind the sternum, the mediastinum separates the lungs. Its major contents include the heart and its vessels, trachea, esophagus, thymus, and lymph nodes. Examination of the nodes, which receive lymphatic drainage from the lungs, can detect lymphoma (including Hodgkin's disease) and sarcoidosis, and can aid in staging lung cancer. A surgical procedure, mediastinoscopy is indicated when such tests as sputum cytology, lung scans, radiography, and bronchoscopic biopsy fail to confirm a diagnosis.

The mediastinum's right side allows easy exploration. Because mediastinoscopy can diagnose bronchogenic carcinoma at an early stage, this procedure is replacing the scalene fat-pad biopsy. Exploration of the left side proves less satisfactory and more hazardous because of the aorta's close proximity. Test complications, although rare, may include pneumothorax, esophageal perforation, infection, hemorrhage, and recurrent left laryngeal nerve damage.

Purpose
• To detect bronchogenic carcinoma, lymphoma, and sarcoidosis
• To stage lung cancer

Procedure
Describe the procedure to the patient and answer any questions he may have. Explain that this test evaluates the lymph nodes and other chest structures. Instruct the patient to fast after midnight before the test. Tell him who will perform the procedure and where, that he'll receive a general anesthetic, and that the procedure will take approximately 1 hour.

Tell him he may temporarily experience chest pain, tenderness at the incision site, or a sore throat (from intubation). Reassure him that the procedure rarely causes complications.

Make sure the patient or a responsible family member has signed a consent form. Check the patient's history for hypersensitivity to the anesthetic. As ordered, administer a sedative the night before the test and just before the procedure.

To begin the mediastinoscopy, after the patient has an endotracheal tube in place, the doctor makes a small transverse suprasternal incision. Using finger dissection, he forms a channel and palpates the lymph nodes. Then he inserts a mediastinoscope into the mediastinum and collects tissue specimens for frozen section examination. (See *Positioning the Mediastinoscope*.) If analysis confirms a resectable cancerous tumor, a thoracotomy and pneumonectomy may follow immediately.

Document the procedure.

Positioning the Mediastinoscope

The mediastinoscope shown here has been inserted suprasternally to inspect the paratracheal and carinal lymph nodes. The path of the mediastinoscope is cleared digitally before the scope is introduced. If the scope meets resistance while it's being advanced, a blunt dissection may be performed to clear the path.

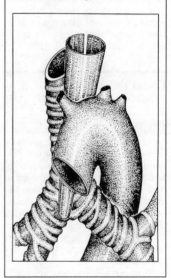

Precautions
Scarring of the affected area from previous mediastinoscopy contraindicates this test.

Post-test care
Monitor the patient's vital signs and check the dressing for bleeding or fluid drainage. Observe for signs of the following complications: fever (mediastinitis); crepitus (subcutaneous emphysema); dyspnea, cyanosis, and diminished breath sounds on the affected side (pneumothorax); tachycardia and hypo-

tension (hemorrhage). Administer the prescribed analgesic, as needed.

Normal findings

Normally, lymph nodes appear as small, smooth, flat oval bodies of lymphoid tissue.

Implications of abnormal results

Cancerous lymph nodes usually indicate inoperable—but not always untreatable—lung or esophageal cancer or lymphoma (such as Hodgkin's disease). Lung cancer staging helps determine the therapeutic regimen. Multiple nodular involvement, for example, may contraindicate surgery.

Chest radiography
(Chest roentgenography)

In this test, X-rays or gamma rays penetrate the chest and react on specially sensitized film. Because normal pulmonary tissue's radiolucent (appearing as black areas on the X-ray), foreign bodies, infiltrates, fluids, tumors, and other abnormalities appear as densities (white areas) on the chest film. A chest radiograph's most useful when compared with the patient's previous films, allowing the radiologist to detect changes.

Although chest radiography was once routinely performed on admission to the hospital and as a cancer screening test, the associated expense and exposure to radiation has caused many authorities to question its usefulness.

Purpose

• To detect pulmonary disorders, such as pneumonia, atelectasis, pneumothorax, pulmonary bullae, and tumors
• To detect mediastinal abnormalities, such as tumors, and cardiac disease
• To determine lesion location and size
• To help assess pulmonary status

Procedure

Describe the procedure to the patient, and explain that this test assesses his respiratory status. Inform him that he needn't restrict food or fluids. Tell him who will perform the test and where and when the X-ray film will be taken.

Provide a gown without snaps and instruct the patient to remove all jewelry in the X-ray field. Tell him that he'll be asked to take a deep breath and to hold it momentarily while the film's being taken to provide a clearer view of pulmonary structures.

If the procedure involves a *stationary X-ray machine,* the patient stands or sits in front of the machine so that films can be taken of the posteroanterior and left lateral views. (See *Common Radiographic Views.*)

When the radiograph is taken by a *portable X-ray machine* at the patient's bedside, assist with patient positioning. An upright chest radiograph is preferable, so move the patient to the top of the bed if he can tolerate it. Elevate the head of the bed for maximum upright positioning. Move cardiac monitoring cables, I.V. tubing from subclavian lines, pulmonary artery catheter lines, and safety pins as far from the X-ray field as possible. Document the procedure.

Precautions

• Chest radiography is usually contraindicated during the first trimester of pregnancy; however, when it's absolutely necessary, a lead apron placed over the patient's abdomen can shield the fetus.
• If the patient is intubated, check that no tubes have been dislodged during positioning.
• To avoid exposure to radiation, leave the room or the immediate area while the films are being taken. If you must stay in the area, wear a lead-lined apron or protective clothing.
• Be as specific as possible about the reason for chest X-ray when filling out the requisition slip; this will assist the

Common Radiographic Views

Frontal

Performed with the X-ray beam positioned posteriorly and anteriorly and with the patient in an upright position. The posteroanterior (PA) view is the most common frontal view and is preferred over the anteroposterior (AP) view because the heart is anteriorly situated in the thorax and magnified less in a PA view than in an AP view. The frontal views show greater lung area than the other views because of the lower diaphragm position.

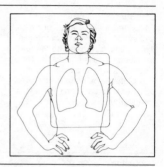

Lateral

Performed with the X-ray beam directed toward the patient's side. The left lateral (LL) view is the most common lateral view and is preferred over the right lateral (RL) view because the heart is left of midline and magnified less in an LL view than in an RL view. Lateral views visualize lesions not apparent on a PA view.

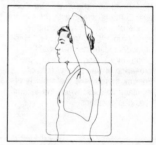

Recumbent

Performed with the X-ray beam overhead and with the patient supine. This view helps distinguish free fluid from encapsulated fluid and from an elevated diaphragm.

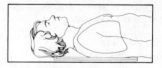

Oblique

Performed with the X-ray beam angled between the frontal and lateral views. This view helps evaluate intrathoracic disorders, pleural disease, esophageal abnormalities, hilar masses, and mediastinal masses (rarely, it also is used to localize lesions within the chest).

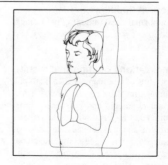

(continued)

Common Radiographic Views (continued)

Lordotic
Performed with the X-ray beam directed through the axis of the middle thoracic lobe and with the patient leaning back against the film plate. This view evaluates the apices of the lungs (usually obscured by bony structures) and helps localize tuberculosis sites.

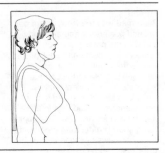

Decubitus
Performed with the X-ray beam parallel to the floor and with the patient in one of several horizontal positions (supine, prone, or side). This view demonstrates the extent of pulmonary abscess or cavity, the presence of free pleural fluid or pneumothorax, and the mobility of mediastinal mass when the patient changes positions.

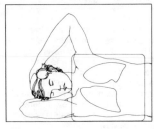

technician in setting the X-ray machine to the correct density.

Post-test care
None

Normal findings
For normal chest radiography findings, see *Some Clinical Implications of Chest X-rays.*

Implications of abnormal results
For an accurate diagnosis, radiography findings must be correlated with additional radiologic and pulmonary tests. Pulmonary hyperinflation with low diaphragm and generalized increased radiolucence may suggest emphysema but may also occur in radiographs of healthy persons. (For common radiography findings, see *Some Clinical Implications of Chest X-rays.*)

Interfering factors
• Portable chest radiographs taken in the anteroposterior position may show larger cardiac shadowing than other radiographs because the distance of the anterior structures from the beam is shorter. Portable chest radiographs—primarily those taken to detect atelectasis, pneumonia, pneumothorax, and mediastinal shift or to evaluate treatment—may be less reliable than stationary radiographs.
• Films taken with the patient in a supine position will not show fluid levels.
• Because chest radiographs vary with the patient's age, sex, and habitus, these factors should be considered in X-ray evaluation.
• Film underexposure or overexposure may result in poor-quality radiographs.

Some Clinical Implications of Chest X-Rays

Normal anatomic location and appearance	Possible abnormality	Implications
Trachea Visible midline in the anterior mediastinal cavity; translucent tubelike appearance	Deviation from midline	Tension pneumothorax, atelectasis, pleural effusion, consolidation, mediastinal nodes, or, in children, enlarged thymus
	Narrowing, with hourglass appearance and deviation to one side	Substernal thyroid
Heart Visible in the anterior left mediastinal cavity; solid appearance from blood contents; edges may be clear in contrast with surrounding air density of the lung.	Shift	Atelectasis
	Hypertrophy of right heart	Cor pulmonale, congestive heart failure
	Cardiac borders obscured by stringy densities ("shaggy heart")	Cystic fibrosis
Aortic knob Visible as water density; formed by the arch of the aorta	Solid densities, possibly indicating calcifications	Atherosclerosis
	Tortuous shape	Atherosclerosis
Mediastinum (mediastinal shadow) Visible as the space between the lungs; shadowy appearance that widens at the hilum of the lungs	Deviation to nondiseased side; deviation to diseased side by traction	Pleural effusion or tumor, fibrosis or collapsed lung
	Gross widening	Neoplasms of esophagus, bronchi, lungs, thyroid, thymus, peripheral nerves, lymphoid tissue; aortic aneurysm; mediastinitis; cor pulmonale; cardiac tamponade; bleeding
Ribs Visible as thoracic cavity encasement	Break or misalignment	Fractured sternum or ribs
	Widening of intercostal spaces	Emphysema
Spine Visible midline in the posterior chest; straight bony structure	Spinal curvature	Scoliosis, kyphosis
	Break or misalignment	Fractures

(continued)

Some Clinical Implications of Chest X-Rays *(continued)*

Normal anatomic location and appearance	Possible abnormality	Implications
Clavicles Visible in upper thorax; intact and equidistant in properly centered X-ray films	Break or misalignment	Fractures
Hila (lung roots) Visible above the heart where pulmonary vessels, bronchi, and lymph nodes join the lungs; appear as small, white, bilateral densities	Shift to one side	Atelectasis
	Accentuated shadows	Emphysema, pulmonary abscess, tumor, enlarged lymph nodes
Mainstem bronchus Visible, part of the hila with translucent tubelike appearance	Spherical or oval density	Bronchogenic cyst
Bronchi Usually not visible	Visible	Bronchial pneumonia
Lung fields Usually not visible throughout, except for the blood vessels	Visible	Atelectasis
	Irregular, patchy densities	Resolving pneumonia, silicosis, fibrosis, metastatic neoplasm
Hemidiaphragm Rounded, visible; right side 3/8" to 3/4" (1 to 2 cm) higher than left	Elevation of diaphragm (difference in elevation can be measured on inspiration and expiration to detect movement)	Active tuberculosis, pneumonia, pleurisy, acute bronchitis, active disease of the abdominal viscera, bilateral phrenic nerve involvement, atelectasis
	Flattening of diaphragm	Asthma, emphysema, tension pneumothorax
	Unilateral elevation of either side	Possible unilateral phrenic nerve paresis
	Unilateral elevation of left side only	Perforated ulcer (rare), gas distention of stomach or splenic flexure of colon, free air in abdomen

Chest fluoroscopy

In chest fluoroscopy, a continuous stream of X-rays passes through the patient, casting shadows of the heart, lungs, and diaphragm on a fluorescent screen. Because fluoroscopy reveals less detail than standard chest radiography, it's indicated only when diagnosis requires visualization of physiologic or pathologic motion of thoracic contents, such as to rule out paralysis in patients with diaphragmatic elevation.

Purpose
• To assess lung expansion and contraction during quiet breathing, deep breathing, and coughing
• To assess diaphragm movement and paralysis
• To detect bronchiolar obstructions and pulmonary disease

Procedure
Describe the procedure to the patient and explain that this test assesses respiratory structures and their motion. Tell him who will perform the test and where, and that the test usually takes 5 minutes.

Tell the patient that he'll be asked to follow specific instructions, such as to breathe deeply and cough, while X-ray images depict his breathing. Instruct him to remove all jewelry in the X-ray field.

If necessary, assist with patient positioning. Move cardiac monitoring cables, I.V. tubing from subclavian lines, pulmonary artery catheter lines, and safety pins as far from the X-ray field as possible. During the test, the patient's cardiopulmonary motion is observed on a screen. Special equipment may be used to intensify the images, or a videotape recording of the fluoroscopy may be made for later study.

Document the procedure.

Precautions
• Fluoroscopy is contraindicated during pregnancy.
• If the patient is intubated, check that no tubes have been dislodged during positioning.
• To avoid exposure to radiation, leave the room or the immediate area during the test; if you must stay in the area, wear a lead-lined apron.

Post-test care
None

Normal findings
Normal diaphragm movement is synchronous and symmetrical. Normal diaphragmatic excursion ranges from $3/4''$ to $1 5/8''$ (2 to 4 cm).

Implications of abnormal results
Diminished diaphragm movement may indicate pulmonary disease. Increased lung translucency may indicate elasticity loss or bronchiolar obstruction. In elderly persons, the trachea's lowest part may be displaced to the right by an elongated aorta. Diminished or paradoxical diaphragm movement may indicate diaphragmatic paralysis; however, fluoroscopy may not detect such paralysis in patients who compensate for diminished diaphragm function by using forceful abdominal muscle contraction to aid exhalation.

Interfering factors
Failure to remove jewelry and metal within the X-ray field may interfere with accurate determination of test results.

Chest tomography
(Laminagraphy, planigraphy, stratigraphy, body-section roentgenography)

Tomography provides clearly focused radiographic images of selected body sections otherwise obscured by shadows of overlying or underlying structures. In this procedure, the X-ray tube and film move around the patient (linear tube sweep) in opposite directions, producing exposures in which a selected body plane appears sharply defined and the areas above and below it are blurred. Because tomography emits high radiation levels, it's used only for further evaluation of a chest lesion.

Purpose

To demonstrate pulmonary densities (for cavitation, calcification, and fat detection), tumors (especially those obstructing the bronchial lumen), or lesions (especially those located deep within the mediastinum, such as hilar lymph nodes)

Procedure

Describe the procedure to the patient, and explain that this test helps evaluate chest structures. Inform him that he needn't restrict food or fluids before the test. Tell him who will perform the test and where, and that it takes 30 to 60 minutes.

Warn the patient that the equipment is noisy (from rapidly moving metal-on-metal parts) and that the X-ray tube swings overhead. Advise him to breathe normally during the test but to remain immobile; tell him that foam wedges will be used to help him maintain a comfortable, motionless position. Suggest he close his eyes to prevent involuntary movement. Instruct him to remove all jewelry within the X-ray field.

To begin, the patient is placed in a supine position or in various degrees of lateral rotation on the X-ray table. The X-ray tube then swings over the patient, taking numerous films from different angles. (For lung tomography, the X-ray tube's usually moved in a linear direction but may be moved in a hypocycloid or a circular, elliptic, trispiral, or figure-eight pattern. Pluridirectional films aid diagnosis of mediastinal lesions or tumors.)

Document the procedure.

Precautions

• Tomography is contraindicated during pregnancy.
• To avoid exposure to radiation, leave the room or the immediate area during the test; if you must stay in the area, wear a lead-lined apron.

Post-test care

None

Normal findings

A normal chest tomogram shows structures equivalent to those seen in a normal chest X-ray.

Implications of abnormal results

Central calcification in a nodule suggests a benign lesion; an irregularly bordered tumor suggests cancer; a sharply defined tumor suggests granuloma or nonmalignancy. Hilar evaluation can help differentiate blood vessels from nodes; identify bronchial dilation, stenosis, and endobronchial lesions; and detect tumor extension into the hilar lung area. Tomography can also identify mediastinal lesion extension to the ribs or spine.

Interfering factors

• Failure to remove jewelry and metal within the X-ray field may interfere with accurate determination of test results.
• The patient's inability to lie still may interfere with test results and necessitate additional X-rays, with greater exposure to radiation.

Pulmonary angiography
(Pulmonary arteriography)

Pulmonary angiography involves radiographic examination of the pulmonary circulation after injection of a radiopaque iodine contrast agent into the pulmonary artery or one of its branches. Most commonly, it's used to confirm symptomatic pulmonary emboli when scans prove nondiagnostic, especially before anticoagulant therapy. It also provides accurate preoperative evaluation of patients with congenital heart disease.

Possible complications include arterial occlusion, myocardial perforation or rupture, ventricular dysrhythmias from myocardial irritation, anaphylaxis, and acute renal failure from hypersensitivity to the contrast agent.

Purpose
• To detect pulmonary emboli in a symptomatic patient with a normal or inconclusive lung scan
• To evaluate pulmonary circulation preoperatively in the patient with congenital heart disease

Procedure
Describe the procedure to the patient, and explain that this test permits blood vessel evaluation to help identify the cause of his symptoms. Instruct him to fast for 8 hours before the test, or as ordered. Tell him who will perform the test and where, and that the test takes approximately 1 hour.

Tell the patient that a small incision will be made in the right arm, where blood samples are usually drawn, or in the right groin, and that he'll receive a local anesthetic to numb the area. Inform him that the doctor will then insert a small catheter into the blood vessel and pass it into the heart's right side to the pulmonary artery. Tell him the contrast agent's then injected into this artery to allow visualization of blood flow to the lungs on the X-ray. Warn him that he may experience a sudden urge to cough, a flushed feeling, nausea, or a salty taste for approximately 5 minutes after the injection. Inform him that his heart rate will be monitored continuously during the procedure.

Make sure that the patient or a responsible family member has signed a consent form. Check the patient's history for hypersensitivity to anesthetics, iodine, seafood, or radiographic contrast agents.

After the patient is placed in a supine position, the local anesthetic is injected and a cardiac monitor is attached. The doctor makes an incision and introduces a catheter into the antecubital or femoral vein. As the catheter passes through the right atrium, the right ventricle, and the pulmonary artery, pressures are measured and blood samples are drawn from various regions of the pulmonary circulatory system. The doctor then injects a contrast agent, which circulates through the pulmonary artery and lung capillaries while X-rays are taken.

Document the procedure.

Precautions
• Pulmonary angiography is contraindicated during pregnancy and in patients with hypersensitivity to iodine, seafood, or radiographic contrast agents.
• Monitor for ventricular dysrhythmias caused by myocardial irritation from catheter passage through the heart chambers.
• Observe for signs of hypersensitivity to the contrast agent, such as dyspnea, nausea, vomiting, sweating, increased heart rate, and extremity numbness.
• Keep emergency equipment available in case of an anaphylactic or hypersensitivity reaction to the contrast agent.

Post-test care
Apply a pressure dressing over the catheter insertion site and note any bleeding. Check the catheter insertion site for inflammation or hematoma formation and report symptoms of a delayed hypersensitive response to the contrast agent or local anesthetic (dyspnea, itching, tachycardia, palpitations, hypotension or hypertension, excitation, or euphoria). Check distal pulses.

Monitor the patient's vital signs, as ordered, observing for possible signs of myocardial perforation or rupture.

Stay alert for signs of acute renal failure, such as sudden onset of oliguria, nausea, and vomiting.

Advise the patient about any restriction of activity. He may resume his usual diet after the test.

Normal findings

Normally, the contrast agent flows symmetrically and without interruption through the pulmonary circulatory system.

Implications of abnormal results

Blood flow interruption may result from emboli, vascular filling defects, or stenosis.

Lung perfusion scan
(Lung scan, lung scintiscan)

The lung perfusion scan produces a visual image of pulmonary blood flow after I.V. injection of a radiopharmaceutical—human serum albumin microspheres (particles) or macroaggregated albumin, both of which bond to technetium. This test helps confirm pulmonary vascular obstruction, such as pulmonary emboli. When performed with a ventilation scan, it assesses ventilation-perfusion patterns.

Purpose
• To assess arterial lung perfusion
• To detect pulmonary emboli
• To preoperatively evaluate the pulmonary function of a patient with marginal lung reserves

Procedure

Explain to the patient that this test helps evaluate respiratory function. Inform him he needn't restrict food or fluids before the test. Tell him who will perform the test and where, and that it takes 15 to 30 minutes.

Inform the patient that the radiopharmaceutical will be injected into an arm vein and that it's only minimally radioactive. Tell him he'll either sit in front of the camera or lie under it and that neither the camera nor the uptake probe emits radiation. Reassure him that he'll be comfortable during the test and that he doesn't have to remain perfectly still.

On the test request slip, note such conditions as chronic obstructive pulmonary disease (COPD), vasculitis, pulmonary edema, tumor, sickle cell disease, or parasitic disease.

To begin, the doctor injects half the total amount of radiopharmaceutical I.V. while the patient is in a supine position, then injects the remaining half while the patient is prone. After uptake of the radiopharmaceutical, the gamma camera takes a series of single stationary images in the anterior, posterior, oblique, and both lateral chest views. Images projected onto an oscilloscope screen show radioactive particle distribution.

Document the procedure.

Precautions

A lung scan is contraindicated in patients with hypersensitivity to the radiopharmaceutical.

Post-test care

If a hematoma develops at the injection site, apply warm soaks.

Normal findings

Hot spots—areas with normal blood perfusion—show high uptake of the radiopharmaceutical; a normal lung shows uniform uptake.

Implications of abnormal results

Cold spots—areas of low radioactive uptake—indicate poor perfusion, suggesting an embolism; however, a ventilation scan must confirm the diagnosis. Decreased regional blood flow that occurs without vessel obstruction may indicate pneumonitis.

Interfering factors

• Scheduling the patient for more than one radionuclide test a day (especially if different trace substances are used) can inhibit adequate diffusion of the radioactive substance in the second test.

• I.V. injection of the radiopharmaceutical while the patient is sitting can produce abnormal images because many particles settle to the lung bases.

• Such conditions as COPD, vasculitis, pulmonary edema, tumors, sickle cell disease, or parasitic disease may cause abnormal perfusion, interfering with accurate determination of test results.

Ventilation scan

Ventilation scan—a nuclear scan performed after inhalation of air mixed with radioactive gas—delineates lung areas ventilated during respiration. The scan involves recording of gas distribution during three phases: buildup of radioactive gas (wash-in phase), after the patient rebreathes from a bag and the radioactivity reaches a steady level (equilibrium phase), and after removal of the radioactive gas from the lungs (wash-out phase). Performed with a perfusion scan, a ventilation scan helps distinguish between parenchymal disease (such as emphysema, sarcoidosis, bronchogenic carcinoma, and tuberculosis) and conditions caused by vascular abnormalities (such as pulmonary emboli).

In a patient on mechanical ventilation, krypton gas must be substituted for xenon gas when performing the test.

Purpose

• To help diagnose pulmonary emboli
• To identify lung areas capable of ventilation
• To help evaluate regional respiratory function
• To locate regional hypoventilation, which usually results from excessive smoking or COPD

Procedure

Describe the procedure to the patient, and explain that this test helps evaluate respiratory function. Inform him he needn't restrict food or fluids. Tell him who will perform the test and where, and that the test takes 15 to 30 minutes.

Instruct the patient to remove all jewelry or metal in the X-ray field. Tell him he'll be asked to hold his breath for a short time after inhaling gas and that a machine will scan his chest, at which time he must remain still. Reassure the patient that the test uses only a minimal amount of radioactive gas.

After the patient inhales air mixed with a small amount of radioactive gas through a mask, a nuclear scanner monitors gas distribution in the lungs; the patient's chest is scanned again as he exhales.

Document the procedure.

Precautions

Watch for leaks in the closed system, such as through the mask, which can contaminate the surrounding atmosphere.

Post-test care

None

Normal findings

Normal findings include equal gas distribution in both lungs and normal wash-in and wash-out phases.

Implications of abnormal results

Unequal gas distribution in both lungs indicates poor ventilation or airway obstruction in areas with low radioactivity. When compared with a lung scan (perfusion scan), perfusion to the embolized area decreases in vascular obstructions (such as pulmonary embolism) while ventilation to this area remains normal. In parenchymal disease (such as pneumonia), ventilation is abnormal within consolidated areas.

Interfering factors

Failure to remove jewelry and metal in the X-ray field during scanning may interfere with accurate determination of test results.

Thoracic computed tomography

Thoracic computed tomography (CT) provides cross-sectional views of the chest by passing an X-ray beam from a computerized scanner through the body at different angles. CT scanning may be done with or without an injected radioiodine contrast agent, which is used primarily to highlight blood vessels and allow greater visual discrimination.

This test proves especially useful in detecting small differences in tissue density. With nuclear medicine scanning, thoracic CT serves as one of the most accurate and informative diagnostic tests and may replace mediastinoscopy in the diagnosis of mediastinal masses and Hodgkin's disease. Its clinical application in the evaluation of pulmonary pathology is proven.

Purpose

• To locate suspected neoplasms (such as in Hodgkin's disease), especially with mediastinal involvement
• To differentiate coin-sized calcified lesions (indicating tuberculosis) from tumors
• To distinguish tumors adjacent to the aorta from aortic aneurysms
• To detect neck mass invasion in the thorax
• To evaluate primary cancer that may metastasize to the lungs, especially in patients with primary bone tumors, soft-tissue sarcomas, and melanomas
• To evaluate mediastinal lymph nodes

Procedure

Explain to the patient that this test provides cross-sectional views of the chest and distinguishes small differences in tissue density. If a contrast agent will not be used, inform him that he needn't restrict food or fluids. If the test will be performed with contrast enhancement, instruct the patient to fast for 4 hours before the test. Tell him who will perform the test and where and that the procedure usually takes 1½ hours. Reassure him that it won't cause discomfort.

Tell the patient that he'll be positioned on an X-ray table that moves into the center of a large ring-shaped piece of X-ray equipment. Warn him that the equipment may be noisy. Inform him that a radiographic contrast agent may be injected into an arm vein and may cause sudden nausea, warmth, facial flushing, or a salty taste. Reassure him that he'll be exposed to minimal radiation. Tell him not to move during the test but to breathe normally. Instruct him to remove all jewelry and metal in the X-ray field.

Make sure the patient or a responsible family member has signed a consent form. Check his history for hypersensitivity to iodine or radiographic contrast agents.

After the patient is placed in a supine position on the radiographic table and the contrast agent has been injected, the machine scans the patient at different angles while the computer calculates small differences in densities of various tissues, water, fat, bone, and air. This information is displayed as a printout of numerical values and as a projection on an oscilloscope screen. Images may be recorded for further study.

Document the procedure.

Precautions

Thoracic CT is contraindicated during pregnancy and, if a contrast agent's used, in patients with a history of hypersensitivity reactions to iodine, shellfish, or radiographic contrast agents.

Post-test care

Watch for signs and symptoms of delayed hypersensitivity to the contrast agent, including itching, hypotension or hypertension, and respiratory distress.

Normal findings

Black and white areas on a thoracic CT scan indicate air and bone densities, respectively. Shades of gray indicate water, fat, and soft-tissue densities.

Implications of abnormal results

Abnormal thoracic CT findings include tumors; nodules; cysts; aortic aneurysm; and blood, fluid, or fat accumulations.

Interfering factors

• Failure to remove jewelry or metal from the X-ray field may interfere with an accurate diagnosis.
• The patient's inability to lie still during scanning may interfere with accurate diagnosis or may require test repetition, which increases his exposure to radiation.
• Obese patients may not fit on the X-ray table.

Sputum culture

Bacteriologic examination of sputum—material expectorated from the lungs and bronchi during deep coughing—serves as an important aid to lung disease management. During passage through the throat and oropharynx, sputum is commonly contaminated with indigenous bacterial flora (such as alpha-hemolytic streptococci), *Neisseria* species, diphtheroids, and some hemophili, pneumococci, staphylococci, and yeasts (such as *Candida*).

Pathogenic organisms most commonly found in sputum include *Streptococcus pneumoniae, Mycobacterium tuberculosis, Klebsiella pneumoniae* (and other *Enterobacteriaceae*), *Hemophilus influenzae, Staphylococcus aureus,* and Pseudomonas aeruginosa. Other organisms, such as *Pneumocystitis carinii, Legionellae, Mycoplasma pneumoniae,* and respiratory viruses, may exist in the sputum and can cause lung disease, but they usually require serologic or histologic diagnosis rather than diagnosis by sputum culture.

Expectoration, the usual method of specimen collection, may necessitate ultrasonic nebulization, hydration, physiotherapy, or postural drainage. Other methods include tracheal suctioning or bronchoscopy. A Gram stain of expectorated sputum must be examined to ensure that the sputum is representative of lower respiratory tract secretions (as indicated by many white blood cells [WBCs] and few epithelial cells) rather than contaminated by oral flora (as indicated by few WBCs and many epithelial cells). Careful examination of an acid-fast sputum smear may provide presumptive evidence of a mycobacterial infection, such as tuberculosis.

Purpose

• To isolate and identify the cause of a pulmonary infection, thus aiding diagnosis of respiratory disease (most frequently, bronchitis, tuberculosis, lung abscess, and pneumonia)

Procedure

Explain to the patient that this test helps identify the organism causing respiratory tract infection. Inform him that the test requires a sputum specimen, and tell him who will perform the procedure. If the suspected organism is *M. tuberculosis,* tell the patient that at least three morning specimens may be required.

Test results are usually available in 48 to 72 hours. However, because tuberculosis cultures take up to 2 months, diagnosis of this disorder usually depends on clinical symptoms, a sputum smear for acid-fast bacilli, chest X-ray, and response to a purified protein derivative (PPD) skin test.

For expectoration

If the specimen will be collected by expectoration, encourage fluid intake the night before to promote sputum production. Teach the patient how to expectorate by taking three deep breaths and forcing a deep cough. Emphasize that sputum isn't the same as saliva, which will be rejected for culturing. Tell him not to brush his teeth or use mouthwash before the specimen collection, although he may rinse his mouth with water.

To begin, instruct the patient to cough deeply and expectorate into the container. If the cough is nonproductive, use chest physiotherapy, heated aerosol spray (nebulization), or intermittent positive pressure breathing (IPPB) with prescribed aerosol to induce sputum, as ordered. Using aseptic technique, close the container securely. Dispose of equipment properly; seal the container in a leak-proof bag before sending it to the laboratory.

For tracheal suctioning

If the specimen will be collected by tracheal suctioning, tell the patient that he'll experience discomfort as the catheter passes into the trachea.

To begin, administer oxygen to the patient before and after the procedure, if necessary. Attach the sputum trap to the suction catheter. Using sterile gloves, lubricate the catheter with normal saline solution and pass the catheter through the patient's nostril without suction. (The patient will cough when the catheter passes through the larynx.) Advance the catheter into the trachea. Apply suction for no longer than 15 seconds to obtain the specimen. Stop suctioning, and gently remove the catheter. Discard the catheter and gloves in the proper receptacle. Then detach the in-line sputum trap from the suction apparatus and cap the opening. If you can't get enough sputum into the trap (for example, with newborns), suction through an artificial airway using sterile technique. The catheter tip usually contains some sputum; using sterile scissors and maintaining sterile technique, let the tip fall into a sterile specimen cup. A swab may then be taken from the tip.

For bronchoscopy

If the specimen will be collected by bronchoscopy, instruct the patient to fast for 6 hours before the procedure. Make sure he or a responsible family member has signed a consent form. Tell him he'll receive a local anesthetic just before the test to minimize discomfort during tube passage.

After the local anesthetic is sprayed into the patient's throat or the patient gargles with a local anesthetic, the doctor inserts the bronchoscope through the pharynx and trachea into the bronchus. He then collects secretions either with a bronchial brush or by aspirating them through the scope's inner channel, using an irrigating solution, such as normal saline, if necessary. After obtaining the specimen, he removes the bronchoscope.

For all three sputum collection methods, document the procedure and label the container with the patient's name. On the test request form, include the specimen's nature and origin, collection date and time, initial diagnosis, and any current antibiotic therapy.

Precautions

• Tracheal suctioning is contraindicated in patients with esophageal varices, cardiac disease, bleeding disorders, or liver disease.
• Before sending the specimen to the laboratory, examine it to make sure it's sputum and not saliva, which can cause misleading results.
• In a patient with asthma or chronic bronchitis, check for aggravated bronchospasms with use of more than 10%

concentration of sodium chloride or acetylcysteine in an aerosol.

• During tracheal suctioning, suction for only 5 to 10 seconds at a time. Never suction longer than 15 seconds. If the patient becomes hypoxic or cyanotic, remove the catheter immediately and administer oxygen.

• Because the patient may cough violently during suctioning, wear a mask to avoid exposure to respiratory pathogens.

• Don't use more than 20% propylene glycol with water as an inducer for a specimen scheduled for tuberculosis culturing; higher concentrations inhibit *M. tuberculosis* growth. (If propylene glycol isn't available, use 10% to 20% acetylcysteine with water or sodium chloride.)

• Send the specimen to the laboratory immediately after collection.

Post-test care

Provide good mouth care. After tracheal suctioning, offer the patient a drink of water.

After bronchoscopy, observe the patient carefully for signs and symptoms of hypoxemia (cyanosis), laryngospasm (laryngeal stridor), bronchospasm (paroxysms of coughing or wheezing), pneumothorax (dyspnea, cyanosis, pleural pain, tachycardia), tracheal or bronchial perforation (subcutaneous crepitus), or trauma to respiratory structures (bleeding). Also check for breathing or swallowing difficulty. Don't give liquids until the gag reflex returns.

Normal findings

Flora commonly found in the respiratory tract include alpha-hemolytic streptococci, *Neisseria* species, and diphtheroids. However, presence of normal flora doesn't rule out infection.

Implications of abnormal results

Because sputum is invariably contaminated with normal oropharyngeal flora, interpretation of a culture isolate must be correlated with the patient's overall clinical condition. Isolation of *M. tuberculosis* is always a significant finding.

Interfering factors

• Improper specimen collection or handling may interfere with accurate determination of results.

• Failure to report current or recent antibiotic therapy prevents the laboratory from correctly interpreting decreased bacterial growth.

• Sputum collected over an extended period may allow pathogen deterioration or overgrowth by commensals; such sputum will not be accepted as a valid specimen by most laboratories.

Examination of sputum for ova and parasites

This test evaluates a sputum specimen for ova and parasites. Parasitic infestation is occurring more frequently in the United States because of the influx of immigrants from Southeast Asia. Infestation may result from exposure to *Entamoeba histolytica*, *Ascaris lumbricoides*, *Echinococcus granulosus*, *Strongyloides stercoralis*, *Paragonimus westermani*, or *Necator americanus*. The specimen is obtained by expectoration or tracheal suctioning.

Purpose

To identify pulmonary parasites

Procedure

Explain to the patient that this test helps identify parasitic pulmonary infection. Tell him that the test requires a sputum specimen or, if necessary, tracheal suctioning. Inform him that early morning collection is preferred because secretions accumulate overnight.

For expectoration

Encourage fluid intake the night before collection to help sputum production. Teach the patient how to expectorate by taking three deep breaths and forcing a deep cough.

To begin, instruct the patient to breathe deeply a few times and then to deep cough and expectorate into the container. If the cough is nonproductive, use chest physiotherapy, heated aerosol spray (nebulization), or intermittent positive pressure breathing with prescribed aerosol to induce sputum, as ordered. Close the container securely and clean the outside. Dispose of equipment properly; take appropriate precautions in sending the specimen to the laboratory.

For tracheal suctioning
Warn the patient that he'll experience some discomfort from the catheter.

To begin, administer oxygen before and after the procedure, if necessary. Attach a sputum trap to the suction catheter. While wearing a sterile glove, lubricate the catheter tip and pass the catheter through the patient's nostril without suction. (The patient will cough when the catheter passes into the larynx.) Advance the catheter into the trachea. Apply suction for no longer than 15 seconds to obtain the specimen. Stop suctioning, and gently remove the catheter. Discard the catheter and glove in a proper receptacle. Then detach the sputum trap from the suction apparatus and cap the opening.

For both methods, label all specimens carefully, including specimen nature and origin, collection date and time, initial diagnosis, patient's name, body temperature at collection time, current antibiotic therapy, and doctor's name.

Precautions
• Tracheal suctioning is contraindicated in patients with esophageal varices, cardiac disease, bleeding disorders, or liver disease.
• Before sending the specimen to the laboratory, examine it to make sure it's sputum and not saliva, which can cause misleading results.

• In a patient with asthma or chronic bronchitis, check for exacerbation of bronchospasms with use of more than 10% concentration of sodium chloride or acetylcysteine in an aerosol.
• During tracheal suctioning, suction for only 5 to 10 seconds at a time. Never suction longer than 15 seconds. If the patient becomes hypoxic or cyanotic, remove the catheter immediately and administer oxygen.
• If helminth infection is suspected, refrigerate the specimen up to 4 hours; if *E. histolytica,* send the specimen to the laboratory immediately.

Post-test care
Provide good mouth care. After tracheal suctioning, offer the patient a drink of water, and monitor vital signs every hour until they're stable.

Normal findings
Normally, sputum contains no parasites or ova.

Implications of abnormal results
The parasite identified in the specimen (usually in its migratory larval stage) indicates the pulmonary infection type and an adult-stage intestinal infection.
• *E. histolytica* trophozoites: pulmonary amebiasis
• *A. lumbricoides* larvae and adults: pneumonitis
• *Toxocara:* visceral larva migrans
• *E. granulosus* cysts of larval stage: hydatid disease
• *P. westermani* larval lung flukes and adults: paragonimiasis
• *S. stercoralis* larvae: strongyloidiasis
• *N. americanus* larvae: hookworm disease

Interfering factors
• Recent therapy with anthelmintics or amebicides may decrease the number of parasites.
• Improper collection may produce a nonrepresentative specimen.

Nasopharyngeal culture

This test evaluates nasopharyngeal secretions for pathogenic organisms. Direct microscopic inspection of a Gram-stained specimen smear provides preliminary organism identification that may guide clinical management and determines the need for additional testing. By streaking a culture plate with the swab and allowing organisms to grow, pathogens can be isolated and identified. Culture pathogens may then require sensitivity testing to determine appropriate antibiotic therapy. Nasopharyngeal cultures sometimes prove useful for identifying *Bordetella pertussis* and *Neisseria meningitidis*, especially in very young, elderly, or debilitated patients.

Nasopharyngeal culture also can be used to isolate viruses, especially to identify carriers of influenza virus A and B. However, this test is rarely performed because of its costly, complex, and time-consuming laboratory procedure.

Purpose
• To identify pathogens causing upper respiratory tract signs and symptoms
• To identify proliferation of normal nasopharyngeal flora, which may prove pathogenic in debilitated and other immunologically vulnerable persons
• To detect asymptomatic carriers of such infectious organisms as *N. meningitidis* and *B. pertussis*

Procedure
Describe the procedure to the patient, and explain that this test isolates the cause of nasopharyngeal infection and allows organism identification and testing for antibiotic sensitivity. Inform him that secretions will be obtained from the back of the nose and the throat using a cotton-tipped applicator. Tell him who will perform this procedure. Warn him that he may experience slight discomfort and may

Obtaining a Nasopharyngeal Specimen

When the swab passes into the nasopharynx, gently but quickly rotate it to collect a specimen. Then remove the swab, taking care not to injure the nasal mucous membrane.

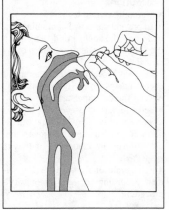

gag, but reassure him that obtaining the specimen takes less than 15 seconds. Inform him that initial test results are usually available in 48 to 72 hours but that viral test results take longer to obtain.

First, ask the patient to cough before you begin specimen collection. Then position the patient with his head tilted back. (See *Obtaining a Nasopharyngeal Specimen*.) Using a penlight and tongue depressor, inspect the nasopharyngeal area. Next, gently pass the applicator through the nostril and into the nasopharynx, keeping the applicator near the septum and nasal floor. Rotate the applicator quickly; then remove it. Or place the Pyrex tube in the patient's nostril and carefully pass the applicator through the tube into the nasopharynx. Rotate the applicator for 5 seconds; then place it in the culture tube with transport medium. Remove the Pyrex tube. Label the specimen appropriately, including collection date and time and origin of the material. Also indicate the suspected organism.

If the specimen is being collected for viral isolation, check with the laboratory for the recommended collection techniques.

Document the procedure.

Precautions
• Maintain aseptic technique.
• To prevent specimen contamination, make sure the applicator doesn't touch the patient's tongue or the sides of his nostril.
• Note any recent antibiotic therapy or chemotherapy on the laboratory slip.
• Keep the container upright.
• Because certain organisms, such as *Corynebacterium diphtheriae* and *B. pertussis*, require special growth media, inform the laboratory if they're suspected.
• Refrigerate or freeze a viral specimen according to your laboratory's procedure.

Post-test care
None

Normal findings
Flora commonly found in the nasopharynx include nonhemolytic streptococci, alpha-hemolytic streptococci, *Neisseria* species (except *N. meningitidis* and *Neisseria gonorrhoeae*), coagulase-negative staphylococci (such as *Staphylococcus epidermidis*), and occasionally the coagulase-positive *Staphylococcus aureus*.

Implications of abnormal results
Pathogens include group A beta-hemolytic streptococci; occasionally, groups B, C, and G beta-hemolytic streptococci; *B. pertussis; C. diphtheriae; S. aureus;* and large amounts of *H. influenzae*, pneumococci, or *C. albicans*.

Interfering factors
• Recent antibiotic therapy decreases bacterial growth.

• Improper collection technique may contaminate the specimen.
• Failure to place the specimen in transport medium allows it to dry out and permits bacteria to deteriorate.
• Failure to send the specimen to the laboratory immediately after collection permits organisms to proliferate.
• Failure to keep a viral specimen cold allows viruses to deteriorate.

Tuberculin skin tests

These skin tests, which screen for previous infection by the tubercle bacillus, are routinely performed in children, young adults, and patients whose radiographic findings suggest this infection. In both the old tuberculin (OT) and purified protein derivative (PPD) tests, intradermal tuberculin antigen injection causes a delayed hypersensitivity reaction in patients with active or dormant tuberculosis; sensitized lymphocytes gather at the injection site, causing erythema, vesiculation, or induration that peaks within 24 to 48 hours and persists for at least 72 hours.

The most accurate tuberculin test method, the Mantoux test, uses a single-needle intradermal injection of PPD, permitting precise dosage measurement. Multipuncture tests—such as the Tine test, Mono-Vacc tests, and Aplitest—involve intradermal injections using tines impregnated with OT or PPD. Because multipuncture tests require less skill and can be done more rapidly than the Mantoux test, they're usually used for screening. However, a positive multipuncture test usually requires a Mantoux test for confirmation.

Purpose
• To distinguish tuberculosis from blastomycosis, coccidioidomycosis, and histoplasmosis
• To identify persons requiring diagnostic investigation for tuberculosis

Procedure

Explain to the patient that this test helps detect tuberculosis. Tell him it requires an intradermal injection, which may cause transient discomfort. Check the patient's history for active tuberculosis, previous skin test results, or hypersensitivities. If the patient has had tuberculosis, don't perform a skin test; if he's had a positive reaction to previous skin tests, consult the doctor or follow hospital policy; if he's had an allergic reaction to acacia, don't perform an OT test because this product contains acacia.

If you're performing a tuberculin test on an outpatient, instruct him to return at the specified time so that test results can be read. Inform the patient that a positive reaction to a skin test appears as a red, hard, raised area at the injection site. Although the area may itch, instruct him not to scratch it. Stress that a positive reaction doesn't always indicate active tuberculosis.

To begin, the patient is placed in a sitting position with his arm extended and supported on a flat surface. Cleanse the volar surface of the upper forearm with alcohol; allow the area to dry completely.

Mantoux test

Perform intradermal injection.

Multipuncture tests

Remove the protective cap on the injection device to expose the four tines. Hold the patient's forearm in one hand, stretching forearm skin tightly. Then, with your other hand, firmly depress the device into the patient's skin (without twisting it). Hold the device in place for at least 1 second before removing it. If you've applied sufficient pressure, you'll see four puncture sites and a circular depression made by the device on the patient's skin. Record where the test was given, the date and time, and when it's to be read. Depending on hospital policy, a circle may be marked on the skin to ensure site identification. Tuberculin skin tests are usually read 48 to 72 hours after injection; however, the Mono-Vacc test can be read 48 to 96 hours after the test. (See *Reading Tuberculin Test Results,* page 84.) Tell the patient not to wash the area; he may shower, but he should not rub it or use soap on it.

For both methods, document the procedure.

Precautions

• Tuberculin skin tests are contraindicated in patients with current reactions to smallpox vaccinations or any rash, skin disorder, or active tuberculosis. These tests are not performed in anergic patients (who don't react to skin tests).

• Don't perform a skin test in areas with excess hair, acne, or insufficient subcutaneous tissue, such as over a tendon or bone. If the patient has a known hypersensitivity to skin tests, use a first-strength dose in the Mantoux test to avoid necrosis at the puncture site.

• Have epinephrine available to treat a possible anaphylactoid or acute hypersensitivity reaction.

Post-test care

If ulceration or necrosis develops at the injection site, apply cold soaks or a topical steroid, as ordered.

Normal findings

In tuberculin skin tests, normal findings show negative or minimal reactions.

• *Mantoux test:* no induration or induration less than 5 mm in diameter
• *Tine and Aplitest:* no vesiculation; no induration or induration less than 2 mm in diameter
• *Mono-Vacc test:* no induration

Implications of abnormal results

A positive tuberculin reaction indicates previous exposure to tubercle ba-

Reading Tuberculin Test Results

You should read the Mantoux, Tine, and Aplitest skin tests 48 to 72 hours after injection; the Mono-Vacc test, after 48 to 96 hours.

In a well-lighted room, flex the patient's forearm slightly. Observe the injection site for erythema and vesiculation. Then gently rub your finger over the site to detect induration. If induration is present, measure the diameter in millimeters, preferably using a plastic ruler marked in concentric circles of a specific diameter. In multipuncture tests, you may find separate areas of induration developed around individual punctures, or induration involving more than one puncture site. If so, measure the diameter of the largest single area of induration or coalesced induration.

mm in diameter without induration, invalidates the test.

• Corticosteroids and other immunosuppressants and live vaccine viruses (measles, mumps, rubella, or polio) given within the past 4 to 6 weeks may suppress skin reactions.

• Elderly patients and those with viral infection, malnutrition, febrile illness, uremia, immunosuppressive disorders, or miliary tuberculosis may have suppressed skin reactions.

• The skin reaction may be suppressed if less than 10 weeks has passed since tuberculosis infection.

• Improper tuberculin dilution, dosage, or storage interferes with accurate testing.

Pulmonary artery catheterization
(Swan-Ganz catheterization, balloon flotation catheterization of the pulmonary artery, right heart catheterization)

cilli. It does not distinguish between an active and dormant infection or provide a definitive diagnosis. If a positive reaction occurs, sputum smear and culture and chest radiography are necessary for further evaluation.

In the Mantoux test, induration between 5 and 9 mm in diameter indicates a borderline reaction; a larger induration, a positive reaction. Because patients infected with atypical myobacteria other than tubercle bacilli may have borderline reactions, they require repeat testing.

In the Tine or Aplitest, vesiculation indicates a positive reaction; induration of 2 mm in diameter without vesiculation requires confirmation by the Mantoux test. Any induration in the Mono-Vacc test indicates a positive reaction; however, it requires confirmation by the Mantoux test.

Interfering factors
• Subcutaneous injection, usually indicated by erythema greater than 10

Pulmonary artery catheterization uses a balloon-tipped, flow-directed catheter to provide intermittent occlusion of the pulmonary artery. Once the catheter is in place, this procedure permits measurement of pulmonary artery pressure (PAP) and pulmonary capillary wedge pressure (PCWP). The PCWP reading accurately reflects left atrial pressure and left ventricular end-diastolic pressure, although the catheter itself never enters the heart's left side. Such a reading is possible because the heart momentarily relaxes during diastole as it fills with blood from the pulmonary veins; at this instant, the pulmonary vasculature, left atrium, and left ventricle act as a single chamber and all have identical pressures. Thus, PAP and PCWP changes reflect changes in left ventricular filling pressure, permitting detection of left ventricular impairment.

In this procedure, usually performed at the bedside in an intensive care unit, the doctor inserts the catheter through the cephalic vein in the antecubital fossa or the subclavian (or, sometimes, femoral) vein. After threading the catheter into the right atrium, he inflates the balloon. The catheter then follows the blood through the tricuspid valve into the right ventricle and out into the pulmonary artery.

Besides measuring atrial and pulmonary arterial pressures, this procedure evaluates pulmonary vascular resistance and tissue oxygenation, as indicated by mixed venous oxygen content. Thermodilution also allows cardiac output measurement. Pulmonary artery catheterization should be performed cautiously in patients with left bundle branch block or implanted pacemakers.

Purpose

• To help assess right and left ventricular failure
• To monitor therapy for complications of acute myocardial infarction, such as cardiogenic shock, pulmonary edema, fluid-related hypovolemia and hypotension, systolic murmur, unexplained sinus tachycardia, and various cardiac dysrhythmias
• To help assess and monitor therapy for pulmonary hypertension
• To assess hemodynamic effects of high positive end-expiratory pressure
• To assess pulmonary artery pressures in children with congenital heart disease and shunting
• To monitor fluid status in patients with serious burns, renal disease, or acute respiratory distress syndrome after open heart surgery
• To monitor the effects of cardiovascular drugs, such as nitroglycerin and nitroprusside

Procedure

Explain to the patient that this test evaluates heart function and vascular changes occurring from pulmonary disease and provides information for determining appropriate therapy or management of fluid status.

Advise the patient that he needn't restrict food or fluids before the test. Tell him who will perform the test and where.

Inform the patient that he'll be conscious during catheterization, and warn him that he may feel transient local discomfort from local anesthetic administration. Tell him that although catheter insertion takes about 30 minutes, the catheter will remain in place, causing little or no discomfort, for 48 to 72 hours. His activity may be slightly restricted. Instruct him to report any discomfort immediately. Make sure the patient or a responsible family member has signed a consent form.

The flexible catheter used in this procedure comes in two-, three-, and four-lumen (thermodilution) modes and in various lengths. (See *Four-Lumen Pulmonary Artery Catheter,* page 87.) In the two-lumen catheter, one lumen contains the balloon, 1 mm behind the catheter tip; the other lumen, which opens at the tip, measures pressure in front of the balloon. The two-lumen catheter measures PAP and PCWP and can be used to sample mixed venous blood and to infuse I.V. solutions. The three-lumen catheter has an additional proximal lumen that opens 30 cm behind the tip; when the tip is in the main pulmonary artery, the proximal lumen lies in the right atrium, permitting fluid administration or monitoring of right atrial pressure (central venous pressure). The four-lumen type includes a transistorized thermistor for monitoring blood temperature and allows cardiac output measurement.

Before catheterization, the equipment is set up and primed according to manufacturer instructions and hospital procedure. Balloon patency and integrity must be checked. Then, if the insertion site is being prepared for a cutdown procedure, the patient's skin is prepared and covered with a sterile drape. Alternatively, a sterile stockinette can be pulled over the patient's arm from wrist to elbow and a hole cut in the stockinette at the insertion site.

The patient is helped to the supine position. For antecubital insertion, his arm is abducted with palm upward on an overbed table for support; for subclavian insertion, he's placed in the supine position with his head and shoulders slightly lower than his trunk to make the vein more accessible. If he can't tolerate the supine position, assist him to semi-Fowler's position. During the test, all pressures are monitored with the patient in the same position.

With the balloon deflated, the catheter is introduced into the vein percutaneously or by cutdown. The catheter is directed to the right atrium and the catheter balloon is partially inflated so that venous flow carries the catheter tip through the right atrium and tricuspid valve into the right ventricle and into the pulmonary artery. While the catheter is being directed, the oscilloscope screen is observed for characteristic waveform changes and the catheter tip's location. (Catheter insertion may also be done under fluoroscopic guidance.) A printout of each catheter insertion stage is obtained for baseline information. (See *Pulmonary Artery Catheter Insertion*, pages 88 and 89.) Monitor the patient's hemodynamic status during insertion by observing vital signs and cardiac rhythm. During insertion, also assess for changes in ventilatory status caused by the patient's position and facial drapes. Talk to the patient during the procedure to provide reassurance and to assess for mental status changes.

As the catheter is passed into the right heart chambers, the oscilloscope screen is observed for frequent premature ventricular contractions (PVCs) and tachycardia—the result of catheter irritation of the right ventricle. If irritation oc-

curs, the catheter may be partially withdrawn or medication administered to suppress the dysrhythmia or right bundle branch block.

To record PCWP, the catheter balloon is carefully inflated with the specified amount of air or carbon dioxide—not fluid—using the smallest syringe possible; the catheter tip will float into the wedge position, as indicated by an altered (dampened) waveform on the oscilloscope screen. If a PCWP waveform occurs with less than the recommended inflation volume, do not inflate the balloon further. After balloon inflation, wedge pressure is recorded. Then balloon air is withdrawn into a syringe, permitting the catheter to float back into the pulmonary artery. The oscilloscope screen is observed for a PA waveform. Next, the system is flushed and recalibrated. Don't overinflate the balloon catheter—overinflation could distend the pulmonary artery, causing vessel rupture. If the balloon can't be fully deflated after recording PCWP, don't reinflate it unless the doctor is present—balloon rupture may cause a life-threatening air embolism. Check all connections for air leaks that may have prevented balloon inflation, particularly if the patient is confused or uncooperative.

When correct catheter positioning and function have been established, the catheter is sutured to the skin and antibiotic ointment and an airtight dressing are applied to the insertion site. A chest X-ray is obtained, as ordered, to verify catheter placement. (Before the procedure, the radiology department is notified that a catheter insertion will take place.) Set alarms on the EKG and pressure monitors. Monitor vital signs as ordered. Make sure PAP waveforms are documented at the beginning of each shift and monitored frequently throughout each shift. Check PCWP and cardiac output, as

Four-Lumen Pulmonary Artery Catheter

Pulmonary artery catheters are made of pliable, radiopaque polyvinyl-chloride. This illustration shows a 110-cm (about 43¼″) catheter, marked in 10-cm increments. It has distal and proximal lumens, which are fluid-filled for pressure monitoring; a thermistor lumen, which holds the wires connecting the thermistor to the cardiac output computer; and a balloon inflation lumen with valve. As a result, this catheter can measure several pressures, as well as cardiac output.

Because catheters vary depending on their manufacturer, consult the manufacturer's manual for additional details.

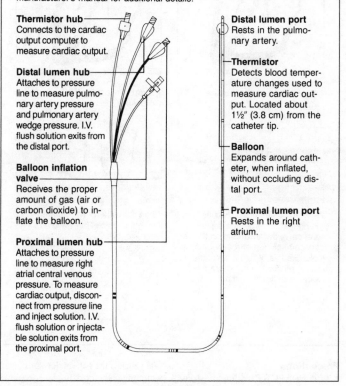

Thermistor hub
Connects to the cardiac output computer to measure cardiac output.

Distal lumen hub
Attaches to pressure line to measure pulmonary artery pressure and pulmonary artery wedge pressure. I.V. flush solution exits from the distal port.

Balloon inflation valve
Receives the proper amount of gas (air or carbon dioxide) to inflate the balloon.

Proximal lumen hub
Attaches to pressure line to measure right atrial central venous pressure. To measure cardiac output, disconnect from pressure line and inject solution. I.V. flush solution or injectable solution exits from the proximal port.

Distal lumen port
Rests in the pulmonary artery.

Thermistor
Detects blood temperature changes used to measure cardiac output. Located about 1½″ (3.8 cm) from the catheter tip.

Balloon
Expands around catheter, when inflated, without occluding distal port.

Proximal lumen port
Rests in the right atrium.

ordered (usually every 6 hours), according to hospital policy. Take routine aseptic precautions to prevent infection.

When the catheter is no longer needed, the patient's blood pressure and radial pulse are taken. Then the doctor deflates the balloon, removes the dressing, and slowly withdraws the catheter. The EKG is monitored for dysrhythmias.

Pressure, an antibiotic ointment, and a sterile dressing are applied to the insertion site after catheter withdrawal. Blood pressure and radial pulse are checked.

Document the procedure and how the patient tolerated it.

Pulmonary Artery Catheter Insertion

As the catheter is directed through the right heart chambers to its wedge position, it produces distinctive waveforms on an oscilloscope screen. These waveforms indicate the catheter's position.

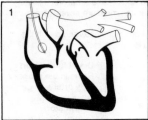

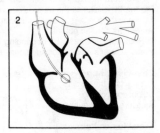

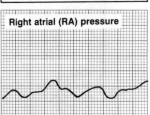

Right atrial (RA) pressure

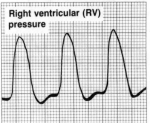

Right ventricular (RV) pressure

When the catheter tip reaches the right atrium from the superior vena cava, the waveform on the oscilloscope screen or readout strip looks like this. When it does, the doctor inflates the catheter's balloon, which floats the tip through the tricuspid valve into the right ventricle.

When the catheter tip reaches the right ventricle, the waveform looks like this.

Precautions

• After each PCWP reading, flush and recalibrate the monitoring system and make sure the balloon is completely deflated; if you have problems flushing the system, notify the doctor. Maintain 300 mm Hg pressure in the pressure bag to permit fluid flow of 3 to 6 ml/hour. Instruct the patient to extend the appropriate arm (or leg, if the catheter is inserted into the femoral vein). If the patient develops fever while the catheter is in place, remove the catheter and send the catheter tip to the laboratory for culture.

• Make sure all stopcocks are properly positioned and all connections are secure. Loose connections during the test may allow rapid, massive arterial blood loss.

• Be sure the lumen hubs are properly identified to serve the appropriate cath-

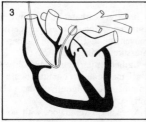

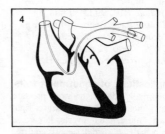

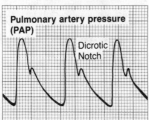

Pulmonary artery pressure (PAP)

Dicrotic Notch

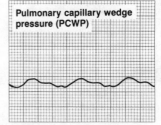

Pulmonary capillary wedge pressure (PCWP)

A waveform like this one indicates that the balloon has floated the catheter tip through the pulmonic valve into the pulmonary artery. A dicrotic notch should be visible in the waveform, indicating the closing of the pulmonic valve.

Blood flow in the pulmonary artery then carries the catheter balloon into one of the pulmonary artery's many smaller branches. When the vessel becomes too narrow for the balloon to pass through, the balloon wedges in the vessel, occluding it. The monitor then displays a pulmonary capillary wedge pressure (PCWP) waveform like this one.

eter ports. Don't add or remove fluids from the distal pulmonary artery port; this may cause pulmonary extravasation or may damage the artery.

• If the catheter has not been sutured to the skin, tape it securely to prevent dislodgment.

• Change the sterile dressing every 24 hours (more often if soiled), according to hospital policy.

Post-test care

Observe the catheter insertion site for signs of infection—redness, swelling, and discharge. Apply a sterile, airtight dressing over the site.

For 24 hours, check for complications, such as pulmonary emboli, pulmonary artery perforation, murmurs, thrombi, and dysrhythmias. Document any changes in the patient's condition.

Normal findings

Normal pressures are as follows:
- *Right atrial:* 1 to 6 mm Hg
- *Systolic right ventricular:* 20 to 30 mm Hg
- *End-diastolic right ventricular:* less than 5 mm Hg
- *Systolic PAP:* 20 to 30 mm Hg
- *Diastolic PAP:* about 10 mm Hg
- *Mean PAP:* less than 20 mm Hg
- *PCWP:* 6 to 12 mm Hg
- *Left atrial:* about 10 mm Hg

Implications of abnormal results

Abnormally high right atrial pressure may indicate pulmonary disease, right heart failure, fluid overload, cardiac tamponade, tricuspid stenosis and regurgitation, or pulmonary hypertension.

Elevated right ventricular pressure can result from pulmonary hypertension, pulmonary valvular stenosis, right ventricular failure, pericardial effusion, constrictive pericarditis, chronic congestive heart failure, or ventricular septal defects.

An abnormally high PAP typically accompanies increased pulmonary blood flow, such as in a left-to-right shunt secondary to ventricular septal defect; increased pulmonary arteriolar resistance, such as in pulmonary hypertension or mitral stenosis; chronic obstructive pulmonary disease; pulmonary edema or embolus; and left ventricular failure from any cause. Under normal conditions, pulmonary artery systolic pressure is identical to right ventricular systolic pressure. Pulmonary artery diastolic pressure is identical to left atrial pressure, except in patients with severe pulmonary disease causing pulmonary hypertension; in such patients, catheterization still provides important diagnostic information.

Elevated PCWP may result from left ventricular failure, mitral stenosis and regurgitation, cardiac tamponade, or cardiac insufficiency; depressed PCWP may result from hypovolemia or other causes of shock.

Interfering factors

- Malfunctioning of monitoring and recording devices, loose connections, clot formation at the catheter tip, air in the fluid column, or balloon rupture may interfere with accurate testing. (See *Solving Problems with Pulmonary Artery Lines.*)
- Incorrect catheter placement causes catheter fling—excessive catheter movement that leads to a dampened pressure tracing.
- Catheter migration against a vessel wall may cause constant occlusion (permanent wedging) of the pulmonary artery.
- Mechanical ventilators with positive pressure cause increased intrathoracic pressure, which raises catheter pressure.

Continuous SvO₂ monitoring

Of the various hemodynamic monitoring techniques now available, few appear more promising than continuous monitoring of mixed venous oxygen saturation (SvO₂). Done through a fiberoptic flow-directed thermodilution pulmonary artery (PA) catheter (Opticath), SvO₂ measurements reflect the body's ability to meet tissue oxygen demands. Two primary factors—oxygen transport and tissue oxygen consumption—affect SvO₂. Oxygen transport, in turn, is affected by cardiac output, hemoglobin (Hb), and arterial oxygen saturation (SaO₂). The following equation best reflects this relationship:

O_2 consumption = cardiac output x Hb x 13.8 (SaO_2-SvO_2)

where 13.8 is the carrying constant.

Purpose

- To detect hemodynamic instability
- To evaluate rapidly the response to drug administration, endotracheal tube suctioning, ventilator setting changes, and positive end-expiratory pressure

Solving Problems with Pulmonary Artery Lines

Problem	Possible causes	Solution
Dampened pressures	Air in system	Check intraflow valves, stopcock, and transducer for bubbles.
	Blood on transducer	Flush off or change transducer.
	Clot in system	Aspirate blood until it thins; notify doctor.
	Catheter kinked	Instruct patient to cough or extend his arm in a 90-degree angle from his body, and gently flush the catheter. If problem, obtain X-ray film.
	Loose connection	Check connections for security.
	Incorrect stopcock position	Correct stopcock position.
	Pressure tubing too long	Shorten distance between patient and transducer.
Transducer imbalance	Damaged transducer	Try another transducer.
	Wrong amplifier	Check transducer connection to amplifier.
	Broken amplifier	Change the amplifier.
	Set at wrong level (mid-chest)	Readjust the transducer.
Waveform drifting	Short warm-up time	Allow recommended time for warm-up.
	Cable air vents kinked or coiled	Unkink or decompress cable air vents.
False-low reading	Dampened waveform	See section on dampened pressures.
	Transducer imbalance	Place transducer at heart level.
	Wrong calibration	Recalibrate the monitor.
False-high reading	Transducer imbalance	Rebalance the transducer.
	Flush solution administered too quickly	Pour slow continual flush (3 to 6 ml/hr).
Configuration	Improper catheter placement	Try to wedge catheter. Obtain PCWP. If problem, obtain X-ray film.

(continued)

Solving Problems with Pulmonary Artery Lines *(continued)*

Problem	Possible causes	Solution
Configuration *(continued)*	Transducer needs to be calibrated	Recalibrate the transducer.
	Transducer not at RA level	Reposition and recalibrate the transducer.
	Transducer loosely connected to catheter	Secure the transducer.
Drifting wedge pressure (with inflated balloon)	Balloon overinflation	Watch scope while inflating balloon. When waveform changes from a PA to a wedge shape, stop inflating.
	Air in system	Remove air from tubing and/or transducer.
PCWP pressure trace unobtainable	Incorrect amount of balloon air	Deflate, start again slowly. Check for air to refill syringe during balloon deflation.
	Ruptured balloon	With no resistance to inflation, stop inflation. Notify doctor.
	Catheter moved proximally	Notify doctor to change catheter; catheter may not be advanced because proximal end is no longer sterile.

- To reduce the need for repeated measurement of arterial blood gases, cardiac output, and other hemodynamic indices
- To help detect and prevent complications associated with traditional pulmonary artery catheters, such as clot formation at the catheter tip

Procedure

Prepare the patient for insertion of the Opticath PA catheter. First, explain the procedure to him and his family. Make sure that they understand the procedure's risks and expected outcomes. Also make sure that the patient or a responsible family member has signed a consent form. Inform him that the procedure takes 15 to 30 minutes and that during this time he must lie still. Inform him that after catheter placement, his activity will be restricted.

Before catheter insertion, the equipment is set up and primed according to manufacturer instructions and hospital procedure. Balloon patency and integrity must be checked. Both the oximeter and pressure module should be turned on for at least 10 minutes beforehand to allow them to warm up.

Assist the doctor with catheter insertion. Monitor the patient's hemodynamic status during insertion by observing vital signs and cardiac rhythm. Also assess for changes in ventilatory status during insertion caused by the patient's dependent position and facial drapes. Talk to the patient during the procedure to provide reassurance and to assess for mental status changes. Document the pressure readings obtained during insertion and any changes in the patient's condition.

Once inserted, the Opticath can be connected to the Optical Module. (See *The SvO₂ Monitoring System.*) This may also be done before insertion, if the doctor prefers. Record the initial SvO₂ reading and calibrate the CO-oximeter to ensure accurate values. Document hourly SvO₂ readings along with vital signs and attach selected strips to the chart as ordered or according to hospital policy.

Precautions

• Complications of this procedure may include pneumothorax, pulmonary artery perforation, air emboli, infection, and cardiac dysrhythmias.

• Help prevent complications by:

—changing the sterile dressing every 24 hours (more often if dressing is soiled) according to hospital policy

—inspecting the site for signs of infection with each dressing change

—changing the I.V. tubing every 24 hours

—maintaining a heparin flush system to prevent clot formation

—maintaining an airtight system (check for air bubbles and make sure that all connections are tight)

—closely monitoring the patient's hemodynamic status

—using gentle technique when wedging the catheter to prevent balloon rupture and pulmonary artery damage

The SvO₂ Monitoring System

The SvO₂ monitoring system includes a fiberoptic catheter, an optical module, and an oximeter. On the CO-oximeter, a panel displays a continuous digital SvO₂ value, and a strip recorder provides a permanent record of SvO₂ measurements.

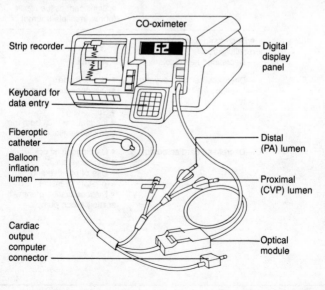

CO-oximeter

Strip recorder

Keyboard for data entry

Fiberoptic catheter

Balloon inflation lumen

Cardiac output computer connector

Digital display panel

Distal (PA) lumen

Proximal (CVP) lumen

Optical module

Interpreting SvO_2 Measurements

High or low SvO_2 levels reflect problems with oxygen delivery and/or oxygen demand. This chart lists the physiologic problems that can alter SvO_2 levels, with their possible causes.

SvO_2 range	Physiologic state	Possible causes
High (80% to 95%)	• Increased oxygen delivery	• Increased FlO_2 from mechanical ventilation
	• Artifact	• Wedged catheter in pulmonary artery
	• Decreased oxygen uptake	• Hypothermia • Septic shock • Anesthesia • Left-to-right shunting
	• Increased cardiac output	• Inotropic drug administration
Normal (60% to 80%)	• Normal oxygen delivery and normal oxygen demand	• Adequate tissue perfusion
Low (below 60%)	• Increased oxygen demands	• Hyperthermia • Seizures • Severe pain and anxiety • Shivering • Significant tissue repair (burns, multiple trauma)
	• Decreased oxygen delivery resulting from: —Decreased hemoglobin	• Anemia
	—Decreased arterial oxygen saturation	• Hemorrhage • Disconnection from ventilator • Suctioning • Inadequate FlO_2 from mechanical ventilation
	—Decreased cardiac output	• Cardiogenic shock • Hypovolemia • Use of positive end-expiratory pressure • Discontinuation of intra-aortic balloon pump

—observing for cardiac dysrhythmias and keeping resuscitation equipment readily available.

• If the SvO_2 level falls below 60% or varies by more than 10% above or below the baseline value, reassess the patient immediately and, if necessary, troubleshoot the monitoring system.

• The CO-oximeter must be calibrated on initial insertion, any time the catheter is disconnected from the Optical Module, and routinely once a day. To do this, draw a mixed venous blood sample for laboratory analysis; then compare the sample's SvO_2 value to the SvO_2 value on the CO-oximeter at the time of sampling. More than 4% difference between the two values necessitates recalibration according to manufacturer instructions.

• Using the keyboard, set alarm parameters—usually at a range of 10% above and below the displayed SvO_2 level. Update these parameters with any SvO_2 change greater than 5% and whenever recalibration alters SvO_2 readings.

• The strip recorder, consisting of graph paper and marking pens, records the SvO_2 level every 5 seconds. At the paper's lower edge, intensity bars measure data transmission intensity every 2 minutes. Inadequate signal intensity, such as from a small clot at the catheter tip or from wedging of the tip against the vessel wall, causes the alarm to sound.

• If the intensity alarm sounds, SvO_2 readings are invalidated and system troubleshooting must begin. Troubleshooting involves checking catheter placement and patency. Remove any air bubbles and kinks from the catheter. Flush the catheter only if you can easily withdraw blood first to prevent dislodging a clot. If blood does not flow easily, reposition the patient—the catheter may be kinked under the skin.

Post-test care

Auscultate the patient's breath sounds and obtain a chest X-ray to verify proper catheter placement and to check for pneumothorax or hemothorax.

Apply a sterile, airtight dressing over the site. Document any changes in the patient's condition.

Normal values

In a healthy adult, an SvO_2 level between 60% and 80% usually indicates adequate tissue perfusion. However, normal values vary in critically ill patients, depending on the disorder; thus, for each patient, baseline SvO_2 values should be established and monitored for trends.

Implications of abnormal results

Usually, an SvO_2 level below 60% indicates cardiac decompensation; below 53%, lactic acidosis; below 32%, unconsciousness; and below 20%, permanent cellular damage. SvO_2 values above 80% occur with increased oxygen delivery, reduced oxygen demands, or decreased oxygen extraction by the tissues. (See *Interpreting SvO_2 Measurements* for disorders associated with above- and below-normal SvO_2 levels.) Although this chart provides a guide for interpreting *individual* SvO_2 values, you must also assess for trends to obtain a complete, accurate clinical picture. For example, a slowly decreasing SvO_2 value may indicate bleeding as hematocrit and hemoglobin levels decline and impair tissue oxygenation.

Oximetry

Oximetry, a noninvasive procedure, continuously monitors arterial oxygen saturation (SaO_2). It involves light transmission through tissue and analysis of differences in light absorption between reduced "blue" hemoglobin and "red" oxyhemoglobin. This spectrophotoelectric technique allows for continuous *in vivo* monitoring. The computed SaO_2 values appear on a monitor; a printout of the resulting waveforms can be obtained to provide a permanent record.

Two forms of oximetry are currently in widespread use—ear oximetry and pulse oximetry. *Ear oximetry* monitors SaO_2 by computing the relative absorption of two to eight wavelengths of light directed through ear or finger vessels. To eliminate venous, capillary, and tissue bed artifacts, the site must be slightly warmed to 102° to 104° F. (39° or 40° C.) and massaged to dilate the vascular bed.

Because use of such an artificially arterialized site presents limitations, oximetry techniques have evolved into measurement of changes in light absorption simultaneously with arterial pulsation—a method called *pulse oximetry*, which works by positioning any pulsating arterial vascular bed between a two- or three-wavelength light source and a detector. Thus, it eliminates the need to warm and massage the site. Sites used include the nasal bridge, finger, palms, great toe, Achilles tendon, and ear. (See *How Pulse Oximetry Works.*)

Newer pulse oximetry units lock the signal onto the R wave of the patient's EKG to pinpoint the pulse of every beat. This permits pulse detection in patients with poor peripheral perfusion. Also, three-light wavelengths are used to detect fractional rather than functional SaO_2, to permit differentiation of oxyhemoglobin and carboxyhemoglobin; theoretically, this should help obtain more accurate readings in smokers and others with abnormal carboxyhemoglobin levels. Wireless telemetry units are also available; these display readings from several units simultaneously on a central monitor.

Both oximetry methods involve similar, although not interchangeable, equipment—a sensor device (the light source and detector), monitor (display panel, printer, settings, and alarms), electrodes, and a microcomputer that approximates the SaO_2 measurement by analyzing data with the appropriate equations.

Oximetry's convenience, simplicity, reliability, low risk of complications, and noninvasive nature represent a major advance in respiratory care. New developments continue to increase the technique's reliability and applicability. Although oximetry doesn't replace arterial blood sampling, it can permit continuous evaluation, even under unstable conditions.

Purpose
• To determine SaO_2 values and monitor trends in patients with such respiratory conditions as respiratory failure, chronic obstructive pulmonary disease (COPD), hypoxia, sleep apnea, and interstitial pulmonary disease
• To determine SaO_2 values and monitor trends during exercise testing, fiberoptic bronchoscopy, general anesthesia and surgery, ventilator therapy, oxygen therapy, ventilator weaning, transport monitoring, and sleep

Procedure
Explain the procedure and describe the equipment to the patient. Tell the patient that the equipment will show how much oxygen his blood contains. Reassure the patient that it's painless. Show him the sensor device and where you will fasten it. Explain that food or fluids need not be restricted. If this is an exercise test, explain what the patient should do. Otherwise, tell him to remain as still as possible to prevent the sensor from slipping. Set up the equipment.

Ear oximetry
Following manufacturer instructions, attach the power cord. Connect either the finger probe or ear probe to the monitor box. Turn on the power switch, allowing time for it to warm up. If alarms

are indicated, set both low and high alarms. Turn on the alarm volume if it's turned off or down. If calibration is required, follow manufacturer instructions or push the calibration button. If test values don't fall within the appropriate range, obtain another oximetry unit. If you use the strip chart recorder, plug in the recorder, set the speed and voltage according to directions, turn it on, zero the recording pen, and adjust recorder input sensitivity.

Massage the patient's earlobe with an alcohol sponge for 10 to 20 seconds. Mild erythema indicates adequate vascularization. For the finger probe, make sure the patient doesn't have long or false fingernails; remove any nail polish. If the index finger is obese, select a smaller finger. (Although the finger probe is slightly more accurate than the ear probe, both produce readings that fall within an acceptably reliable range in most situations.)

Be sure to attach the ear probe to the patient's ear lobe or pinna according to manufacturer instructions. (See *Ear Probe Placement,* page 98.) Use an ear probe stabilizer for prolonged use or exercise testing if one comes with the unit. Finding and maintaining a good contact on the ear may be difficult, but it is important because slippage will set off the low perfusion alarm.

After a few seconds, a saturation reading and pulse waveform will appear on the screen. You may leave the ear probe in place for 3 or more minutes until the readings stabilize at the highest point, or average three separate readings, revascularizing the patient's ear lobe each time. The probe may be left on as a monitoring device.

When the probe is no longer needed, remove it, turn the power off, and unplug the power cord. Clean the probe by rubbing it gently with alcohol. Do not immerse. After use in an isolation setting, sterilize the entire unit in ethylene oxide or follow manufacturer instructions.

How Pulse Oximetry Works

As shown below, two diodes send red (visible) and infrared light beams through tissue. A photodetector determines the relative amount of color absorbed by arterial blood; this data indicates arterial hemoglobin saturation.

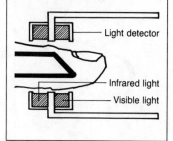

Document the date, time, procedure, oximetric measurement, and any action taken. Use appropriate flow sheets if indicated. If strips were taken, paste selected ones on the chart and note the trends during that time period.

Pulse oximetry

Patient preparation is essentially the same as with ear oximetry except that arterialization isn't necessary.

When setting up the equipment, set high and low pulse alarms in addition to high and low SaO_2 parameters. On some units, some alarm limits are preset and can be adjusted according to hospital policy, patient condition, or doctor's order. Adult and neonate settings differ, with high oxygen saturation preset at 100% SaO_2 for adults and 95% SaO_2 for neonates; low oxygen saturation is preset at 85% SaO_2 for adults and 80% SaO_2 for neonates. Pulse settings differ markedly by age: high pulse rate is preset at 140 beats/minute for adults and 200 beats/min-

Ear Probe Placement

Earlobe placement

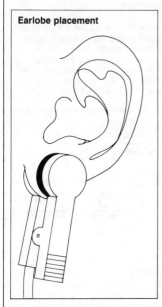

Pinna placement

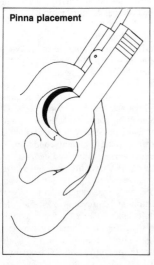

ute for neonates; low pulse rate is preset at 55 beats/minute for adults and 100 beats/minute for neonates.

Some units also offer a choice of modes to adjust response times:
• *fast,* for sleep and other special studies with inactive patients
• *moderate,* for relatively inactive patients
• *slow,* for active patients, as in stress testing or continuous monitoring of small children.

Place the transducer/sensor over the patient's finger so that light beams and light sensors oppose each other. Select the appropriate site. In adults, the index finger is usually best unless the patient is obese. If the patient has long nails, you may position the sensor perpendicular to the finger, depending on sensor type. With neonates and infants, you can wrap the sensor around the foot so that light beams and light sensors oppose each other. The foot is preferred because it's less active. A sensor that fits on the great toe is best used for larger infants. Protect the sensor by putting a sock on the foot. If the foot is inaccessible, wrap the sensor around the palm of the hand or across the Achilles tendon. Check circulation to the distal extremity frequently, and inspect skin under the sensor for irritation at least once a day. *Note:* Choose the appropriate sensor for the module and apply it correctly to maintain good adhesion.

Following manufacturer instructions, attach the power cord to the monitor and connect the patient module to the oximeter. Then connect the transducer/sensor to the patient module.

Turn on the power switch and set the alarm limits, if necessary. If the device is working properly, you'll hear a beep and see the displays light momentarily and the pulse searchlight flash. The SaO_2 and pulse rate displays should show stationary zeros. After four to six heartbeats, the SaO_2 and pulse rate displays will begin to show information with each beat, and the pulse amplitude indicator will begin tracking the pulse. You'll also hear a beep rising in pitch as SaO_2 increases and falling as SaO_2 decreases with each beat. When the SaO_2 level or pulse rate exceeds or drops below the alarm limits, the corresponding indicator light and SaO_2 display on the front panel flash and the audio alarm sounds steadily (unless you've turned it off). *Note:* Loss of pulse signal or transducer connection also causes the audio alarm to sound. In this case, however, the SaO_2 and pulse rate displays go blank and the pulse search indicator flashes.

Document the date, time, procedure, oximetric measurement, and any action taken. Use appropriate flow sheets, if indicated.

Precautions
• With ear oximetry, the low perfusion light indicates a loose probe or insufficient arterial perfusion. Check the connections, rearterialize the ear, reposition the probe, or select another site. If the problem persists, notify the doctor.
• Never turn the audio alarm off if doing so would compromise patient safety.
• With pulse oximetry, the wide range of available sensors helps to eliminate patient activity artifacts and allow more accurate readings. However, all sensors must be applied according to manufacturer instructions. Before reusing a sensor, make sure that its backing has sufficient adhesive. *Note:* Some sensors, such as the nasal sensor, can't be reused.
• The nasal sensor, applied over the nasal bridge, makes oximetric readings possible even with extremes of perfusion. Pulsation of the nasal septal anterior ethmoid artery supplied by the internal carotid can be sensed long after the finger pulse disappears. However, this sensor can be used only on

immobile, anesthetized, or paralyzed patients because it's highly sensitive to motion and respiration. It proves especially helpful during surgery, when severe vasoconstriction makes other sites nonpulsatile.
• A larger pulse oximetry sensor, designed for the great toe, is available for infants weighing 7 to 33 lb (3 to 15 kg). This minimizes motion artifact in sleeping and quiet infants; however, for more active infants, you may need to switch to a slower operating mode.
• Because of decreased reliability at PaO_2 levels greater than 100 mm Hg (which can cause retrolental fibroplasia), pulse oximeter SaO_2 values probably should not exceed 90%. Consider a value of 85% to 90% a safer range in neonates and patients receiving oxygen therapy.
• Pulse oximetry proves more accurate than transcutaneous oxygen monitoring in patients with wide ranges in SaO_2 values (57% to 100%), hematocrit values (20% to 67%), fetal hemoglobin concentration (1.3% to 60%), and peripheral temperatures (79.7° to 97.7° F. [26.5° to 36.5° C.]). (See *Transcutaneous PO_2 Monitoring*, page 100.)

Post-test care
Take appropriate action based on the readings.

Normal values
Normal SaO_2 values with ear and pulse oximetry are as follows:
• *Adults:* 95% to 100% (expected values may be lower with certain diseases, such as COPD, and in elderly patients)
• *Healthy term neonates:* 93.8% to 100% by 1 hour after birth.

Implications of abnormal results
Significant changes from normal values or the patient's usual values indi-

Transcutaneous PO$_2$ Monitoring

Transcutaneous PO$_2$ (tcPO$_2$) monitoring is a noninvasive method of measuring oxygen pressure (unlike oximetry, which measures oxygen saturation). Like oximetry, however, tcPO$_2$ monitoring can be used continuously or intermittently to identify hypoxemia and to monitor response to oxygen therapy.

tcPO$_2$ monitoring has been used mostly on neonates in intensive care units. However, it has several drawbacks. Because it measures the amount of oxygen diffusing through the capillaries just below the skin surface, the cutaneous site must be arterialized (heated to at least 111° F. [44° C.]) to increase capillary permeability and oxygen diffusion; this increases the risk of skin burns. Also, tcPO$_2$ monitoring does not always yield accurate readings because of difficulty in maintaining good skin contact. In addition, conditions causing elevated bilirubin levels, shock, and low cardiac output give false results. Because of these problems, the technique has been replaced by pulse oximetry in many hospitals. Normal tcPO$_2$ values for the neonate range from 50 to 90 mm Hg, depending on the equipment and the patient. Sudden and significant tcPO$_2$ decreases call for immediate resuscitation (unless the neonate is crying). Values below the expected range warrant an increase in oxygen therapy, an equipment check, or a call to the doctor.

cate hypoxemia and warrant intervention. According to hospital policy or doctor's orders, increase oxygen therapy. A sudden SaO$_2$ decrease calls for immediate resuscitation. Notify the doctor of any significant change in the patient's condition. Keep in mind that oximetry is an adjunct to arterial blood gas (ABG) measurements and doesn't replace them. For example, oximetry doesn't measure pH and PCO$_2$. When oximetry SaO$_2$ readings differ significantly from ABG measurements, notify the doctor—oximetry may be inaccurate in certain situations.

Interfering factors

• Falsely low ear SaO$_2$ readings may occur in jaundiced neonates with elevated bilirubin values.
• Falsely elevated ear SaO$_2$ readings may result when carboxyhemoglobin (COHb) values exceed 4%, such as in heavy smokers.
• Intralipids and certain intravascular dyes prevent accurate readings.
• Phototherapy, surgical lamps, direct sunlight, and excessive ambient lighting interfere with sensors and can cause inaccurate or erratic measurements. Cover sensors with foil or bed linens.
• Patient activity may interfere with readings. If necessary, move the sensor to a less active site. It also may be necessary to select a different sensor.
• With ear oximetry, large amounts of pigment on the ear may reduce the intensity of light reaching the photodetector and may signal the alarm. Reposition the probe to the pinna, revascularize the site, or move the probe to the finger.
• Mild hypothermia, hypotension, and vasoconstrictive drug infusion decrease finger pulsation with pulse oximetry, and thus reduce measurement accuracy.

Selected References

Bordow, R.A., et al. *Manual of Clinical Problems in Pulmonary Medicine,* 2nd ed. Boston: Little, Brown & Co., 1985.

Boutros, A., and Lee, C. "Value of Continuous Monitoring of Mixed Venous Blood Oxygen Saturation in the Management of Critically Ill Patients," *Critical Care Medicine* 14(2):132-34, February 1986.

Brunner, L.S., and Suddarth, D.S. *Textbook of Medical-Surgical Nursing,* 5th ed. Philadelphia: J.B. Lippincott Co., 1984.

Cecil, W.T., et al. "Clinical Evaluation of the Biox IIA Ear Oximeter in the Critical Care Environment," *Respiratory Care* 30(3):179-83, March 1985.

"Controlling External Optical Interference in Pulse Oximetry," *Pulse Oximetry Note Number 5.* Nellcor Incorporated, 25495 Whitesell St., Hayward, Calif., 94545.

Diagnostics, 2nd ed. Nurse's Reference Library. Springhouse, Pa.: Springhouse Corp., 1986.

Deckardt, R., and Steward, D.J. "Noninvasive Arterial Hemoglobin Oxygen Saturation Versus Transcutaneous Oxygen Tension Monitoring in the Preterm Infant," *Critical Care Medicine* 12(11):935-39, November 1984.

Durand, M., and Ramanathan, R. "Pulse Oximetry for Continuous Oxygen Monitoring in Sick Newborn Infants," *The Journal of Pediatrics* 109(6):1052-56, December 1986.

Fanconi, S., et al. "Pulse Oximetry in Pediatric Intensive Care: Comparison with Measured Saturations and Transcutaneous Oxygen Tension," *The Journal of Pediatrics* 107(3):362-66, September 1985.

Fletcher, B.J. *Quick Reference to Critical Care Nursing.* Philadelphia: J.B. Lippincott Co., 1982.

Grossman, Z.D., et al. *The Clinician's Guide to Diagnostic Imaging: Cost-Effective Pathways,* 2nd ed. New York: Raven Press Pubs., 1987.

Henry, J.B., ed. *Todd-Sanford-Davidsohn: Clinical Diagnosis and Management by Laboratory Methods,* 17th ed. Philadelphia: W.B. Saunders Co., 1984.

Hess, D., et al. "An Evaluation of the Nellcor N-10 Portable Pulse Oximeter," *Respiratory Care* 31(9):796-802, 1986.

Hudak, C.M., and Gallo, B.M. *Critical Care Nursing: A Holistic Approach,* 4th ed. Philadelphia: J.B. Lippincott Co., 1985.

Mok, J.Y., et al. "Transcutaneous Monitoring of Oxygenation: What is Normal?" *The Journal of Pediatrics* 108(3):365-71, March 1986.

Nursing87 Yearbook. Nurse's Reference Library. Springhouse, Pa.: Springhouse Corp., 1987.

Ohmeda Biox IV Pulse Oximeter Operating/Service Manual. Ohmeda, P.O. Box 914, Boulder, Colo., 80306-0914, 1983.

Petersdorf, R.G., and Adams, R.D., eds. *Harrison's Principles of Internal Medicine,* 10th ed. New York: McGraw-Hill Book Co., 1983.

Respiratory Disorders. Nurse's Clinical Library. Springhouse, Pa.: Springhouse Corp., 1984.

Ries, A.L., et al. "Accuracy of Two Ear Oximeters at Rest and During Exercise in Pulmonary Patients," *American Review of Respiratory Disease* 132(3):685-89, September 1985.

Shively, M., and Clark, A. "Continuous Monitoring of Mixed Venous Oxygen Saturation: An Instrument for Research," *Nursing Research* 35(1):56-58, January/February 1986.

Smoker, J.M., et al. "A Protocol to Assess and Administer Aerosol Bronchodilator Therapy," *Respiratory Care* 31(9):780-85, September 1986.

User's Manual for the Nellcor Pulse Oximeter Model N-100C. Nellcor Incorporated, 25495 Whitesell St., Hayward, Calif., 94545.

4 RESTRICTIVE DISORDERS

Introduction

Restrictive lung disease is rapidly gaining attention as a significant health problem. Although this chronic condition usually lends itself to home treatment, noncompliance may pose a major obstacle to maintaining optimal respiratory function. The patient may feel discouraged at the prospect of adhering to a lifelong treatment plan or making necessary life-style changes.

You can play a critical role in caring for these patients and promoting compliance by teaching them and their families about the disease, its potential complications, and the rationale for treatment. To provide such teaching, you'll need to understand the disease's pathophysiology, characteristic signs and symptoms, and current treatments.

Definition

Restrictive lung disease refers to a varied group of disorders that restrict lung expansion and sometimes prevent adequate pulmonary ventilation. Usually, it results from underlying interstitial or extrapulmonary disease. (See *Restrictive Lung Disease: Interstitial Causes;* and *Restrictive Lung Disease: Extrapulmonary Causes,* page 104.)

More than 100 interstitial lung diseases have been identified. These diseases gradually obliterate normal lung elasticity, causing the lung to become stiff and noncompliant. In about 70% of patients, the underlying cause of interstitial lung disease remains un-

known. Rarely, toxins may cause acute interstitial disease. For example, use of marijuana tainted with the herbicide paraquat can cause lung fibrosis within 2 weeks. Certain chemotherapeutic drugs, such as bleomycin, may also cause fibrosis.

In extrapulmonary restrictive lung disease, lung structures are normal but expansion is limited. For example, skeletal disorders can increase thoracic cage rigidity, impairing lung expansion.

Prognosis

Prognosis and mortality of patients with restrictive lung disease usually depend on the disease's underlying cause. Death may result from respiratory failure caused by infection or from the primary disease. Infection poses the greatest threat to respiratory function in these patients. Because of limited lung expansion, these patients can't cough productively. Secretions remain in the airways, causing obstruction, ventilation-perfusion mismatch, and sometimes respiratory failure.

Pathophysiology

The hallmarks of restrictive lung disease are reduced air volume and capacity (especially vital capacity and total lung capacity) and lung noncompliance.

Interstitial restrictive disease

All chronic interstitial lung diseases share certain pathologic features. The major feature is accumulation of fluid and various inflammatory and immune effector cells within extravascular lung tissues and spaces. During inflammation, interstitial collagen becomes abnormal, accumulates in interstitial spaces, and undergoes fibrosis. Stiff, fibrotic scar tissue then replaces normal elastic tissue, decreasing lung compliance. Fibrotic changes mainly affect the alveolar septa but may also affect the bronchioles—presumably because areas with uneven elasticity exert variable tension on them.

In advanced interstitial disease stages, fibrotic tissue constriction may cause alveolar dilation. Dilated areas alternate with constricted fibrotic areas, giving the lung a honeycomb appearance. In addition, fibrosis may narrow the pulmonary capillaries and impair blood flow to the affected areas. Infiltration of the interstitial spaces by cells, fluids, or fibrotic tissue alters the alveolar-capillary membrane by widening the space between the basement membranes. Normally, alveolar cells and pulmonary capillaries lie so close together that their basement membranes appear fused. Fibrous tissue may also thicken the interlobar septa and visceral pleurae.

Extrapulmonary restrictive disease
Lung dysfunction in extrapulmonary restrictive disease results from neurologic, neuromuscular, skeletal, or pleural disorders.

Neurologic and neuromuscular disorders cause loss of respiratory muscle tone or function, preventing muscles from contracting sufficiently to expand the lungs. Because they don't expand fully, the lungs can't maintain sufficient alveolar ventilation. As a result, atelectasis may occur in underventilated areas, stiffening the lungs. Although acute, such atelectasis can be reversed.

Skeletal disorders, such as kyphoscoliosis, may increase thoracic cage rigidity, which, in turn, reduces chest-wall compliance and restricts lung expansion.

Pleural disorders may also restrict lung expansion. In inflammatory pleural disorders, inspiration causes so

Restrictive Lung Disease: Interstitial Causes

Fibrotic disorders
- Idiopathic pulmonary fibrosis
- Bronchiolitis with interstitial pneumonitis
- Desquamative, giant cell, or lymphocytic interstitial pneumonitis

Granulomatous disorders
- Sarcoidosis
- Wegener's granulomatosis

Collagen-vascular disorders
- Progressive systemic sclerosis
- Rheumatoid arthritis
- Sjögren's syndrome
- Systemic lupus erythematosus

Lymphocytic infiltration disorders
- Immunoblastic lymphadenopathy
- Lymphangitic metastatic cancer
- Lymphomatoid granulomatosis

Vascular disorders
- Hypersensitivity angiitis
- Idiopathic pulmonary hemosiderosis
- Pulmonary veno-occlusive disease

Renal disorders
- Goodpasture's syndrome

Inherited disorders
- Familial pulmonary fibrosis
- Neurofibromatosis
- Tuberous sclerosis

Occupational disorders
- Hypersensitivity pneumonitis (extrinsic allergic alveolitis)
- Pneumoconiosis such as silicosis and asbestosis

Drugs and toxins
- Paraquat
- Bleomycin

Restrictive Lung Disease: Extrapulmonary Causes

Neuromuscular and neurologic disorders
- Amyotrophic lateral sclerosis
- Guillain-Barré syndrome
- Multiple sclerosis
- Muscular dystrophy
- Myasthenia gravis
- Poliomyelitis

Thoracic cage disorders
- Ankylosing spondylitis
- Chest-wall deformity
- Kyphosis
- Pickwickian syndrome
- Scoliosis

Pleural disorders
- Hemothorax
- Pleural effusion
- Pleurisy
- Pleuritis

much pain that the patient takes shallow breaths to avoid discomfort. This may lead to alveolar underventilation. In pneumothorax, hemothorax, and pleural effusion, the pleural space fills with air or fluid, preventing lung expansion and decreasing the surface area available for gas exchange.

Altered breathing patterns
Reduced lung compliance changes normal breathing patterns. First, respiratory muscles contract more forcefully to maintain tidal volume, thereby increasing the work of breathing. Then the respiratory system tries to compensate through shallow, rapid breathing, which reduces tidal volume and eases breathing labor. Minute volume and alveolar ventilation increase sharply, however, resulting in greater carbon dioxide exhalation. Supposedly, alveolar hyperventilation results from increased transmission of afferent nerve impulses in the diseased lung—not from hypoxemia. As a result, oxygen therapy doesn't completely reverse hyperventilation.

As restrictive lung disease progresses, compensatory mechanisms fail, lung compliance decreases, and respiratory muscle fatigue occurs. All these factors may lead to inadequate alveolar ventilation and carbon dioxide retention.

Ventilation-perfusion mismatch
In most restrictive lung diseases, ventilation-perfusion mismatch is apparently the primary cause of hypoxemia. It results from variable lung compliance caused by fibrosis, atelectasis, chest-wall deformity, or neuromuscular dysfunction, and leads to altered gas movement into the affected areas. Mismatch also results from impaired blood flow to ventilated alveoli caused by fibrotic narrowing of pulmonary capillaries or lung tissue compression by a chest-wall deformity.

Ventilation-perfusion mismatch causes shunting of blood from underventilated to ventilated alveoli; this, in turn, increases pulmonary vascular pressure. Resulting chronic pulmonary hypertension may eventually lead to right ventricular failure and cor pulmonale.

Hypoxemia mechanisms
Many patients with restrictive lung disease don't experience hypoxemia at rest until a late disease stage. However, they may experience hypoxemia during exercise, when ventilation exceeds cardiac output.

Also, pulmonary vascular resistance increases from fibrotic narrowing of pulmonary capillaries. Thus, with increased cardiac output, red blood cells flow too rapidly through narrowed capillaries, allowing insufficient oxygenation time.

Hypoxemia may also result from fibrosis and interstitial collagen accumulation, which widens the interstitial spaces, thereby increasing the distance that oxygen must diffuse from the alveolus to the capillary bed; this leads to poor diffusion or impaired gas exchange.

Treatment

Detecting the underlying cause of restrictive lung disease is essential to setting treatment goals. The patient's history, physical examination, and diagnostic test results can provide crucial information about the cause and extent of restrictive lung disease. Treatment's directed at the underlying cause. Depending on the patient's condition, treatment measures may also include oxygen administration, mechanical ventilation, and drugs. For patients with severe restrictive disease limited to the lungs, a lung transplant may be the only option (even though this procedure hasn't been refined to the extent of other organ transplants).

Pneumonia

Description

An acute infection of the lung parenchyma, pneumonia commonly impairs gas exchange. Patients with normal lungs and an adequate immune system before disease onset have a good prognosis. In debilitated patients, however, bacterial pneumonia ranks as the fifth leading cause of death. (See *Risk Factors for Pneumonia;* and *Common Respiratory Syndromes in AIDS,* pages 106 and 107.)

Pneumonia can be classified in several ways. Based on microbiologic etiology, it may be viral, bacterial, fungal, protozoal, mycobacterial, mycoplasmal, or rickettsial in origin. Based on location, it may be classified as bronchopneumonia, lobular pneumonia, or lobar pneumonia. By type, it can be classified as primary, secondary, or aspiration pneumonia. (See Chapter 7 for more details on aspiration pneumonia.)

Risk Factors for Pneumonia

Predisposing factors for pneumonia include:
- chronic illness and debilitation
- cancer (particularly lung cancer)
- abdominal or thoracic surgery
- atelectasis
- common colds or other viral respiratory infections
- chronic respiratory disease (chronic obstructive pulmonary disease, asthma, bronchiectasis, cystic fibrosis)
- influenza
- smoking
- malnutrition
- alcoholism
- rib fractures
- sickle cell disease
- pleural diseases that limit chest excursion
- tracheostomy
- prolonged bed rest
- exposure to noxious gases
- aspiration
- immunosuppressive therapy

For more information on pneumonia types, see *Classifying Pneumonia,* pages 108 to 111.

Causes

- Inhalation of a pathogen
- Lung damage from noxious chemical exposure or other insult (superinfection)
- Hematogenous spread of bacteria from a distant focus

Pathophysiology

When caused by bacterial infection, pneumonia may involve the distal airways and alveoli (*bronchopneumonia*), part of a lobe (*lobular pneumonia*), or an entire lobe (*lobar pneumonia*). Bacterial infection initially triggers alveolar inflammation and edema. Capillaries become engorged with blood, causing stasis. As the alveolar-capil-

Common Respiratory Syndromes in AIDS

Infection	Signs and symptoms
Cytomegalovirus (CMV) infection CMV, a herpesvirus, may result in serious, widespread infection in AIDS patients. The most common sites for CMV infection include the lungs, adrenal glands, eyes, central nervous system, GI tract, male genitourinary tract, and blood.	Unexplained fever, malaise, GI ulcers, swollen lymph nodes, enlarged liver and spleen, and blurred vision are common signs and symptoms associated with CMV infection. Vision changes leading to blindness may also occur.
***Pneumocystis carinii* pneumonia (PCP)** A protozoan infection found in the lung's air sacs, PCP is the most common lung infection in AIDS patients.	The three most common signs and symptoms of PCP are fever, shortness of breath, and a dry, nonproductive cough.
***Mycobacterium avium-intracellulare* (MAI) infection** MAI infection is caused by bacteria commonly found in the environment. The bacteria rarely cause infection in the healthy individual. However, in AIDS, bacteria spread throughout the patient's lungs, blood, lymph nodes, bone marrow, liver, and GI tract.	The four most common signs and symptoms of MAI infection are fever, diarrhea, weight loss, and debilitation. These are typically masked by or confused with those of other opportunistic infections.

lary membrane breaks down, alveoli fill with blood and exudate, resulting in atelectasis. In several bacterial infections, the lungs assume a heavy, liverlike appearance, as in adult respiratory distress syndrome (ARDS).

Viral infection, which typically causes diffuse pneumonia, first attacks bronchiolar epithelial cells, causing interstitial inflammation and desquamation. It then spreads to the alveoli, which fill with blood and fluid. In advanced infection, a hyaline membrane may form. As with bacterial infection, severe viral infection may clinically resemble ARDS.

Aspirated hydrocarbons trigger similar inflammatory changes and also in-activate surfactant over a large alveolar area; decreased surfactant leads to alveolar collapse.

Signs and symptoms

The five cardinal signs and symptoms of early bacterial pneumonia are coughing; production of thick yellow, green, or bloody sputum; pleuritic chest pain; shaking chills; and fever. Physical findings vary widely, ranging from diffuse, fine crackles to signs of localized or extensive consolidation and pleural effusion.

Complications include hypoxemia, respiratory failure, pleural effusion, empyema, lung abscess, and bacter-

Treatment and related care

Currently, no effective therapy for CMV infection exists. Ganciclovir, also known as DHPG, an experimental drug, may help slow the virus, particularly with eye involvement.

Treatment for PCP includes co-trimoxazole (sulfamethoxazole-trimethoprim) or pentamidine isethionate; antileprosy drugs, such as dapsone; and trimetrexate gluconate.

Oxygen therapy may be used continuously or as needed. An oxygen concentrator may be more cost-effective for long-term home intervention. Oral morphine solution may be ordered to reduce respiratory rate and anxiety.

Treatment involves a multidrug regimen, including isoniazid, ethambutol, and rifampin. The experimental drugs ansamycin and clofazimine may be added to this regimen. (This regimen has shown poor results, however.) Other experimental protocols to treat MAI infection may be available.

emia; infection spread to other body regions may result in meningitis, endocarditis, and pericarditis.

Diagnosis
• Clinical features, chest X-ray showing infiltrates, and a sputum smear showing acute inflammatory cells support the diagnosis.
• Positive blood cultures in a patient with pulmonary infiltrates strongly suggest pneumonia produced by organisms isolated from blood cultures.
• Pleural effusions, if present, should be tapped and the fluid analyzed for evidence of pleural space infection (empyema).

• Occasionally, transtracheal aspirate of tracheobronchial secretions or bronchoscopy with brushings may be done to obtain material for smear and culture.
• The patient's response to antimicrobial therapy also provides important evidence of pneumonia.

Treatment
Antimicrobial therapy varies with the causative agent. Therapy should be re-evaluated early in the course of treatment. Supportive measures include humidified oxygen therapy for hypoxia, mechanical ventilation for respiratory failure, a high-calorie diet, adequate fluid intake, bed rest, and an analgesic to relieve pleuritic chest pain. Patients with severe pneumonia who are receiving mechanical ventilation may require positive end-expiratory pressure to facilitate adequate oxygenation.

Clinical considerations
Proper supportive care can increase patient comfort, avoid complications, and speed recovery.

Throughout the illness
• Maintain a patent airway and adequate oxygenation. Take arterial blood gas measurements, especially in hypoxic patients. Administer supplemental oxygen if PO_2 is less than 55 mm Hg. Give oxygen cautiously if the patient has underlying chronic lung disease.
• Teach the patient how to cough and perform deep-breathing exercises to clear secretions; encourage him to do this often. In severe pneumonia that requires endotracheal intubation or tracheostomy with or without mechanical ventilation, provide thorough respiratory care and suction often (as indicated by breath sounds) to remove secretions.
• Obtain sputum specimens, as needed, by suctioning if the patient can't produce specimens himself.
• Administer antibiotics and pain medication, as ordered and needed; record the patient's response.

Classifying Pneumonia

Type	Signs and symptoms
Viral	
Influenza Prognosis poor even with treatment; 50% mortality	• Cough (initially nonproductive; later, purulent sputum), marked cyanosis, dyspnea, high fever, chills, substernal pain and discomfort, moist crackles, frontal headache, myalgia • Death results from cardiopulmonary collapse
Adenovirus Insidious onset; generally affects young adults	• Sore throat, fever, cough, chills, malaise, small amounts of mucoid sputum, retrosternal chest pain, anorexia, rhinitis, adenopathy, scattered crackles, and rhonchi
Respiratory syncytial virus (RSV) Most prevalent in infants and children	• Listlessness; irritability; tachypnea with retraction of intercostal muscles; slight sputum production; fine, moist crackles; fever; severe malaise; and possibly cough or croup
Measles (rubeola)	• Fever, dyspnea, cough, small amounts of sputum, coryza, skin rash, and cervical adenopathy
Chicken pox (varicella) Uncommon in children, but present in 30% of adults with varicella	• Cough, dyspnea, cyanosis, tachypnea, pleuritic chest pain, hemoptysis and rhonchi 1 to 6 days after onset of rash • May lead to adult respiratory distress syndrome
Cytomegalovirus (CMV)	• Difficult to distinguish from other nonbacterial pneumonias • Fever, cough, shaking chills, dyspnea, cyanosis, weakness, and diffuse crackles • Occurs in neonates as devastating multisystemic infection; in normal adults resembles mononucleosis; in immunocompromised hosts, varies from clinically inapparent to devastating infection
Bacterial	
Streptococcus (Diplococcus pneumoniae)	• Sudden onset of a single, shaking chill, and sustained temperature of 102° to 104° F. (38.9° to 40° C.); commonly preceded by upper respiratory tract infection • Production of thick green or yellow sputum

strep gram +

Diagnosis	Intervention
• *Chest X-ray:* diffuse bilateral broncho-pneumonia radiating from hilus • *White blood cell (WBC) count:* normal to slightly elevated • *Sputum smears:* no specific organisms	• *Supportive:* for respiratory failure, endotracheal intubation and ventilator assistance; for fever, hypothermia blanket or antipyretics; for influenza A, amantadine
• *Chest X-ray:* patchy distribution of pneumonia; more severe than indicated by physical examination • *WBC count:* normal to slightly elevated	• Intervene for symptoms only • Mortality low; usually clears with no residual effects
• *Chest X-ray:* patchy bilateral consolidation • *WBC count:* normal to slightly elevated	• *Supportive:* humidified air, oxygen, antimicrobials typically given until viral etiology confirmed • Complete recovery in 1 to 3 weeks
• *Chest X-ray:* reticular infiltrates, sometimes with hilar lymph node enlargement • *Lung tissue specimen:* characteristic giant cells	• *Supportive:* bed rest, adequate hydration, antimicrobials; assisted ventilation, if necessary
• *Chest X-ray:* shows more extensive pneumonia than indicated by physical examination, and bilateral, patchy, diffuse, nodular infiltrates • *Sputum analysis:* predominant mononuclear cells and characteristic intranuclear inclusion bodies with characteristic skin rash confirm diagnosis	• *Supportive:* adequate hydration, oxygen therapy in critically ill patients • May warrant mechanical ventilation
• *Chest X-ray:* in early stages, variable patchy infiltrates; later, bilateral, nodular, and more predominant in lower lobes • *Percutaneous aspiration of lung tissue, transbronchial biopsy or open lung biopsy:* microscopic examination shows typical intranuclear and cytoplasmic inclusions; virus can be cultured from lung tissue	• Usually, benign and self-limiting in mononucleosis-like form • *Supportive:* adequate hydration and nutrition, oxygen therapy, bed rest • In immunosuppressed patients, disease is more severe and may be fatal.
• *Chest X-ray:* areas of consolidation, commonly lobar • *WBC count:* elevated • *Sputum culture:* may show gram-positive *S. pneumoniae;* this organism not always recovered	• *Antimicrobial therapy:* penicillin G (or erythromycin, if patient's allergic to penicillin) for 7 to 10 days. Such therapy begins after obtaining culture specimen but without waiting for results.

(continued)

Classifying Pneumonia *(continued)*

Type	Signs and symptoms
Bacterial *(continued)*	
Klebsiella *gram +* *aminoglycoside cephalosporin*	• Fever and recurrent chills; cough producing rusty, bloody, viscous sputum (currant jelly); cyanosis of lips and nail beds from hypoxemia; shallow, grunting respirations • Likely in patients with chronic alcoholism, pulmonary disease, and diabetes
Staphylococcus *gram + r*	• Temperature of 102° to 104° F. (38.9° to 40° C.), recurrent shaking chills, bloody sputum, dyspnea, tachypnea, and hypoxemia • Should be suspected with viral illness, such as influenza or measles, and in patients with cystic fibrosis
Legionnaires' disease *(Legionella pneumophila)* *gram –*	• Prodromal signs and symptoms: diarrhea, anorexia, malaise, diffuse myalgias, generalized weakness, headache, recurrent chills, and fever that develops within 12 to 48 hours and may reach 105° F. (40.5° C.) • Cough initially nonproductive but eventually may produce grayish, mucopurulent, blood-streaked sputum • Nausea, vomiting, disorientation, mental sluggishness, confusion, temporary amnesia, pleuritic chest pain, dyspnea, tachypnea, crackles, and bradycardia

• Administer parenteral fluids, as ordered, to loosen secretions so that the patient can expectorate them.
• Administer additional I.V. fluids and electrolyte replacement if fever and dehydration warrant.
• Maintain adequate nutrition to offset high calorie expenditure secondary to infection. Arrange for a high-calorie, high-protein diet consisting of soft, easy-to-eat foods. Encourage the patient to eat. As necessary and ordered, provide nasogastric (NG) tube feedings or parenteral nutrition. Monitor fluid intake and output.
• Provide a quiet, calm environment and frequent rest periods.

• Provide emotional support and be sure to explain all procedures (especially intubation and suctioning) to the patient and his family. Encourage family visits. Provide diversionary activities appropriate to the patient's age.
• To control infection spread, dispose of secretions properly.

To prevent pneumonia
• Advise patients to avoid using antibiotics indiscriminately for minor viral infections, because this may result in upper airway colonization with antibiotic-resistant bacteria. If the patient then develops pneumonia, the causative organisms may require treatment with more toxic antibiotics.

Diagnosis	Intervention
• *Chest X-ray:* typically, but not always, consolidation in the upper lobe that causes bulging of fissures • *WBC count:* elevated • *Sputum culture and Gram stain:* may show gram-positive cocci *Klebsiella*	• *Antimicrobial therapy:* aminoglycoside and, in serious infections, a cephalosporin
• *Chest X-ray:* multiple abscesses and infiltrates; high incidence of empyema • *WBC count:* elevated • *Sputum culture and Gram stain:* may show gram-positive staphylococci	• *Antimicrobial therapy:* nafcillin or oxacillin for 14 days if staphylococci are penicillinase-producing • Chest tube drainage of empyema
• *Chest X-ray:* patchy, localized infiltration, which progresses to multilobar consolidation, pleural effusion, and in fulminant disease, opacification of entire lung • *WBC count:* elevated • *Culture of respiratory tract secretions:* gram-negative bacilli *L. pneumophila* • *Serum antibody test:* convalescent serum sample confirms diagnosis, showing fourfold or greater rise in antibody titer for legionnaires' disease bacterium	• *Antimicrobial therapy:* erythromycin is the drug of choice; if it's ineffective, rifampin may be added. If erythromycin is contraindicated, rifampin or rifampin with tetracycline may be used. Such therapy begins after obtaining test specimens but without waiting for results. • *Supportive:* antipyretics; adequate hydration; circulatory support with pressor drugs; oxygen therapy, assisted ventilation, if necessary

• Encourage annual influenza vaccinations and Pneumovax for high-risk patients, such as those with chronic obstructive pulmonary disease, chronic heart disease, and sickle cell disease.

• Urge all bedridden and postoperative patients to perform deep-breathing and coughing exercises frequently. Properly position such patients to promote full aeration and drainage of secretions.

• To prevent aspiration during NG tube feedings, elevate the patient's head, check tube position, and administer the feeding slowly. Don't give large volumes at one time because this could cause vomiting. If the patient has an artificial airway, inflate the tube cuff. Keep his head elevated for at least 30 minutes after the feeding.

Tuberculosis

Description

An acute or chronic infection caused by *Mycobacterium tuberculosis* (and, in some cases, other mycobacteria strains), tuberculosis (TB) is characterized by pulmonary infiltrates, formation of granulomas with caseation, fibrosis, and cavitation. Active TB reportedly occurs in nearly 14 out of every 100,000 people. Those living in crowded, poorly ventilated conditions have the highest risk. With correct treatment, prognosis is excellent.

Cause
Exposure to *M. tuberculosis*

Pathophysiology
After exposure to *M. tuberculosis*, roughly 5% of infected persons develop active TB within 1 year; in the remainder, microorganisms cause a latent infection. The infected person's immune system usually controls the tubercle bacillus by killing or restricting it to a tiny nodule (tubercle). However, the bacillus may lie dormant within the tubercle for years, then become reactivated, spread, and cause active infection.

Although the primary infection focus is the lungs, mycobacteria commonly exist in other body parts, such as the kidneys and lymph nodes. Various factors increase the risk of reactivation: gastrectomy, serious illness that compromises immune mechanisms, treatment with corticosteroids and immunosuppressants, and silicosis.

Transmission occurs by droplet nuclei produced when an infected person coughs or sneezes. If a tubercle bacillus settles in the alveolus of a person who inhales the droplet, infection occurs, with alveolar capillary dilation and endothelial cell swelling. Alveolitis results, with tubercle bacilli replication and influx of polymorphonuclear leukocytes. These bacilli disseminate through the lymphatic system to the circulatory system, then throughout the body. Cell-mediated immunity to the mycobacteria, which develops about 3 to 6 weeks later, usually contains the infection and arrests the disease. If the infection later becomes reactivated, the body's response characteristically leads to caseation—conversion of necrotic tissue to a cheese-like material. The caseum may localize, undergo fibrosis, or form cavities; multiplying tubercle bacilli stud cavity walls. If this happens, infected caseous debris may spread throughout the lungs via the tracheobronchial tree. Extrapulmonary TB sites include the pleura, meninges, joints, lymph nodes, peritoneum, genitourinary tract, and intestines.

Signs and symptoms
In primary TB infection, after an incubation period from 4 to 8 weeks, most patients are asymptomatic. Some, however, may have nonspecific symptoms, such as fatigue, weakness, anorexia, weight loss, night sweats, and low-grade fever.

In patients with TB reactivation, symptoms may include cough that produces mucopurulent sputum, occasional hemoptysis, and chest pains.

Diagnosis
Diagnostic tests include physical examination, chest X-ray, tuberculin skin test, and sputum smears and cultures to identify tubercle bacilli. Because such diseases as lung cancer, lung abscess, pneumoconiosis, and bronchiectasis may mimic TB, diagnosis must be definitive. Diagnostic techniques include the following:

• *Auscultation:* detects crepitant crackles, bronchial breath sounds, wheezes, and whispered pectoriloquy.

• *Chest percussion:* detects dullness over the affected area, indicating consolidation or pleural fluid.

• *Chest X-ray:* shows nodular lesions, patchy infiltrates (mainly in upper lobes), cavity formation, scar tissue, and calcium deposits. However, an X-ray may not distinguish active from inactive TB.

• *Tuberculin skin test:* detects previous exposure to TB but doesn't distinguish between an active and a dormant infection and doesn't provide a definitive diagnosis. In this test, intermediate-strength purified protein derivative of 5 tuberculin units (0.1 ml) is injected intradermally into the forearm and read 48 to 72 hours later. If a positive reaction (equal to or exceeding a 10-mm induration) occurs, a sputum smear and culture and a chest X-ray must be done for further information.

• *Stains and cultures (of sputum, cerebrospinal fluid, urine, abscess drainage, or pleural fluid):* show heat-sensitive, nonmotile, aerobic, acid-fast bacilli; these confirm the diagnosis.

Treatment

Antitubercular therapy with daily oral doses of isoniazid or rifampin (with ethambutol added in some cases) for at least 9 months usually cures TB. After 2 to 4 weeks, the disease usually is no longer infectious and the patient can resume his normal life-style while continuing to take medication. The patient with atypical mycobacterial disease or drug-resistant TB may require second-line drugs, such as capreomycin, streptomycin, para-aminosalicylic acid, pyrazinamide, and cycloserine.

Clinical considerations

• Isolate the infectious patient in a quiet, well-ventilated room until he's no longer contagious. Teach him to cough and sneeze into tissues and to dispose of all secretions properly. Instruct him to wear a mask when leaving his room. Make sure that visitors and hospital personnel wear masks in the patient's room.

• Remind the patient to get plenty of rest. Stress the importance of eating balanced meals to promote recovery. If the patient's anorexic, urge him to eat frequent small meals. Record weight weekly.

• Stay alert for adverse medication effects. Because isoniazid sometimes leads to hepatitis or peripheral neuritis, monitor serum glutamic-oxaloacetic transaminase (SGOT) and serum glutamic-pyruvic transaminase (SGPT) levels. To prevent or treat peripheral neuritis, give pyridoxine (vitamin B_6), as ordered. If the patient's receiving ethambutol, watch for optic neuritis; discontinue the drug if this problem develops. If he's receiving rifampin, watch for purpura and signs of hepatitis. Observe him for other complications, such as hemoptysis.

• Before discharge, instruct the patient to watch for adverse medication effects and to report these immediately. Emphasize the importance of regular follow-up examinations, and teach the patient and family to watch for signs and symptoms of recurring TB. Stress the need for compliance with long-term treatment.

• Advise persons who've been exposed to infected patients to receive tuberculin tests and, if ordered, to take prophylactic isoniazid and have a chest X-ray done.

• Because health care professionals may care for a patient with TB even if the disease isn't suspected, they have an increased exposure risk. In many institutions, all employees have tine tests every 6 to 12 months. A staff member who responds positively after a previous negative response may receive therapy regardless of documented exposure to an infected patient.

Lung abscess

Description

A lung infection accompanied by pus accumulation and tissue destruction, lung abscess may be putrid (caused by anaerobic bacteria) or nonputrid (caused by anaerobic or aerobic bacteria). It often has a well-defined border. The availability of effective antibiotics has made lung abscess much less common than before.

Causes

• Necrotizing pneumonia (commonly the result of aspiration of oropharyngeal contents)
• Poor oral hygiene, with dental or gingival (gum) disease
• Septic pulmonary emboli

Pathophysiology

When bacteria localize in the lungs, usually from obstruction, lung destruction can result from liquefaction necrosis. The abscess may initially appear as a solid mass on X-ray until the liquefied material drains into a bronchus; then an air-fluid level may be identified. Hematogenous bacterial spread may result in multiple abscesses throughout the lungs.

Signs and symptoms

Clinical effects of lung abscess include a cough that may produce bloody, purulent, or foul-smelling sputum; pleuritic chest pain; dyspnea; excessive sweating; chills; fever; headache; malaise; diaphoresis; and weight loss. Complications include abscess rupture into the pleural space, resulting in empyema and, rarely, massive hemorrhage. Chronic lung abscess may cause localized bronchiectasis. An abscess that doesn't respond to antibiotic treatment suggests a possible underlying neoplasm or other cause of obstruction.

Diagnosis

• Chest auscultation may reveal crackles and decreased breath sounds.
• Chest X-ray shows a localized infiltrate with one or more clear spaces, usually containing air-fluid levels.
• Percutaneous aspiration of an abscess may be attempted or bronchoscopy used to obtain cultures to identify the causative organism. Bronchoscopy is used only if abscess resolution is eventful and the patient's condition permits it.
• Blood and sputum cultures and Gram stain help detect the causative organism; leukocytosis (white blood cell count above 10,000/mm^3) is common.

Treatment

Treatment consists of prolonged antibiotic therapy, commonly lasting for months, until radiographic resolution or definite stability occurs. Symptoms usually disappear in a few weeks. Postural drainage may facilitate discharge of necrotic material into upper airways where expectoration's possible; however, care must be taken not to spread infection. Oxygen therapy may relieve hypoxemia. Poor response to therapy warrants lesion resection or removal of the diseased lung portion. All patients need rigorous follow-up and serial chest X-rays.

Clinical considerations

Help the patient perform chest physiotherapy (including coughing and deep breathing). Encourage him to increase fluid intake to loosen secretions. Provide a quiet, restful atmosphere.

To prevent lung abscess in the unconscious patient and in the patient with seizures, first prevent aspiration of secretions. Do this by suctioning the patient and positioning him to promote secretion drainage. Give good mouth care and encourage the patient to practice good oral hygiene.

Sarcoidosis

Description

This multisystemic granulomatous disorder characteristically produces lymphadenopathy, pulmonary infiltration, and skeletal, liver, eye, or skin lesions. It's most common in young adults (aged 20 to 40). In the United States, sarcoidosis occurs predominantly among blacks and affects twice as many women as men. Acute sarcoidosis usually resolves within 2 years. Chronic, progressive sarcoidosis, an uncommon disorder, is associated with pulmonary fibrosis and progressive pulmonary disability.

Causes

The cause of sarcoidosis remains unknown. The following possible causes have been considered:
• hypersensitivity response to such agents as atypical mycobacteria, fungi, and pine pollen, possibly from T cell

imbalance. (For information on other hypersensitivity diseases, see *Pneumoconiosis Diseases*, pages 118 and 119, and *Hypersensitivity Diseases*, pages 120 and 121.)

- genetic predisposition (suggested by a slightly higher-than-normal incidence of sarcoidosis within the same family)
- immune system abnormalities, such as lymphopenia with decreased T cells, impaired lymphocyte function, anergy, and panhypergammaglobulinemia
- exposure to such chemicals as zirconium or beryllium; this can lead to illnesses resembling sarcoidosis, suggesting an extrinsic cause for this disease.

Pathophysiology

Although the exact mechanism of sarcoidosis is unknown, research suggests a T cell problem and perhaps, more specifically, a lymphokine production problem. In other granulomatous diseases, such as tuberculosis, granuloma formation occurs from inadequate pathogen clearance by macrophages. These macrophages require the help of T cells that secrete lymphokines, which, in turn, activate less effective macrophages to become aggressive phagocytes. Lack of lymphokine secretion by T cells may help explain granuloma formation in sarcoidosis.

Signs and symptoms

Initial signs and symptoms of sarcoidosis include arthralgia (in wrists, ankles, and elbows), fatigue, malaise, and weight loss. Other clinical features vary according to fibrosis extent and location:

- *Respiratory:* breathlessness, cough (usually nonproductive), substernal pain; in advanced pulmonary disease, complications may include pulmonary hypertension and cor pulmonale
- *Cutaneous:* erythema nodosum, subcutaneous skin nodules with maculopapular eruptions, extensive nasal mucosal lesions
- *Ophthalmic:* anterior uveitis (common); glaucoma, blindness (rare)

- *Lymphatic:* bilateral hilar and right paratracheal lymphadenopathy, splenomegaly
- *Musculoskeletal:* muscle weakness, polyarthralgia, pain, punched-out lesions on phalanges
- *Hepatic:* granulomatous hepatitis (usually asymptomatic)
- *Genitourinary:* hypercalciuria
- *Cardiovascular:* dysrhythmias (premature beats, bundle branch block, or complete heart block), cardiomyopathy (rare)
- *CNS:* cranial or peripheral nerve palsies, basilar meningitis, seizures, pituitary and hypothalamic lesions causing diabetes insipidus.

Diagnosis

Typical clinical features and laboratory and X-ray findings help diagnose sarcoidosis. A positive Kveim-Siltzbach skin test supports the diagnosis. In this test, the patient receives an intradermal injection of an antigen prepared from human sarcoidal spleen or lymph nodes from patients with sarcoidosis. If the patient has active sarcoidosis, granuloma develops at the injection site in 2 to 6 weeks. The reaction's considered positive when a biopsy of skin at the injection site shows discrete epithelioid cell granuloma. Other relevant findings include:

- *Chest X-ray:* bilateral hilar and right paratracheal adenopathy with or without diffuse interstitial infiltrates; occasionally, large nodular lesions in lung parenchyma
- *Lymph node, skin, or lung biopsy:* noncaseating granulomas with negative cultures for mycobacteria and fungi
- *Other laboratory data:* rarely, increased serum calcium level, mild anemia, leukocytosis, hyperglobulinemia
- *Pulmonary function tests:* decreased total lung capacity and compliance, decreased diffusing capacity
- *Arterial blood gas measurements:* decreased arterial oxygen tension.

Treatment

Asymptomatic sarcoidosis requires no treatment. Sarcoidosis that causes hypercalcemia or destructive skin lesions or that leads to ocular, respiratory, central nervous system, cardiac, or systemic symptoms (such as fever and weight loss) requires treatment with systemic or topical steroids. Such therapy usually continues for 1 to 2 years, although some patients may need lifelong therapy. Patients with hypercalcemia may need to maintain a low-calcium diet and avoid direct exposure to sunlight.

Clinical considerations

• Watch for and report any complications. Monitor laboratory results for findings that could necessitate changes in patient care (for example, anemia).
• If the patient has arthralgia, administer analgesics, as ordered. Record signs of progressive muscle weakness.
• Provide a nutritious high-calorie diet and plenty of fluids. If the patient has hypercalcemia, suggest a low-calcium diet. Weigh the patient regularly to detect any weight loss.
• Monitor respiratory function. Check chest X-rays for extent of lung involvement; note and record any bloody sputum or sputum increase. If the patient has pulmonary hypertension or end-stage cor pulmonale, check arterial blood gas measurements. Watch for dysrhythmias, and administer oxygen, as needed.
• Because steroids may cause or worsen diabetes mellitus, test urine for glucose and acetone at least every 12 hours at the beginning of steroid therapy. Also, watch for other adverse steroid effects, such as fluid retention, electrolyte imbalance (especially hypokalemia), moon face, hypertension, and personality change. During or after steroid withdrawal (particularly if the patient has an infection or is experiencing any other stress-producing condition or situation), watch for and report any vomiting, orthostatic hy-

potension, hypoglycemia, restlessness, anorexia, malaise, and fatigue. Keep in mind that the patient receiving long-term or high-dose steroid therapy is vulnerable to infection.
• When preparing the patient for discharge, stress the need for compliance with prescribed steroid therapy, regular follow-up examinations, and other treatment. Refer the patient with failing vision to community support and resource groups, including the American Foundation for the Blind, if necessary.

Silicosis

Description

In this progressive disease—the most common pneumoconiosis form—nodular lesions develop and commonly progress to fibrosis. (For more information on this and other pneumoconiosis forms, see *Pneumoconiosis Diseases,* pages 118 and 119, and *Hypersensitivity Diseases,* pages 120 and 121.) Silicosis can be classified according to pulmonary disease severity and rapidity of onset and progression; it usually occurs as a simple asymptomatic illness. Acute silicosis develops after 1 to 3 years in such persons as sand blasters and in tunnel workers who are exposed to high concentrations of respirable silica. Accelerated silicosis appears after 10 years' exposure (on average) to lower concentrations of free silica. Chronic silicosis develops after 20 or more years' exposure to lower free silica concentrations. Prognosis is good, unless the disease progresses into the complicated fibrotic form, which causes respiratory insufficiency and cor pulmonale, and is associated with pulmonary tuberculosis.

Cause

Inhalation of crystalline silica dust, mostly from quartz.

Pathophysiology

Nodules result when alveolar macrophages ingest silica particles, which they can't process. As a result, the macrophages die and release proteolytic enzymes into surrounding tissue. Subsequent inflammation attracts other macrophages and fibroblasts into the affected region to produce fibrous tissue and wall off the reaction. The resulting nodule has an onionskin appearance when viewed under a microscope.

Nodules develop adjacent to terminal and respiratory bronchioles. Although frequently accompanied by bullous changes in both lobes, nodules concentrate in upper lung lobes. If the disease doesn't progress, only minimal physiologic disturbances occur and no disability results. Occasionally, however, the fibrotic response accelerates, engulfing and destroying a large lung area (progressive massive fibrosis or conglomerate lesions). Fibrosis may continue despite termination of dust exposure.

Signs and symptoms

Silicosis initially may be asymptomatic or it may produce dyspnea on exertion, typically attributed to poor physical conditioning or aging. If the disease progresses to the chronic, complicated stage, dyspnea on exertion worsens and other symptoms appear—usually tachypnea and an insidious dry cough (most pronounced in the morning) appear. Progression to the advanced stage causes dyspnea on minimal exertion, worsening cough, and pulmonary hypertension, which in turn leads to right ventricular failure and cor pulmonale. Patients with silicosis have a high incidence of active tuberculosis, which should be considered when evaluating a patient with this disease. CNS changes—confusion, lethargy, decreased respiratory rate and depth as PCO_2 increases—also occur in advanced silicosis. Other clinical features include malaise, disturbed sleep, and hoarseness. (*Note:*

Symptom severity may not correlate with chest X-ray findings or pulmonary function test results.)

Diagnosis

Patient history reveals occupational exposure to silica dust. With simple silicosis, findings are normal; with chronic silicosis with conglomerate lesions, findings may include decreased chest expansion, diminished intensity of breath sounds, areas of hyporesonance and hyperresonance, faint to medium crackles, and tachypnea. With simple silicosis, chest X-rays show small, discrete, nodular lesions distributed throughout both lung fields but typically concentrated in the upper lung zones: hilar lung nodes may be enlarged and exhibit "eggshell" calcification. In complicated silicosis, X-rays show one or more conglomerate masses of dense tissue.

Pulmonary function tests typically yield the following results:
- *Forced vital capacity (FVC):* reduced in complicated silicosis
- *Forced expiratory volume in the 1st second (FEV_1):* reduced in obstructive disease (emphysematous silicosis areas); reduced in complicated silicosis, but FEV_1 to FVC ratio is normal or high
- *Maximal voluntary ventilation:* reduced in both restrictive and obstructive diseases
- *Diffusing capacity for carbon monoxide:* reduced when fibrosis destroys alveolar walls and obliterates pulmonary capillaries or when it thickens the alveolar-capillary membrane.

In addition, arterial blood gas measurements show:
- PaO_2: normal in simple silicosis: may be significantly below normal in late stages of chronic or complicated disease, when the patient breathes room air
- $PaCO_2$: normal in early stages but may drop below normal from hyperventilation; may rise above normal as restric-

Pneumoconiosis Diseases

Pneumoconiosis	Causative pollutant	High-risk occupations
Antimony pneumoconiosis	Antimony	• Mining and crushing antimony ore • Cleaning extraction chambers • Alloy production
Baritosis	Barium	• Mining crude barium ore • Drying and bagging ground ore
Carbon pneumoconioses	Carbon, carbon black	• Handling carbon black (used as a filler and coloring agent in rubber, plastics, printing inks, paints, or enamels) • Manufacturing carbon electrodes and carbon paper
	Graphite	• Mining and handling graphite • Manufacturing refractory ceramics and crucibles, pencils, lubricants, electrodes, and neutron moderators in atomic reactors
Anthracosilicosis	Coal	• Mining and handling coal
Siderosis	Iron	• Iron and steel rolling, steel grinding • Electric arc and steel welding • Silver and steel polishing with iron oxide • Scouring, chipping, and dressing castings in iron foundries • Boiler scaling (cleaning fireboxes) • Mining and crushing iron ores • Mining, milling, and mixing emery
Stannosis	Tin	• Milling, grinding, and handling tin ore • Tipping ore into and raking out refinery furnaces
Asbestosis	Asbestos	• Mining asbestos • Manufacturing asbestos-cement products (tiles and roofing) • Manufacturing and installing insulating and fireproofing materials • Maintaining equipment in asbestos-processing factories
Diatomite silicosis	Diatomite	• Mining and processing diatomite • Manufacturing filters for inorganic and organic liquids • Manufacturing bricks and cement used for heat and sound insulation • Handling diatomite (used as a filler for plastics, rubber, insecticides, paints, varnishes, floor coverings, or fertilizers)

Pneumoconiosis Diseases *(continued)*

Pneumoconiosis	Causative pollutant	High-risk occupations
Fuller's earth lung	Fuller's earth (type of clay)	• Mining and processing fuller's earth • Clarifying mineral, animal, or vegetable oils • Manufacturing herbicides, insecticides, paints, and cosmetics • Refining mineral oils
Kaolin pneumoconiosis	Kaolin (china clay)	• Processing kaolin • Manufacturing paper, rubber, or plastics
Silicosis	Free silica	• Mining gold, tin, copper, platinum, and mica • Quarrying granite, slate, and pumice • Tunneling for sewers and roads; excavating sandstone • Stonecutting and polishing, cleaning, and carving masonry • Manufacturing abrasives using crushed sand, sandstone, or quartzite; abrasive blasting • Manufacturing glass, enameling • Processing products that use rock-containing quartz • Working in iron and steel foundries • Manufacturing china, porcelain, stoneware, and earthenware • Building and dismantling kilns, steel furnaces, ovens in gas-making plants, and boiler houses • Cleaning and scaling boiler flues and fireboxes
Talc pneumoconiosis	Talc	• Mining and processing talc • Manufacturing cosmetic powders or paints

tive pattern develops, particularly if the patient's hypoxic and has severe alveolar ventilatory impairment.

Treatment

Treatment aims to relieve respiratory symptoms, manage hypoxia and cor pulmonale, and prevent respiratory tract irritation and infections. Treatment also includes careful observation for development of tuberculosis. Respiratory symptoms may be relieved through daily use of bronchodilating aerosols and increased fluid intake (at least 3 liters daily). Steam inhalation and chest physiotherapy techniques (such as controlled coughing and segmental bronchial drainage) with chest percussion and vibration help clear secretions. In severe cases, the patient with chronic hypoxia may need oxygen by cannula, mask, or mechanical ventilation (if arterial oxy-

Hypersensitivity Diseases

Hypersensitivity disease	Pathogen	Environmental source
Bagassosis	*Thermoactinomyces sacharii*	Moldy sugarcane
Bird fancier's disease	Avian dust or serum	Birds
Byssinosis (brown lung)	Flax, hemp, or cotton dust	Textiles
Cheese washer's disease	*Penicillium, Aspergillus clavatus*	Cheese mold
Chicken handler's disease	Feathers, serum	Chickens
Coffee worker's lung	Unknown	Coffee dust
Coptic disease	Mold	Mummies
Duck fever	Serum	Ducks
Farmer's lung	*Micropolyspora faeni; Thermoactinomyces candidus, virdis*, and *vulgaris*	Moldy hay
Furrier's lung	Unknown	Hair dust
Humidifier or forced-air-system lung	*Thermoactinomyces candidus* and *vulgaris*	Fungal spores
Malt worker's disease	*Aspergillus clavatus* and *fumigatus*	Malt and barley dusts
Maple bark stripper's disease	*Cryptostroma corticale*	Moldy maple bark
Mushroom worker's disease	*Micropolyspora faeni, Thermoactinomyces vulgaris*	Mushroom compost
New Guinea lung	*Streptomyces olivaceous*	Thatched roof dust
Paprika splitter's lung	*Mucor stolonifer*	Moldy pods
Pituitary snuff taker's disease	Bovine and porcine proteins	Pituitary powder
Rodent worker's lung	Dried rat serum	Laboratory rats
Sauna taker's disease	*Pullularia* species	Moldy water and bucket

Hypersensitivity Diseases (continued)

Hypersensitivity disease	Pathogen	Environmental source
Sequoiosis	Graphium aureobasidium pullulans	Moldy redwood sawdust
Turkey handler's disease	Serum	Turkeys
Wheat weevil disease	Sitophilus granarius	Wheat flour
Wood dust disease	Unknown	Mahogany and oak dust
Wood pulp worker's disease	Alternaria tenuis	Moldy logs

genation can't be maintained). Respiratory infection warrants prompt antibiotic administration.

Clinical considerations
• Teach the patient to prevent infection by avoiding crowds and persons with respiratory infections and by receiving influenza and pneumococcal vaccines.
• Increase the patient's exercise tolerance by encouraging regular activity. Advise him to plan his daily activities to decrease the work of breathing and to pace himself, rest often, and move slowly through his daily activities.

Asbestosis

Description
This pneumoconiosis form, characterized by diffuse interstitial fibrosis, can develop up to 20 years after regular exposure to asbestos has ended. High-risk industries include asbestos mining, milling, construction (in which asbestos is used in a prefabricated form), fireproofing, and textiles. Asbestos also is used in the production of paints, plastics, and brake and clutch

linings. Exposure may also occur in public buildings during asbestos insulation removal.

Asbestos-related diseases may occur in families of asbestos workers from exposure to fibrous dust shaken off the worker's clothing at home. Such diseases may develop in the general population from exposure to fibrous dust or waste piles from nearby asbestos plants.

Asbestos also causes pleural plaques and mesotheliomas of the pleura and the peritoneum. A potent co-carcinogen, it increases the risk of lung cancer in cigarette smokers.

Cause
Inhalation of respirable asbestos fibers (50 μ or more in length; 0.5 μ or less in diameter)

Pathophysiology
Inhaled asbestos fibers take on a longitudinal placement in the airway, move in the direction of airflow, and penetrate respiratory bronchioles and alveolar walls. They become encased in a brown, iron-rich, protein-like sheath (ferruginous bodies or asbestos bodies) found in sputum and lung tissue. Interstitial fibrosis develops in lower lung zones,

causing obliterative changes in lung parenchyma and pleurae. Raised hyaline plaques may form in the parietal pleura, diaphragm, and pleura contiguous with the pericardium.

Signs and symptoms

Clinical features may appear before chest X-ray changes. The first symptom—usually dyspnea on exertion—typically occurs after 10 years of asbestos exposure. As fibrosis extends, dyspnea on exertion increases until it eventually occurs even at rest. Advanced disease also causes a dry cough (which may be productive in smokers), chest pain (commonly pleuritic), recurrent respiratory infections, and tachypnea.

Cardiovascular complications include pulmonary hypertension, right ventricular hypertrophy, and cor pulmonale. Finger clubbing commonly occurs.

Diagnosis

Patient history reveals occupational, family, or neighborhood exposure to asbestos fibers. Physical examination reveals characteristic dry crackles at the lung bases. Chest X-rays show fine, irregular, linear diffuse infiltrates; extensive fibrosis results in a honeycomb or ground-glass appearance. X-rays may also show pleural thickening and calcification, with bilateral obliteration of costophrenic angles and, in later stages, an enlarged heart with a classic shaggy heart border.

Pulmonary function studies show:
• *Vital capacity, forced vital capacity (FVC), and total lung capacity:* decreased
• *Forced expiratory volume in 1 second (FEV_1):* normal or decreased
• *FEV_1 to FVC ratio:* usually normal
• *Diffusing capacity for carbon monoxide:* below normal when fibrosis destroys alveolar walls and thickens the alveolar-capillary membrane.

Arterial blood gas measurements reveal:
• *PaO_2:* decreased
• *$PaCO_2$:* decreased from hyperventilation.

Treatment

Treatment aims to relieve respiratory symptoms and, in advanced disease, to manage hypoxia and cor pulmonale. Respiratory symptoms may be relieved by chest physiotherapy techniques, such as controlled coughing and segmental bronchial drainage, with chest percussion and vibration. Aerosol therapy, inhaled mucolytics, and increased fluid intake (at least 3 liters daily) may also help relieve respiratory symptoms. Diuretics, digitalis preparations, and salt restrictions may be indicated for patients with cor pulmonale. Hypoxia necessitates oxygen administration by cannula or mask, or by mechanical ventilation if arterial oxygenation can't be maintained. Respiratory infection warrants prompt antibiotic administration.

Clinical considerations

• Teach the patient to prevent infection by avoiding crowds and persons with infections and by receiving influenza and pneumococcal vaccines.
• Improve the patient's ventilatory efficiency by encouraging physical reconditioning, energy conservation in daily activities, and relaxation techniques.

Berylliosis
(Beryllium poisoning, beryllium disease)

Description

A form of pneumoconiosis, berylliosis is a systemic granulomatous disorder with dominant pulmonary manifestations. This disease occurs among beryllium alloy workers, cathode-ray tube makers, gas mantle makers, missile technicians, and nuclear reactor workers. It's usually associated with beryllium milling and use, not with beryl ore mining. Berylliosis may also affect families of these workers, as a result of dust shaken off a worker's clothing at home, as well as people living near plants using beryllium alloy.

Berylliosis occurs in two forms: acute nonspecific pneumonitis and chronic noncaseating granulomatous disease with interstitial fibrosis, which may cause death from respiratory failure and cor pulmonale. Most patients with chronic interstitial disease become only slightly to moderately disabled by impaired lung function and other symptoms; however, with each acute exacerbation, the prognosis worsens.

Cause
Inhalation of beryllium dust, fumes, or mist, with the disease pattern related to the amount inhaled. Beryllium may also be absorbed through the skin.

Pathophysiology
The mechanism by which beryllium exerts its toxic effect is unknown.

Signs and symptoms
Beryllium absorption through broken skin produces an itchy rash, which usually subsides within 2 weeks after exposure. A "beryllium ulcer" results from accidental implantation of beryllium metal in the skin.

Respiratory signs and symptoms of acute berylliosis include swelling and ulceration of nasal mucosa, which may progress to septal perforation, tracheitis, and bronchitis (dry cough). Acute pulmonary disease may develop rapidly (within 3 days) or weeks later, producing a progressive dry cough, chest tightness, substernal pain, tachycardia, and signs and symptoms of bronchitis. This disease form has a significant mortality related to respiratory failure.

About 10% of patients with acute berylliosis develop chronic disease 10 to 15 years after exposure. The chronic form causes increasing dyspnea that becomes progressively unremitting, along with mild chest pain, dry unproductive cough, and tachypnea. Pneumothorax may occur, with pulmonary scarring and bleb formation.

Cardiovascular complications include pulmonary hypertension, right ventricular hypertrophy, and cor pulmonale. Other clinical features include hepatosplenomegaly, renal calculi, lymphadenopathy, anorexia, and fatigue.

Diagnosis
Patient history reveals occupational, family, or neighborhood exposure to beryllium dust, fumes, or mist. In acute berylliosis, chest X-rays may suggest pulmonary edema, showing an acute miliary process or a patchy acinous filling, and diffuse infiltrates with prominent peribronchial markings. In chronic berylliosis, X-rays show reticulonodular infiltrates and hilar adenopathy and large coalescent infiltrates in both lungs.

Pulmonary function tests show decreased vital capacity, forced vital capacity, residual volume to total lung capacity ratio, diffusing capacity for carbon monoxide, and compliance as lungs stiffen from fibrosis. Arterial blood gas analysis shows decreased PaO_2 and $PaCO_2$.

The in vitro lymphocyte transformation test diagnoses berylliosis and monitors workers for occupational exposure to beryllium. A positive beryllium patch test establishes only hypersensitivity to beryllium—it doesn't confirm the disease. Tissue biopsy and spectrographic analysis results are positive for most exposed workers, although these tests aren't absolutely diagnostic. Urinalysis may show beryllium in urine; however, this indicates only exposure. Differential diagnosis must rule out sarcoidosis and granulomatous infections.

Treatment
Beryllium ulcers call for excision or curettage. Acute berylliosis warrants prompt corticosteroid therapy. Hypoxia may necessitate oxygen administration by nasal cannula or mask.

Severe respiratory failure calls for mechanical ventilation if arterial oxygenation can't be maintained.

Chronic berylliosis is usually treated with corticosteroids, although doctors don't know whether steroids alter disease progression. Lifelong maintenance therapy may be necessary.

Respiratory symptoms may be treated with bronchodilators, increased fluid intake (at least 3 liters daily), and chest physiotherapy. Diuretics, digitalis preparations, and salt restriction may be useful in patients with cor pulmonale.

Clinical considerations
• Teach the patient to prevent infection by avoiding crowds and persons with infection and by receiving influenza and pneumococcal vaccines.
• Encourage the patient to practice physical reconditioning, energy conservation in daily activities, and relaxation techniques.

Coal worker's pneumoconiosis
(Black lung disease, coal miner's disease, miner's asthma, anthracosis, anthracosilicosis)

Description
A progressive nodular pulmonary disease, coal worker's pneumoconiosis (CWP) occurs in two forms. In simple CWP, lung capacities are characteristically small. Patients with simple CWP may develop complicated CWP (also known as progressive massive fibrosis), characterized by fibrous tissue mass formation in the lungs. The risk for developing CWP depends on the duration of exposure to coal dust (usually 15 years or longer), intensity of exposure (dust count, particle size), mine location, silica content of the coal (highest in anthracite coal), and the worker's susceptibility. CWP incidence is highest among anthracite coal miners in the eastern United States.

Prognosis varies. Simple asymptomatic disease is self-limiting. Complicated CWP may be disabling, resulting in severe ventilatory failure and right-sided heart failure secondary to pulmonary hypertension.

Cause
Inhalation and prolonged retention of respirable coal dust particles (less than 5 μ in diameter)

Pathophysiology
Simple CWP results in formation of macules (accumulations of macrophages laden with coal dust) around terminal and respiratory bronchioles, surrounded by a halo of dilated alveoli. Macule formation leads to atrophy of supporting tissue, causing permanent small airway dilation (focal emphysema).

Simple disease may progress to complicated CWP; this is most likely if CWP begins after a relatively short exposure period. Complicated CWP may involve one or both lungs; fibrous tissue masses enlarge and coalesce, causing gross distortion of pulmonary structures (destruction of vessels, alveoli, and airways).

Signs and symptoms
Simple CWP is asymptomatic, especially in nonsmokers. In complicated CWP, signs and symptoms include exertional dyspnea and a cough that occasionally produces inky-black sputum, when fibrotic changes undergo avascular necrosis and their centers cavitate. Other clinical features include increasing dyspnea and a cough that produces milky, gray, clear, or coal-flecked sputum. Recurrent bronchial and pulmonary infections produce yellow, green, or thick sputum. Possible complications include pulmonary hypertension, right ventricular hypertrophy and cor pulmonale, and pulmonary tuberculosis. In

cigarette smokers, chronic bronchitis and emphysema may also complicate the disease.

Diagnosis

Patient history reveals exposure to coal dust. Physical examination reveals barrel chest, hyperresonant lungs with dull areas, diminished breath sounds, crackles, rhonchi, and wheezes. In simple CWP, chest X-rays show small opacities (less than 10 mm in diameter), possible in all lung zones but more prominent in the upper ones. In complicated CWP, one or more large opacities (1 to 5 cm in diameter) appear, possibly with cavitation.

Pulmonary function test results include:

• *Vital capacity:* normal in simple CWP; decreased in complicated CWP

• *Forced expiratory volume in 1 second* (FEV_1): decreased in complicated CWP

• FEV_1 *to forced vital capacity (FVC) ratio:* usually normal

• *Residual volume to total lung capacity ratio:* normal in simple CWP; decreased in complicated CWP

• *Diffusing capacity for carbon monoxide:* significantly below normal in complicated CWP (reflecting alveolar septal destruction and pulmonary capillary obliteration).

Arterial blood gas analysis reveals:

• PaO_2: normal in simple CWP; decreased in complicated CWP

• $PaCO_2$: normal in simple CWP (possibly decreased from hyperventilation); may be increased if the patient's hypoxic and has severely impaired alveolar ventilation.

Treatment

Treatment aims to relieve respiratory symptoms, manage hypoxia and cor pulmonale, and avoid respiratory tract irritants and infections. Observe the patient closely for development of tuberculosis. Respiratory signs and symptoms may be relieved by bronchodilator therapy with theophylline or aminophylline (if bronchospasm's reversible), oral or inhaled sympathomimetic amines (metaproterenol), corticosteroids (oral prednisone or an aerosol beclomethasone form), or cromolyn sodium aerosol. Chest physiotherapy techniques, such as controlled coughing and segmental bronchial drainage, with chest percussion and vibration, help remove secretions.

Other measures include increased fluid intake (at least 3 liters daily) and respiratory therapy techniques, such as aerosol therapy, inhaled mucolytics, and perhaps intermittent positive pressure breathing. Diuretics, digitalis preparations, and salt restriction may be indicated in cor pulmonale. In severe cases, the patient may need oxygen by cannula or mask (1 to 2 liters/ minute) if he has chronic hypoxia, or by mechanical ventilation if arterial oxygenation can't be maintained. Respiratory infection requires prompt antibiotic administration.

Clinical considerations

• Teach the patient to prevent infection by avoiding crowds and persons with respiratory infection and by receiving influenza and pneumococcal vaccines.

• Encourage the patient to stay active to prevent his physical condition from deteriorating, but to pace his activities and practice relaxation techniques.

Lung cancer

Description

Lung cancer usually develops within the bronchial tree wall or epithelium. Its most common types are squamous cell carcinoma, small cell carcinoma, adenocarcinoma, and large cell carcinoma.

Smokers over age 40—especially those who started smoking before age 15, who've smoked one pack or more daily for 20 years, or who work with or near asbestos—have the highest risk. Lung cancer's 10 times more common in smokers than in nonsmokers. Cancer risks depend on the number of cigarettes smoked daily, depth of smoke inhalation, when the person started smoking, and the nicotine content of cigarettes. Hereditary factors and exposure to carcinogenic industrial and air pollutants (such as asbestos, uranium, arsenic, nickel, iron oxides, chromium, radioactive dust, and coal dust) also increase the risk.

Although prognosis usually is poor, it varies with the extent of spread at time of diagnosis and the growth rate of the cell type. Only 13% of patients survive 5 years after diagnosis.

The most common cause of cancer death in men, lung cancer's fast becoming the most common cause in women, even though it's largely preventable.

Cause
Inhalation of carcinogenic pollutants by a susceptible host

Pathophysiology
Squamous cell carcinoma
This lung cancer, the most common type, usually arises in the central airway's ciliated epithelium. Initially, the epithelium shows atypical changes, then appears prickly with whorls or nests of keratinous cells. These tumorous cells usually cause metaplastic or dysplastic changes in adjacent bronchial mucosa. Squamous cell carcinoma causes early local signs and symptoms. The patient commonly develops airway occlusion with lung collapse distal to the occlusion. The tumor spreads first to intrathoracic sites and tends to cavitate more than other lung cancer types. Because metastasis to distant sites occurs relatively late, early treatment improves patient prognosis.

Adenocarcinoma
Unlike squamous cell carcinoma, adenocarcinoma usually arises in peripheral lung tissue or in areas scarred by pulmonary infarction, infection, or idiopathic fibrosis. Characterized by acinar or papillary structures, this tumor may also contain mucin-secreting glands. Because primary adenocarcinoma resembles metastatic adenocarcinoma, it's difficult to identify. Compared with squamous cell carcinoma, adenocarcinoma metastasizes to the pleura easily. Bronchoalveolar carcinoma, an uncommon adenocarcinoma form, develops from peripheral bronchioles or the alveolar epithelium. (In many cases, this tumor erupts in alveolar walls and several areas simultaneously. Expect hypoxemia as the cardinal sign, with right-to-left shunting of blood to bypass alveoli blocked by the tumor or by copious mucoid secretions.)

Large cell anaplastic carcinoma
This tumor has large, poorly differentiated, polygonal cells with abundant cytoplasm and variably sized nuclei. By light microscopy, large cell carcinoma resembles poorly differentiated squamous cell carcinoma or adenocarcinoma. This aggressive tumor spreads early and extensively.

Small cell carcinoma
Unlike other lung cancers, this tumor type arises from Kulchitsky's cells of the airways or from neuroendocrine cells elsewhere in the body. Containing dense hyperchromatic nuclei and relatively little cytoplasm, those cells are classified as fusiform, polygonal, or oat cells (resembling an unusually large lymphocyte).

Because this tumor typically spreads to regional nodes, other intrathoracic structures, and distant sites before it's diagnosed, the usual lung cancer staging classification doesn't apply. Instead, it's classified as limited-stage or extensive-stage disease. In limited-stage disease, carcinoma spreads to structures in the ipsilateral hemothorax, mediastinum, and ipsilateral supraclavicular nodes. Only a third of small cell carcinomas fall into this category at diagnosis. In extensive-stage disease, carcinoma spreads to distant sites. Although chemotherapy and radiation therapy may help prolong survival time for patients in either stage, few live more than 5 years after diagnosis.

Signs and symptoms

Because early-stage lung cancer usually produces no signs and symptoms, this disease is commonly diagnosed in an advanced stage. The following late-stage symptoms typically lead to diagnosis:
• *Epidermoid and small cell carcinomas:* smoker's cough, hoarseness, wheezing, dyspnea, hemoptysis, and chest pain
• *Adenocarcinoma and large cell carcinoma:* fever, weakness, weight loss, anorexia, and shoulder pain.

Besides obvious interference with respiratory function, a lung tumor may alter production of hormones that regulate body function or homeostasis. Clinical conditions that result from such changes are called hormonal paraneoplastic syndromes, which include:
• *Gynecomastia:* may result from large cell carcinoma
• *Hypertrophic pulmonary osteoarthropathy (bone and joint pain from cartilage erosion caused by abnormal production of growth hormone):* may result from large cell carcinoma and adenocarcinoma
• *Cushing's and carcinoid syndromes:* may result from small cell carcinoma
• *Hypercalcemia:* may result from epidermoid tumors.

Metastatic signs and symptoms vary greatly, depending on the tumor's effect on intrathoracic and distant structures:
• *Bronchial obstruction:* hemoptysis, atelectasis, pneumonitis, dyspnea
• *Recurrent nerve invasion:* hoarseness, vocal cord paralysis
• *Chest wall invasion:* piercing chest pain, increasing dyspnea, severe shoulder pain radiating down the arm
• *Local lymphatic spread:* cough, hemoptysis, stridor, pleural effusion
• *Phrenic nerve involvement:* dyspnea, shoulder pain, unilateral paralyzed diaphragm (with paradoxical motion)
• *Esophageal compression:* dysphagia
• *Vena cava obstruction:* venous distention and edema of the face, neck, chest, and back
• *Pericardial involvement:* pericardial effusion, tamponade, cardiac dysrhythmias
• *Cervical thoracic sympathetic nerve involvement:* miosis, ptosis, exophthalmos, reduced sweating.

Distant metastases may involve any body part, most commonly the central nervous system, the liver, and bone.

Diagnosis

Even if typical clinical findings strongly suggest lung cancer, firm diagnosis requires further evidence.
• Chest X-ray usually shows an advanced lesion but can detect a lesion up to 2 years before symptoms appear. It also delineates tumor size and location.
• Sputum cytology, which is about 75% reliable, requires a specimen expectorated from the lungs and tracheobronchial tree (not postnasal secretions or saliva).
• Bronchoscopy can locate the tumor site and permit direct biopsy. Bronchoscopic washings can also provide material for cytologic and histologic examination. Use of a flexible fiberoptic bronchoscope increases test effectiveness.
• Needle biopsy of the lungs uses biplane fluoroscopic visual control to detect a peripheral tumor. This allows firm diagnosis in about 80% of patients.
• Tissue biopsy of accessible metastatic sites includes supraclavicular and mediastinal node and pleural biopsy.
• Thoracentesis allows chemical and cytologic examination of pleural fluid.

Additional studies include chest tomography, bronchography, esophagography, and angiocardiography (contrast studies of the bronchial tree, esophagus, and cardiovascular tissues). Tests to detect metastases include bone scan (a positive scan may necessitate bone marrow biopsy, which is also recommended in small cell carcinoma), computed tomography brain scan, liver function studies, and gallium scan (noninvasive nuclear scan) of liver, spleen, and bone.

After histologic confirmation, staging determines disease extent, helps plan treatment, and helps determine prognosis. (See *Staging Lung Cancer.*)

Treatment

Recently introduced treatment regimens, which involve combinations of surgery, radiation, and chemotherapy, may improve prognosis and prolong survival.

Surgery is the primary treatment for Stage I, Stage II, or selected Stage III squamous cell carcinoma, adenocarcinoma, and large cell carcinoma, unless the tumor's nonresectable or other conditions (such as cardiac disease) rule out surgery. Surgery may include partial lung removal (wedge resection, segmental resection, lobectomy, radical lobectomy) or total lung removal (pneumonectomy, radical pneumonectomy).

Preoperative radiation therapy, which aims to reduce tumor bulk to allow surgical resection, has questionable value. Radiation therapy's usually recommended for Stage I and Stage II lesions if surgery's contraindicated, and for Stage III lesions when the disease is confined to the involved hemothorax and ipsilateral supraclavicular lymph nodes. Usually, radiation therapy's delayed until 1 month after surgery to allow the wound to heal; it's directed to the chest region most likely to develop metastasis.

Recent improvements in radiation technology allow delivery of high-energy X-ray beams and electron beams using a 25 MeV linear accelerator. High-energy beams deliver radiation doses at great depths, thus avoiding injury to skin and surrounding normal tissue. The electron beam is used to treat superficial lesions.

Several new chemotherapy combinations show promise. For example, combined therapy of fluorouracil, vincristine, and mitomycin induces remission in 40% of patients with adenocarcinomas. Promising combinations for treating small cell carcinomas include cyclophosphamide, doxorubicin, and vincristine (CAV); cyclophosphamide, doxorubicin, vincristine, and etoposide (CAVE); and etoposide and cisplatin (VP-16).

Immunotherapy with such agents as interferon, thymic factors, monoclonal antibodies, and interleukin-2 remains experimental. Nonspecific immunotherapy using Bacillus Calmette-Guerin (BCG) vaccine or possibly *Corynebacterium parvulum* appears the most promising.

In photodynamic therapy (PDT), also largely experimental, laser energy's directed through a bronchoscope to destroy local tumors. PDT has been used mainly as a palliative treatment for obstructive endobronchial tumors unresponsive to conventional treatment.

Clinical considerations

Comprehensive supportive care and patient teaching can minimize complications and speed recovery from surgery, radiation, and chemotherapy.

For preoperative patients

• Supplement and reinforce what the doctor has told the patient about the disease and the surgical procedure.
• Explain expected postoperative care, such as Foley catheter insertion, endotracheal tube placement, dressing changes, and I.V. therapy. Teach the patient how to cough, deep breathe, and perform range-of-motion exercises. Reassure him that analgesics and proper positioning will help control postoperative pain.
• Inform the patient that he shouldn't take food or fluids after midnight the night before surgery; that he'll take a povidone-iodine shower the night or morning before surgery; and that he'll

Staging Lung Cancer

Primary tumor (T)
- *TO:* No evidence of primary tumor.
- *TX:* Tumor proven by the presence of malignant cells in bronchopulmonary secretions but not visualized by X-ray or bronchoscopy.
- *TIS:* Carcinoma in situ.
- *T1:* Tumor 3 cm or less in diameter, surrounded by normal lung or visceral pleura.
- *T2:* Tumor more than 3 cm in diameter, or tumor of any size that invades the visceral pleura or extends to the hilar region. Tumor lies within a lobar bronchus or at least 2 cm from the carina. Any associated atelectasis or obstructive pneumonitis involves less than an entire lung.
- *T3:* Tumor of any size that extends into the neighboring structures, such as the chest wall, diaphragm, or mediastinum, that involves a main bronchus less than 2 cm from the carina, or that occurs with atelectasis or obstructive pneumonitis of an entire lung or with pleural effusion.

Regional lymph nodes *(N)*
- *NO:* No metastasis to regional lymph nodes.
- *N1:* Metastasis to peribronchial and/or ipsilateral hilar lymph nodes.
- *N2:* Metastasis to mediastinal lymph nodes.

Distant metastasis *(M)*
- *MO:* No distant metastasis.
- *M1:* Distant metastasis, such as to scalene, cervical, or contralateral hilar lymph nodes; brain; bones; lung; or liver.

These T, N, and M factors may be combined into the following groups or stages:

Occult carcinoma
- *TX NO MO:* Bronchopulmonary secretions contain malignant cells; no other evidence of the primary tumor or of metastasis.

Stage I
- *TIS NO MO:* Carcinoma in situ.
- *T1 NO MO:* Tumor classified as T1 without any metastasis to the regional lymph nodes.
- *T1 N1 MO:* Tumor classified as T1 with metastasis to the ipsilateral hilar lymph nodes only.
- *T2 NO MO:* Tumor classified as T2 without any metastasis to nodes or distant metastasis. (Note: TX N1 MO and TO N1 MO also fall under Stage I, but are difficult, if not impossible, to diagnose.)

Stage II
- *T2 N1 MO:* Tumor classified as T2 with metastasis to ipsilateral hilar lymph nodes only.

Stage III
- *T3 with any N or M:* Any tumor more extensive than T2.
- *N2 with any T or M:* Any tumor with metastasis to mediastinal lymph nodes.
- *M1 with any T or N:* Any tumor with distant metastasis.

be given preoperative medications, such as a sedative and an anticholinergic (to dry secretions).

For postoperative patients
- Maintain a patent airway and monitor chest tubes to reestablish normal intrathoracic pressure and prevent postoperative and pulmonary complications.

- Check vital signs every 15 minutes during the first hour after surgery, every 30 minutes during the next 4 hours, and then every 2 hours. Watch for and report abnormal respiration and other changes.
- Suction the patient often and encourage him to begin deep breathing and coughing as soon as possible. Check secretions frequently. Initially,

sputum will be thick and dark with blood, but it should become thinner and gray-yellow within a day.

• Monitor and record closed chest drainage. Keep chest tubes patent and effectively draining. (Fluctuation in the water-seal chamber on inspiration and expiration indicates tube patency.) Watch for air leaks and report them immediately. Position the patient on the surgical side to promote drainage and lung reexpansion.

• Watch for and report foul-smelling discharge and excessive drainage on the dressing. Usually, the dressing's removed after 24 hours, unless the wound appears infected.

• Monitor intake and output. Maintain adequate hydration.

• Check for signs and symptoms of infection, shock, hemorrhage, atelectasis, mediastinal shift, and pulmonary embolus.

• To prevent pulmonary embolus, apply antiembolism stockings and encourage range-of-motion exercises.

For patients receiving chemotherapy and radiation

• Explain possible side effects of radiation and chemotherapy. Watch for and correct these effects and, when possible, try to prevent them.

• Arrange for soft, nonirritating, high-protein foods, and encourage the patient to eat high-calorie, between-meal snacks.

• Give antiemetics and antidiarrheals, as ordered and needed.

• Schedule care to help the patient conserve energy.

• Implement reverse isolation if the patient develops bone marrow suppression.

• During radiation therapy, give good skin care to minimize skin breakdown. If the patient's receiving radiation therapy as an outpatient, warn him to avoid tight clothing, sunburn, and harsh ointments on his chest. Teach exercises to prevent shoulder stiffness.

For high-risk patients

• Refer smokers who want to quit to local branches of the American Cancer Society, Smoke Enders, I Quit Smoking Clinics, or I'm Not Smoking Clubs; or suggest group therapy, individual counseling, or hypnosis.

• Recommend that all heavy smokers over age 40 have a chest X-ray annually and sputum cytology every 6 months. Also encourage patients with recurring or chronic respiratory infections and those with chronic lung disease who detect any change in the character of a cough to see the doctor promptly for evaluation.

Pleural effusion

Description

Pleural effusion refers to excessive fluid accumulation in the pleural space. Normally, the pleural space contains a small amount of extracellular fluid that lubricates pleural surfaces. Increased production or inadequate removal of this fluid results in pleural effusion. Blood (hemothorax), pus and necrotic tissue (empyema), and lymph (chylothorax) may also collect.

Causes

• Congestive heart failure
• Hepatic disease with ascites
• Peritoneal dialysis
• Hypoalbuminemia
• Disorders resulting in overexpanded intravascular volume
• Tuberculosis
• Subphrenic abscess
• Pancreatitis
• Bacterial or fungal pneumonitis or empyema
• Cancer
• Pulmonary embolism with or without infarction
• Collagen disease (lupus erythematosus and rheumatoid arthritis)
• Inflammatory disorders
• Myxedema
• Chest trauma

Pathophysiology

The balance of osmotic and hydro-static pressures in parietal pleural capillaries normally causes fluid to move into the pleural space. Balanced pressures in visceral pleural capillaries promote reabsorption of this fluid. Excessive hydrostatic pressure or decreased osmotic pressure can cause excessive fluid amounts to pass across intact capillaries. A transudative pleural effusion—a plasma ultrafiltrate containing low concentrations of protein—results. Congestive heart failure is one cause of this effusion.

Exudative pleural effusion occurs when capillary permeability increases, with or without changes in hydrostatic and colloid osmotic pressures, allowing protein-rich fluid to leak into the pleural space. These effusions may occur with such disorders as tuberculosis.

Signs and symptoms

Patients with pleural effusion characteristically have signs and symptoms relating to the underlying pathology. Most patients with large effusions, particularly those who have underlying pulmonary disease, typically complain of dyspnea. Those with effusions associated with pleurisy usually complain of pleuritic chest pain. Other clinical features depend on the cause of effusion. For example, patients with empyema develop fever and malaise.

Diagnosis

Chest X-ray shows radiopaque fluid in dependent regions. Chest auscultation reveals decreased breath sounds; percussion reveals dullness over the effused area, which doesn't change with respiration. Although these tests verify pleural effusion, other tests must be done to distinguish transudative from exudative effusion and determine the underlying disorder. In thoracentesis, the most useful test, analysis of aspirated pleural fluid typically shows the following:

• with transudative effusion, specific gravity usually below 1.015 and protein level below 3 g/dl
• with exudative effusion, ratio of protein in pleural fluid to that in serum is 0.5 or above, pleural fluid lactic dehydrogenase (LDH) level of 200 IU or above, and ratio of LDH in pleural fluid to LDH in serum is 0.6 or above
• with empyema, acute inflammatory white blood cells and microorganisms
• with empyema or rheumatoid arthritis, extremely low pleural fluid glucose level.

With a pleural effusion that results from esophageal rupture or pancreatitis, amylase levels in pleural fluid usually exceed those in serum. Aspirated fluid may be tested for lupus erythematosus cells, antinuclear antibodies, and neoplastic cells. It may also be analyzed for color and consistency; acid-fast bacillus, fungal, and bacterial cultures; and triglycerides (in chylothorax).

Cytology can also be done on pleural fluid. Cell analyis reveals leukocytosis in empyema. A negative tuberculin skin test strongly rules against tuberculosis as the cause. In exudative pleural effusion in which thoracentesis yields inconclusive results, pleural biopsy may be done; this test is particularly useful for confirming tuberculosis or cancer.

Treatment

Depending on the amount and the source of fluid present, symptomatic effusion may warrant thoracentesis to remove fluid or careful monitoring of the patient's fluid reabsorption. Hemothorax calls for drainage to prevent fibrothorax formation. Empyema requires insertion of one or more chest tubes after thoracentesis to allow drainage of purulent material, and possibly decortication (surgical removal of the lung's thick coating) or rib resection to allow open drainage and lung expansion. Empyema also calls for parenteral antibiotics. Associated hypoxia requires oxygen administration.

Clinical considerations
• Explain thoracentesis to the patient. Before the procedure, tell him to expect a stinging sensation from the local anesthetic and pressure when the needle's inserted. Instruct him to tell you immediately if he feels uncomfortable or has trouble breathing during the procedure.
• Allow adequate time between premedication administration and the procedure (postoperative sedatives and analgesics aren't nearly as effective).
• Give reassurance during thoracentesis. Remind the patient to breathe normally and avoid sudden movements, such as coughing or sighing. Monitor vital signs and watch for syncope. If fluid's removed too quickly, the patient may suffer bradycardia, hypotension, pain, pulmonary edema, or even cardiac arrest. Watch for respiratory distress or pneumothorax (sudden onset of dyspnea or cyanosis) after thoracentesis. Observe the removed fluid—if it's bloody and hemothorax isn't suspected, the liver may have been punctured accidentally and complications may occur.
• As ordered, administer oxygen and, in empyema, antibiotics.
• Encourage the patient to breathe deeply to promote lung expansion. Have him use an incentive spirometer to promote deep breathing.
• Provide meticulous chest tube care and use aseptic technique for changing dressings around the tube insertion site if the patient has empyema. To ensure proper tube functioning, look for water in the water-seal chamber to rise and fall with respirations. Record the amount, color, and consistency of any tube drainage.
• If the patient has open drainage through a rib resection or intercostal tube, use hand and dressing precautions. Such drainage is usually necessary for weeks to obliterate the space, so make visiting nurse referrals for patients who will be discharged with the tube in place.
• If pleural effusion was a complication of pneumonia or influenza, advise prompt medical attention for chest colds.

Pleurisy
(Pleuritis)

Description
Pleurisy is inflammation of the visceral and parietal pleurae that line the inside of the thoracic cage and envelop the lungs. This disorder usually begins suddenly.

Causes
Pleurisy develops as a complication of any of the following:
• pneumonia
• tuberculosis
• viruses
• systemic lupus erythematosus
• rheumatoid arthritis
• uremia
• Dressler's syndrome
• cancer
• pulmonary infarction
• chest trauma.

Pathophysiology
With inflammation, the pleurae become swollen and congested, hampering pleural fluid transport. This increases friction between the pleural surfaces and causes sharp, stabbing pain that worsens with inspiration. Pain results from inflammation or irritation of sensory nerve endings in the parietal pleura; it increases during respiration as the pleurae shift against each other. Inflammation may stimulate production or hinder reabsorption of pleural fluid, leading to pleural effusion.

Signs and symptoms
Sharp, stabbing pain that increases with respiration may be so severe that

it limits movement on the affected side during breathing. Dyspnea also occurs. Other symptoms vary with the underlying pathologic process.

Diagnosis

Chest auscultation reveals a characteristic pleural friction rub—a coarse, creaky sound heard during late inspiration and early expiration, directly over the area of pleural inflammation. Palpation over the affected area may reveal coarse vibration.

Treatment

Treatment's generally symptomatic and includes anti-inflammatory agents, analgesics, and bed rest. Severe pain may call for an intercostal nerve block of two or three nerves. Pleurisy with pleural effusion calls for thoracentesis as both a therapeutic and diagnostic measure.

Clinical considerations

• Stress the importance of bed rest and plan your care to allow the patient as much uninterrupted rest as possible.
• Administer antitussives and pain medication, as ordered, but be careful not to overmedicate. If the patient's to be discharged with a narcotic analgesic, warn him to avoid overuse because such medication depresses coughing and respiration.
• Encourage the patient to cough even though this may prove difficult. To minimize pain, apply firm pressure at the pain site during coughing exercises.

Pneumothorax

Description

Pneumothorax is air or gas accumulation between the parietal and visceral pleurae. The amount of air or gas trapped in the intrapleural space determines the degree of lung collapse.

Pneumothorax may be classified in various ways. An open pneumothorax—also called an open or sucking chest wound, a penetrating pneumothorax, or a traumatic pneumothorax—allows atmospheric air (positive pressure) to flow directly into the pleural cavity (negative pressure) through a chest wall opening.

Closed pneumothorax is partial or complete lung collapse occurring when air enters the pleural space from within the lung and causes increased pleural pressure, preventing lung expansion during normal inspiration. Closed pneumothorax may be called traumatic pneumothorax when blunt chest trauma causes lung tissue rupture and resulting air leakage. Spontaneous pneumothorax, another closed pneumothorax type, is more common in men than in women. It's common in older patients with chronic pulmonary disease, but it may occur in healthy, tall, young adults.

In tension pneumothorax, air in the pleural space is under higher pressure than air in adjacent lung and vascular structures. This life-threatening emergency requires immediate treatment to release air trapped in the pleural space because pressure can compress the heart. (See *Tension Pneumothorax: A Crisis Situation*, pages 134 and 135.)

Causes

Open pneumothorax
• Penetrating chest injury, such as a gunshot or knife wound
• Insertion of a central venous catheter
• Chest surgery
• Transbronchial biopsy
• Thoracentesis or a closed pleural biopsy

Closed pneumothorax
• Blunt chest trauma
• Air leakage from ruptures, congenital blebs adjacent to the visceral pleural surface
• Rupture of an emphysematous bulla
• Rupture from barotrauma caused by high intrathoracic pressures during mechanical ventilation

Tension Pneumothorax: A Crisis Situation

The situation

The patient in Room 220 was admitted with dehydration caused by gastroenteritis. Her doctor has just finished placing a central venous pressure (CVP) catheter in her subclavian vein so he can assess her fluid status. Because of her obesity, placing the catheter was difficult, but the doctor succeeded on the third try.

He has ordered a chest X-ray to confirm that the catheter's placed correctly. You hang a bag of normal saline solution, attach it to the catheter, and start the infusion at a keep-vein-open (KVO) rate until catheter placement's confirmed.

While you're waiting for the portable X-ray machine to arrive, the respiratory therapist comes in to give the patient, who also has emphysema, her regularly scheduled intermittent positive-pressure breathing (IPPB) therapy. Suddenly, the patient gasps and tells you her chest hurts and she can't breathe.

You see that the left side of her chest is fixed in an inspiratory position. Her pulse is racing.

The problem

The patient seems to have developed a tension pneumothorax. Apparently, the traumatic catheter insertion punctured her lung; then the IPPB treatment forced air through the hole into the pleural space.

The worst case

The patient's lung collapses, and pressure buildup in the pleural space causes a mediastinal shift, great vessel compression, and circulatory collapse. Cardiopulmonary arrest quickly follows.

The best case

The doctor inserts a chest tube to relieve pressure in the pleural space and the patient's condition improves dramatically.

The assessment

The patient's in severe respiratory distress and pain. The left side of her chest sounds hollow on percussion and you detect no breath sounds. Her trachea's deviated to the right, confirming your initial suspicion of tension pneumothorax. The resultant pressure on the great vessels and heart causes her blood pressure to drop. She's rapidly becoming hypoxic and losing consciousness.

Assessment: If pressure in the pleural space isn't relieved immediately, the patient will suffer cardiopulmonary arrest.

Immediate actions

Page the doctor to return to the patient's room so he can insert a chest tube at once. Reassure the patient that she's going to get immediate help, and put her in Fowler's position. Check her vital signs continuously, especially her pulse. Be prepared to call a code.

Begin giving 100% oxygen through a non-rebreathing mask. If she doesn't already have a peripheral I.V. line in place, insert one so emergency drugs can be administered if necessary.

Have someone get a thoracotomy tray, chest tube, and chest drainage system while you stay with the patient. Open the tray so it's ready when the doctor arrives. If you have time, swab povidone-iodine on the patient's anterior chest along the midclavicular line. The doctor will insert the chest tube in the second intercostal space.

When the doctor arrives, brief him on the patient's status while he inserts the chest tube. (He may choose to first do a needle thoracotomy—as a temporary measure—by inserting a 12G to 16G needle into the chest.)

While the doctor inserts the chest tube, set up the chest drainage system as you continue to monitor the patient's condition. After he connects the chest tube to the drainage system, he'll probably suture it to the patient's chest to secure it. Then you'll apply a dressing.

Tape the dressing to the patient's chest; then tape all junctions of the drainage tubing. Coil the tubing and pin it to the patient's bedclothes, allowing enough slack for her to move.

The patient really needs that chest X-ray now to check placement of the CVP catheter and chest tube and to confirm that the pneumothorax has resolved. Maintain the infusion through the CVP line at a KVO rate until catheter placement's confirmed; then adjust the rate as ordered.

Later actions

Auscultate the patient's lungs and assess her vital signs; then record your findings. Because she didn't suffer an arrest, her condition should improve as quickly as it deteriorated. Once it's stable, the doctor should explain to her what happened. Stay with her during the explanation so you can answer her questions later.

Assess the patient's need for oxygen and draw an arterial blood sample for blood gas analysis if her condition warrants it. Be sure the chest drainage system's operating properly. Restock the thoracotomy tray, and replace any other supplies you used. Then record what happened in the patient's chart.

Evaluate the staff's response to the emergency. Did everyone act quickly and confidently? Were the thoracotomy tray and chest tube readily available on the unit? If not, find out why.

If hospital policy doesn't require that these supplies be stocked on each unit, suggest that the policy be changed. As you've seen from this incident, the time it takes to get the tray and tube could mean the difference between life and death for a patient with a tension pneumothorax.

- Tubercular or cancerous lesions that erode into the pleural space
- Interstitial lung disease, such as eosinophilic granuloma

Tension pneumothorax
- Penetrating chest wound treated with an airtight dressing
- Lung or airway puncture by a fractured rib associated with positive pressure ventilation
- Post-chest injury, mechanical ventilation that forces air into the pleural space through damaged areas
- High levels of positive end-expiratory pressure causing rupture of an alveolar bleb
- Chest tube occlusion or malfunction

Pathophysiology

Open pneumothorax

With an open chest wound, atmospheric air enters the pleural cavity. As air pressure in the pleural cavity becomes positive, the lung totally collapses on the affected side, resulting in substantially decreased total lung capacity, vital capacity, and lung compliance. The resulting ventilation-perfusion imbalances lead to hypoxia.

Closed pneumothorax

Both types of closed pneumothorax—traumatic and spontaneous—can also result in a collapsed lung with hypoxia and decreased total lung capacity, vital capacity, and lung compliance. However, closed pneumothorax can vary greatly, depending on the cause and degree of lung collapse. With closed pneumothorax, lung collapse can range from 5% to 95%. A collapse of less than 25% can be observed and treated without chest tubes; a greater collapse requires further intervention.

Tension pneumothorax

Air enters the pleural space either from within the lung (as the result of lung or airway damage) or from the atmosphere because of a sucking chest wound that can create a one-way valve effect. Whatever the cause, air can't escape, and accumulating pressure causes lung collapse. As air continues to accumulate and intrapleural pressures rise, the mediastinum shifts away from the affected side and decreases venous return. This forces the heart, trachea, esophagus, and great vessels to the unaffected side, compressing the heart and the contralateral lung. Without immediate appropriate intervention, tension pneumothorax rapidly proves fatal. (Because the heart's compressed, cardiopulmonary resuscitation's ineffective; the heart can't expand to accept venous return.)

Signs and symptoms

Cardinal features of pneumothorax include sudden sharp, pleuritic pain (exacerbated by chest movement, breathing, and coughing); asymmetric chest wall movement; shortness of breath; and cyanosis. In moderate to severe pneumothorax, profound respiratory distress may develop with signs of tension pneumothorax: weak and rapid pulse, increased central venous pressure (CVP), decreased blood pressure, pallor, neck vein distention, anxiety, and tracheal deviation away from the affected side. Tension pneumothorax produces the most severe respiratory symptoms; a spontaneous pneumothorax that releases only a small amount of air into the pleural space may cause no symptoms.

Diagnosis

Sudden, sharp chest pain and shortness of breath suggest pneumothorax. Chest X-ray showing air in the pleural space and, possibly, mediastinal shift confirms this diagnosis. Without a definitive chest X-ray, physical examination occasionally reveals the following:

• *Inspection:* overexpansion and rigidity of the affected chest side; in tension pneumothorax, neck vein distention with hypotension and tachycardia
• *Palpation:* crackling beneath the skin, indicating subcutaneous emphysema (air in tissues) and decreased vocal fremitus; in tension pneumothorax, tracheal deviation
• *Percussion:* hyperresonance on the affected side
• *Auscultation:* decreased or absent breath sounds over the collapsed lung.

Treatment

Treatment's conservative for spontaneous pneumothorax with no signs of increased pleural pressure (indicating tension pneumothorax), lung collapse less than 25%, and no signs of dyspnea or other evidence of physiologic compromise. Treatment measures include bed rest; careful monitoring of blood pressure, pulse rate, and respirations; oxygen administration; and possible needle aspiration of air with a large-bore needle attached to a syringe. If more than 25% of the lung's collapsed, treatment to reexpand the lung includes thoracostomy tube placement in the second or third intercostal space in the midclavicular line, connected to an underwater seal with low suction pressures.

Recurring spontaneous pneumothorax may require thoracotomy and pleurectomy; these procedures prevent recurrence by causing the lung to adhere to the parietal pleura. Traumatic open and closed pneumothorax and tension pneumothoraces call for chest tube drainage; traumatic pneumothorax may also warrant surgical repair.

Clinical considerations

• Check for pallor, gasping respirations, and sudden chest pain. Carefully monitor vital signs frequently for indications of shock, increasing respiratory distress, or mediastinal shift. Listen for breath sounds over both lungs. Falling blood pressure and increasing pulse, respiration rates, and CVP may indicate tension pneumothorax, which can prove fatal without prompt treatment.
• Urge the patient to control coughing and gasping during thoracotomy.

However, after the chest tube's in place, encourage him to cough and breathe deeply to facilitate lung expansion.

• In the patient who's undergoing chest tube drainage, watch for continuing bubbling in the water-seal chamber, indicating the lung hasn't healed. (See "Closed chest drainage" in Chapter 14.) Also, watch for increasing subcutaneous emphysema by checking around the patient's neck or at the tube insertion site for crackling beneath the skin.

• Change dressings around the chest tube insertion site, as necessary. Be careful not to reposition or dislodge the tube. If the tube dislodges, place a petrolatum gauze dressing over the opening immediately to prevent rapid lung collapse; however, use extreme caution. If the lung has a hole or tear (evidenced by bubbling in the water-seal chamber), a tension pneumothorax may be created by dressing placement.

• Monitor vital signs frequently after thoracotomy. For the first 24 hours, assess respiratory status by checking breath sounds hourly. Observe the chest tube site for leakage and note the amount and color of drainage. Walk the patient, as ordered (usually on the first postoperative day), to facilitate deep inspiration and lung expansion.

• Reassure the patient, teach him about pneumothorax and its causes, and explain all diagnostic tests and procedures. Make him as comfortable as possible. (The patient with pneumothorax usually is most comfortable sitting upright.)

Hemothorax

Description

In hemothorax, blood from damaged intercostal, pleural, mediastinal, and (infrequently) lung parenchymal vessels enters the pleural cavity. Depending on the amount of bleeding and the underlying cause, hemothorax may be associated with varying degrees of lung collapse. Pneumothorax—air in the pleural cavity—commonly accompanies hemothorax (hemopneumothorax).

Causes

• Blunt or penetrating chest trauma
• Thoracic surgery
• Pulmonary infarction
• Neoplasm
• Dissecting thoracic aneurysm
• Anticoagulant therapy

Pathophysiology

Blood accumulation in the pleural space can cause partial or total lung collapse.

Signs and symptoms

The patient with hemothorax may have some or all of the following signs and symptoms: chest pain; tachypnea; rapid-onset dyspnea; tachycardia; diaphoresis; dusky skin color; hemoptysis; bloody, frothy sputum; and mild to severe hypotension, depending on how much blood has been lost. If respiratory failure results, he may appear anxious, restless, possibly stuporous, and cyanotic; the affected chest side expands and stiffens, whereas the unaffected side rises and falls with gasping respirations. Auscultation reveals diminished or absent breath sounds on the affected side; percussion reveals dullness.

Diagnosis

Characteristic clinical signs with a history of trauma strongly suggest hemothorax. Percussion reveals dullness, and auscultation reveals decreased to absent breath sounds over the affected side. Thoracentesis yields blood or serosanguineous fluid; chest X-rays show pleural fluid with or without mediastinal shift; Arterial blood gas (ABG) measurements may document respiratory failure; hemoglobin concentration may drop below normal, depending on blood loss.

Treatment

Treatment aims to stabilize the patient's condition, stop bleeding, evacuate blood from the pleural space, and reexpand the underlying lung. Mild hemothorax usually clears rapidly in 10 to 14 days, requiring only observation for further bleeding. In severe hemothorax, thoracentesis serves not only as a diagnostic tool but also to remove pleural cavity fluid. Autotransfusion may also be used to treat blood loss (1,000 ml or more). (See "Autotransfusion" in Chapter 14.)

After diagnosis has been confirmed, the doctor quickly inserts a chest tube into the sixth intercostal space in the posterior axillary line. Use of a large-bore tube prevents clot blockage. Suction may be used. If the chest tube doesn't improve the patient's condition, the doctor may perform a thoracotomy to evacuate blood and clots and to control bleeding.

Clinical considerations

• As ordered, give oxygen by face mask or nasal cannula.

• Give I.V. fluids and blood transfusions (monitored by a central venous pressure line), as needed, to treat shock. Monitor ABG measurements often.

• Explain all procedures to the patient to allay his fears. Assist with thoracentesis. Warn him not to cough during this procedure.

• Observe chest tube drainage carefully and record volume drained (at least every hour). If hospital policy permits, gently milk the chest tube as needed to keep it open and clot-free. If the tube's warm and full of blood and the bloody fluid level in the collection bottle is rising rapidly, report this immediately. The patient may need immediate surgery.

• Check the patient closely for pallor and gasping respirations. Monitor his vital signs diligently. Falling blood pressure, increasing pulse rate, and rising respiration rate may indicate shock or massive bleeding.

Flail chest

Description

Flail chest is a thoracic disruption caused by fractures of multiple ribs, fractures of the ribs and sternum, or fractures of two or more adjacent ribs in more than one place.

Cause

Blunt chest trauma

Pathophysiology

A direct blow, such as from assault or a motor vehicle accident, causes the multiple rib fractures seen in flail chest. These injuries cause a segment of the chest wall to detach, allowing it to move inward rather than outward during inspiration. (See *Flail Chest: Paradoxical Breathing.*) As a result, the fractured bone ends may bruise or puncture a lung and cause pneumothorax, tension pneumothorax, or hemothorax.

Signs and symptoms

Bruised skin, extreme pain caused by rib fracture and disfigurement; paradoxical chest movement; rapid, shallow respirations; tachycardia; hypotension; respiratory acidosis; and cyanosis may signal flail chest.

Diagnosis

History of trauma with dyspnea, chest pain, and other typical clinical features suggest a blunt chest injury. To determine the injury's extent, the patient must undergo physical examination and diagnostic tests.

• Chest X-rays confirm rib and sternal fractures, pneumothorax, flail chest, pulmonary contusions, lacerated or ruptured aorta, tension pneumothorax (mediastinal shift), diaphragmatic rupture, lung compression, or atelectasis with hemothorax.

• Serial serum glutamic-oxaloacetic transaminase (SGOT), serum glu-

Flail Chest: Paradoxical Breathing

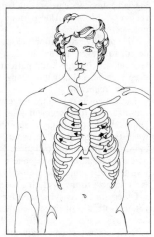 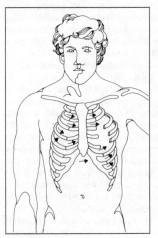

Inhalation
- Injured chest wall collapses in
- Uninjured chest wall moves out

Exhalation
- Injured chest wall moves out
- Uninjured chest wall moves in

tamic-pyruvic transaminase (SGPT), lactic dehydrogenase (LDH), creatine phosphokinase (CPK), and CPK-MB rise above normal.
- Retrograde aortography may reveal aortic laceration or rupture.
- Contrast studies and liver and spleen scans may detect diaphragmatic rupture.
- Other studies, such as echocardiography, computed tomography, and cardiac and lung scans, will show the injury's extent.

Treatment and clinical considerations

Blunt chest injuries call for immediate physical examination, control of bleeding, maintenance of a patent airway, adequate ventilation, and maintenance of fluid and electrolyte balance. Initial care includes establishing an I.V. line for fluid and med-

ication access, drawing blood for arterial blood gas measurements, and connecting the patient to a cardiac monitor. Consider alleviating the patient's respiratory distress your immediate priority.

If you observe paradoxical chest-wall movement, stabilize the segment immediately with tape or a sandbag to prevent broken ribs from puncturing or bruising the lung. (Rescue personnel may have done this already.) For mild respiratory distress, administer oxygen via nasal cannula or mask to prevent hypoxemia.

If the patient has severe respiratory distress, he'll need immediate intubation and mechanical ventilation to treat hypoxemia and possible hypercapnia and to stabilize his flail segment internally. Positive end-expiratory pressure (PEEP) may be ordered to maintain positive pressure within the lung, to prevent alveoli from collapsing, and to maintain internal stabilization. As ordered, give paralyzing agents, such as pancuronium bromide (Pavulon) or succinylcholine chloride (Anectine), to prevent the patient from breathing on his own and to allow the ventilator to control his chest-wall movement during respiration.

Pain relief is another priority. Take your patient's vital signs and administer pain medication, such as meperidine hydrochloride (Demerol) or morphine sulfate, as ordered. Although narcotics may cause respiratory depression, pain control remains the overriding concern because pain may cause voluntary and involuntary splinting, resulting in hypoventilation; this in turn may lead to hypoxemia, hypercapnia, and atelectasis.

For more sustained pain control for the patient with multiple rib fractures, but no flail segments, the doctor may use an intercostal nerve block, particularly if the patient isn't intubated. Provide syringes and needles for this procedure—the doctor will request the appropriate sizes. He'll inject a long-acting local anesthetic, such as bupivacaine (Marcaine), into the affected area, typically in combination with epinephrine to prolong the effect. Reassure your patient that the nerve block will make him more comfortable and better able to tolerate the deep breathing and pulmonary care essential to his recovery. Monitor the patient for pneumothorax.

Give prophylactic antibiotics, as ordered, to prevent pneumonia and infection. Encourage your patient to deep-breathe, and help him change his position frequently.

The patient may require surgery to stabilize the flail segment—for example, when the injury's severe or when the doctor wants to avoid prolonged mechanical ventilation. Prepare the patient for surgery and make sure his chest remains stabilized during transport to the operating room.

Other clinical considerations for the patient with a flail chest include the following:
• To remove secretions, frequently reposition and suction the patient who's on a ventilator.
• Make sure the patient keeps his oxygen apparatus on.
• Monitor the patient for signs and symptoms of such complications as hemothorax or tension pneumothorax. If you detect these, call the doctor and prepare for emergency chest tube insertion.

Selected References

Bordow, R.A., et al. *Manual of Clinical Problems in Pulmonary Medicine*, 2nd ed.Boston: Little, Brown & Co., 1985.

Burton, G.G., and Hodgkin, J.E., eds. *Respiratory Care: A Guide to Clinical Practice*, 2nd ed. Philadelphia: J.B. Lippincott Co., 1984.

Emanuelson, K., and Desmore, M.J. *Acute Respiratory Care*. New York: John Wiley & Sons, 1981.

Emergency Care Handbook. Springhouse, Pa.: Springhouse Corp., 1986.

Frame, P.T. "Acute Infectious Pneumonia in the Adult," *Respiratory Care* 28(1):100-9, January 1983.

Patient Teaching Manual, vol. 2. Springhouse, Pa.: Springhouse Corp., 1987.

Professional Guide to Diseases, 2nd ed. Springhouse, Pa.: Springhouse Corp., 1987.

Respiratory Disorders. Nurse's Clinical Library. Springhouse, Pa.: Springhouse Corp., 1984.

5 OBSTRUCTIVE DISORDERS

Introduction

Obstructive respiratory disorders are a group of diseases characterized by increased resistance, or obstruction, to airflow in the upper or lower airways. They include such acute obstructive conditions as upper airway obstruction and acute bronchitis as well as chronic obstructive pulmonary diseases. Some major symptoms of these disorders include dyspnea, easy fatigability, wheezing, and productive cough.

Pulmonary function tests (PFTs) are routinely used to diagnose obstructive lung diseases and to differentiate them from other lung diseases, such as restrictive disorders. Major PFT findings with obstructive disorders include a decreased forced expiratory volume in 1 second, maximal midexpiratory flow, or expiratory flow rates and increased total lung capacity, functional residual capacity, and residual volume, which indicate airflow obstruction and lung overdistention.

Acute obstructions occur suddenly and, without prompt intervention, can be life-threatening. Unlike chronic disorders, which usually progress even with treatment, acute problems usually resolve completely when promptly treated. For details on severe acute conditions occurring during infancy and childhood, see *Guide to Pediatric Airway Emergencies,* pages 142 to 145.

Chronic obstructive pulmonary disease (COPD) is a diagnostic umbrella that includes asthma, chronic bronchitis, emphysema, and bronchiectasis. Cigarette smoking has been established as a major risk factor for COPD; other risk factors include occupational exposure and air pollution. COPD now ranks as the sixth major cause of disability in this nation and the fifth leading cause of death. Mortality from lung diseases is increasing faster than mortality from any other major disease category.

Chronic obstructive lung diseases, when severe, can have a devastating impact on the patient's life-style. He may be severely disabled, with shortness of breath that prevents him from performing such basic tasks as washing, dressing, and talking. These diseases also can negatively affect other aspects of the patient's health, causing, for example, a decreased appetite resulting in poor nutritional status and weight loss. Treatment of these diseases can also have serious potential side effects. For example, long-term corticosteroid therapy can lead to osteoporosis and increased susceptibility to fractures.

General treatment goals for COPD include:
• providing optimal bronchodilation and decreasing bronchospasm
• preventing or treating hypoxia
• effectively clearing secretions from the airway
• achieving smoking cessation
• increasing activity level in patients with dyspnea on exertion

Guide to Pediatric Airway Emergencies

You know that a child isn't a "small adult"—that his developing body is uniquely susceptible to numerous disorders. For example, a child's at increased risk for respiratory problems, including aspiration of foreign materials, infection, and trauma. In fact, in a child, even an apparently minor respiratory system problem may quickly become life-threatening. Here's why:
• A child's airway is smaller in diameter than an adult's and contains a greater proportion of soft tissue. This makes airway obstruction more likely if excessive mucus formation or edema occurs.
• Because a child's mucous membranes are loosely attached to his airway, they're easily irritated. This may cause edema and coughing.
• An infant's larynx is located two or three cervical vertebrae higher than an adult's, increasing the risk of airway obstruction by aspiration.

Condition	Signs and symptoms
Bronchiolitis A viral infection that inflames the lining of the small bronchioles, bronchiolitis causes airway obstruction and overdistention of the lungs. It's most common in children ages 2 months to 2 years—with a peak incidence at 6 months—and usually follows a mild cold. It occurs most often in the winter and spring and is highly contagious to other young children.	• Rhinitis • Fever • Paroxysmal, hacking cough • Dyspnea and nasal flaring • Tachypnea • Intercostal and subcostal retractions • Crackles, wheezing, and decreasing breath sounds • Hyperexpanded lungs with scattered consolidation seen on X-ray • Lethargy or restlessness and irritability from hypoxemia • Possible dehydration • Impaired ability to eat and sleep
Acute laryngotracheobronchitis (viral croup) Upper airway obstruction results from this viral infection, which causes severe inflammation of the larynx, trachea, and bronchi. It's most common in children ages 3 months to 3 years who've had an upper respiratory infection. It usually occurs in the fall and winter.	• Mild fever or hypothermia • Hoarseness • Barking, brassy cough • Tachycardia • Dyspnea • Laryngitis • Inspiratory stridor and expiratory wheezing • Substernal and suprasternal retractions • Crackles, decreased breath sounds, and rhonchi, usually transmitted from upper airway • Pallor or cyanosis • Restlessness or irritability from hypoxemia • Fatigue

• A child's smaller respiratory tract allows bacteria and other microorganisms to travel easily into his lungs.
• A child's lungs contain fewer alveoli than an adult's, so when his lungs become congested, he suffers a greater loss of oxygen and carbon dioxide exchange. Yet, because of his more rapid metabolism, he needs even more oxygen than an adult needs.
• Besides his increased risk of respiratory problems, a child's more vulnerable to alterations in fluid and electrolyte balance than an adult, and is more likely to become dehydrated and go into shock from excessive diarrhea or vomiting, polyuria, fever, or fluid loss from burns. Because a child's immune system isn't well developed, he has fewer defenses against infection.

This chart helps you identify emergencies and intervene appropriately.

Clinical interventions

• Follow your hospital's isolation procedures to avoid spreading infection.
• Monitor the patient's respiratory rate and pattern; report nasal flaring, retractions, wheezing, tachypnea, or any change in level of consciousness.
• Keep his nostrils open; using cotton-tipped applicators to clear them of mucus will alleviate respiratory difficulty and reduce mouth breathing.
• Prepare him for chest X-rays to determine the presence of pulmonary hyperinflation, and draw venous and arterial blood, as ordered, for laboratory studies.
• Place him in a mist tent on his stomach to aid mucus drainage and to compress his distended lungs during expiration. Or place him in semi-Fowler's position, with his neck slightly extended to open his airway and to aid lung expansion.
• Administer oxygen via the tent if needed.
• Monitor the patient's arterial blood gas (ABG) measurements. Notify the doctor of any decrease in Pao_2 level or increase in $Paco_2$ level, and be prepared to assist with intubation and mechanical ventilation.
• If the patient has increased tachypnea and dyspnea when eating, give him nothing by mouth and expect to administer I.V. fluids.
• Keep an accurate intake and output record, and check the patient's urine specific gravity regularly for evidence of dehydration.
• Begin antibiotic therapy as ordered for secondary bacterial infection.

• Monitor the patient's respirations; place him in a sitting position while you listen for his breath sounds.
• Place the patient in a cool mist tent, administer oxygen, and administer racemic epinephrine by inhalation for temporary relief of respiratory distress, as ordered.
• Draw blood for ABG analysis as ordered.
• Insert an I.V. line and begin fluid replacement as ordered, if the patient can't take liquids orally.
• Prepare to assist with an emergency intubation or tracheotomy if the patient develops these signs of impending respiratory failure: increased heart rate, decreased respiratory rate, and decreased or absent breath sounds.
• Prepare the patient for X-rays of the chest (to rule out bronchiolitis) and cervical trachea (to rule out epiglottitis).

(continued)

Guide to Pediatric Airway Emergencies *(continued)*

Condition	Signs and symptoms
Epiglottitis A bacterial infection of the epiglottis and surrounding area, epiglottitis rapidly causes inflammation, edema, induration, and—if not treated—complete airway obstruction. It's most common in children ages 2 to 7 who've had an upper respiratory infection. It may occur in any season.	• Sudden onset of high fever • Sore throat and sudden dysphagia • Drooling • Unusual body positioning: the child leans forward, head hyperextended, jaw thrust forward, mouth open, and tongue protruding • Severe respiratory distress with inspiratory stridor; nasal flaring; intercostal, suprasternal, supraclavicular, and subcostal retractions; and paradoxical breathing • Rhonchi and diminished breath sounds, usually transmitted from the upper airway • Cherry red, irregularly swollen epiglottis • Apprehension, restlessness, and anxiety from hypoxemia • Pallor or cyanosis

• improving nutritional status in patients with such problems as decreased appetite and weight loss
• providing psychosocial support
• teaching the patient about the disease and treatment.

Upper airway obstruction

Description
A life-threatening condition, an upper airway obstruction results from compromised ventilation and oxygenation caused by partial or complete airway occlusion.

Causes
• Foreign body aspiration (the most common cause of complete airway obstruction in the conscious patient)
• External compression
• Trauma (including burns)
• Laryngospasm (for example, from an allergic reaction)
• Vocal cord edema
• Infection, such as epiglottitis or retropharyngeal abscess
• Tumor

Pathophysiology
If not treated promptly, complete airway obstruction leads—within minutes—from hypoxia to loss of consciousness and subsequent death. With incomplete obstruction, breathing becomes difficult, leading to increased work of breathing, which, in turn, increases the cardiovascular work load. Usually, ventilation's inadequate to sustain the patient. Without intervention, respiratory arrest may occur.

Signs and symptoms
With partial airway obstruction, the patient may exhibit coughing, stridor, wheezing, intercostal muscle retraction, nasal flaring, snoring respirations (if the patient's unconscious), and altered speech.

With complete airway obstruction, the patient may exhibit anxiety or panic, clutching at his throat (if the patient's conscious); inspiratory chest movement, with no air movement heard on auscultation; inability to talk or cough; diaphoresis; tachycardia; and severe hypoxemia, progressing rapidly and leading to cyanosis, lethargy, and, eventually, loss of consciousness.

Clinical interventions

- Don't use a tongue depressor to visualize the epiglottis. Doing so may cause a laryngospasm and complete airway obstruction.
- Place the patient in a sitting position to ease his respiratory difficulty. Assess his vital signs and respirations frequently, and report any changes. Never leave him alone—he may develop total airway obstruction at any time.
- Assemble the equipment for possible intubation or tracheotomy (tracheotomy may be done

prophylactically), and prepare to administer humidified oxygen.
- Calm the patient during X-rays of his chest and cervical trachea.
- Keep external stimuli to a minimum.
- Start an I.V. line for antibiotic therapy and fluid replacement, and draw blood for laboratory studies, as ordered.
- Keep an accurate intake and output record, and monitor the patient's urine specific gravity.

Diagnosis

Clinical manifestations alone may establish the diagnosis; often, the dramatic presentation is unmistakable.

- Radiographic studies (X-rays, computed tomography scans of the neck, contrast tracheograms) may be needed to assess the obstruction.
- Bronchoscopy and laryngoscopy may be performed to define the obstruction's location, size, and nature.
- Arterial blood gas analysis will indicate a decreased PaO_2 level and an increased $PaCO_2$ level, as well as metabolic and respiratory acidosis, if the patient has a complete, or nearly complete, upper airway obstruction.
- Pulmonary function tests may be obtained. The patient with a variable intrathoracic obstruction, such as an aspirated foreign body, may have normal inspiratory flow but abnormal expiratory flow, evidenced by decreased forced expiratory volume in 1 second (FEV_1), maximum voluntary ventilation (MVV), peak expiratory flow rate (PEFR), FEV_1/FVC ratio, and possibly forced vital capacity (FVC). The patient with a variable extrathoracic obstruction, such as epiglottitis or

postintubation edema, has abnormal inspiratory flow, with decreased MVV, PEFR, FEV_1, and FEV_1 to FVC ratio. The patient with a fixed obstruction, such as a tumor, has normal FVC and forced inspiratory capacity, except with severe obstruction. However, his MVV and PEFR decrease with even moderate obstruction.

Treatment and clinical considerations

Treatment for upper airway obstruction aims at opening the airway and restoring baseline respirations.

Partial airway obstruction

If your patient can cough forcefully, inhale, and cough again, let him try to expel the foreign body on his own. These efforts indicate that he still has adequate air exchange. Stay with him at all times, however, because air exchange may stop. Watch for a weak, ineffective cough; high-pitched sounds on inspiration; increased respiratory difficulty; and cyanosis. These signs indicate deteriorating air exchange; intervene as you would for a complete airway obstruction (see page 146).

Complete airway obstruction

Suspect complete airway obstruction if a patient who's eating (or who's just finished eating) suddenly clutches his throat and can't speak or cough. His skin may become dusky, and he may make exaggerated efforts to breathe without any apparent air movement. Intervene immediately by initiating the techniques recommended by the American Heart Association. (See *Basic Life Support*, Appendix 1.) If these techniques prove unsuccessful and you have appropriate equipment on hand, help the doctor remove the object with a bronchoscope, Magill forceps, or suctioning equipment. As a last resort, a cricothyrotomy or percutaneous transtracheal catheter ventilation may be performed. (See *Performing Cricothyrotomy and Percutaneous Transtracheal Catheter Ventilation,* page 262, in Chapter 12.)

Artificial airway placement

If the patient has a partial airway obstruction, you may need to insert an artificial airway or assist the doctor with insertion. Available airways include oropharyngeal, nasopharyngeal, oral endotracheal, nasal endotracheal, and tracheostomy devices. (For associated care, see Chapter 12.)

Other treatments

Removal of an aspirated foreign object may warrant bronchoscopy. Early removal is important because the object may later become surrounded by granulation tissue. If this occurs, thoracotomy or bronchotomy may be necessary. Tracheal stenosis may require bronchoscopic dilation, surgical repair, or laser resection. Vocal cord paralysis may call for surgery or tracheotomy. Tumors may warrant endoscopic or laser resection, surgery, or radiation.

You may need to administer I.V. corticosteroids, such as dexamethasone or methylprednisolone, to decrease edema and swelling if they caused the obstruction. You may also give epinephrine if the obstruction (laryngeal edema) resulted from an allergic reaction.

If massive hemoptysis obstructed your patient's airway, initial endotracheal tube placement and suctioning may have removed tracheal blood and clots. If he's still bleeding, however, he'll need rigid bronchoscopy to locate the bleeding site and to clear additional blood.

You may administer humidified oxygen if your patient's obstruction resulted from inflammation (for example, from diphtheria, allergic reactions, croup, or epiglottitis) or edema (for example, from thermal injury). Unless an artificial airway's in place, the cool mist will help decrease swelling, thereby opening the airway. Continue to provide oxygen until your patient's obstruction has been removed and the swelling and inflammation have been reduced. (See *Preventing Food Aspiration.*)

Asthma

Description

Asthma is a chronic reactive airway disorder that produces episodic airway obstruction via bronchospasms, increased mucus secretion, and mucosal edema. The disorder can be reversed in the acute disease. Signs and symptoms range from mild wheezing and dyspnea to life-threatening respiratory failure. Although this common condition can strike at any age, half of all cases occur in children under age 10.

Asthma can be classified as extrinsic and intrinsic. (See *Classifying Asthma,* page 148.) Most asthma attacks last from a few minutes to several hours, after which the patient seems to recover completely. Some patients experience airway obstruction almost daily. Status asthmaticus occurs when the attack's acutely severe and prolonged and doesn't respond to oral medication.

Asthma may have hereditary origins: about one third of all asthmatic patients share the disease with at least one member of their immediate family, and about 75% of children with two asthmatic parents have asthma.

Causes
Scientists have identified several factors that may contribute to the bronchoconstriction. These include:
• hereditary predisposition
• sensitivity to allergens or to irritants, such as pollutants
• viral infections
• aspirin, beta blockers, and other drugs
• psychological stress
• cold air
• exercise.

Pathophysiology
In this disorder, the trachea and bronchi overreact to various stimuli, giving rise to episodic smooth muscle spasms that severely constrict the airways. Mucosal edema and thickened secretions further block the airways. As a result, expiratory airflow decreases and gas becomes trapped in the airways, causing alveolar hyperinflation. Atelectasis may develop in some areas. Increased airway resistance makes breathing more laborious.

IgE antibodies, attached to histamine-containing mast cells and receptors on cell membranes, initiate extrinsic asthma attacks. When exposed to an antigen, such as pollen, the IgE antibody combines with the antigen. On subsequent exposure to the antigen, mast cells degranulate and release mediators. These mediators—including slow-reacting substance of anaphylaxis, histamine, and eosinophil chemotactic factor of anaphylaxis—cause the bronchoconstriction and edema of an asthma attack.

Some researchers suggest that asthma results from an imbalance between the adrenergic nervous system (which controls bronchodilation) and the cholinergic nervous system (which controls

---

Preventing Food Aspiration

Sudden death from food obstruction (sometimes called café coronary) mimics death by myocardial infarction. To ensure appropriate intervention, consider whether the victim's at risk of choking. Factors that increase the risk include drug and alcohol use, diseases that affect motor coordination (such as Parkinson's disease), and conditions that alter mental function (such as retardation and senility).

Recommend the following precautions to minimize the risk of foreign body aspiration:
• Always cut food into small pieces.
• Chew slowly and thoroughly.
• Avoid laughing and talking while chewing and swallowing.
• Avoid excessive alcohol use before and during meals.
• Keep small objects away from toddlers.
• Don't allow children to run, walk, talk, or play while they're chewing or swallowing.

Encourage patients, co-workers, and others to obtain instruction in basic life-support techniques from the American Heart Association or the American Red Cross.

---

bronchoconstriction). Studies suggest that asthma patients have a defective adrenergic response. Others believe that inhalation of noxious stimuli, such as pollutants, stimulates receptors in the tracheobronchial tree, leading to bronchoconstriction. (See *How Status Asthmaticus Progresses,* page 149.)

Signs and symptoms
An asthma attack may begin dramatically, with simultaneous onset of severe, multiple symptoms, or insidiously, with gradually increasing respiratory distress. Typically, an acute asthma attack causes sudden dyspnea,

Classifying Asthma

Asthma falls into two categories: extrinsic and intrinsic. Extrinsic asthma (also referred to as allergic or immunologic asthma) has an external source, such as an antigen.

A patient with extrinsic asthma may have the following:

• a personal allergy history, shown by a positive skin or serum test to antigens such as ragweed
• positive immediate skin tests
• a family allergy history (usually of multiple allergies such as hay fever, asthma, or eczema)
• eosinophilia detected in serum or sputum samples, or both
• elevated IgE levels
• a symptom onset before age 40.

A patient with intrinsic asthma (also known as nonallergic or non-immunologic asthma) shows the following:

• no known external allergens
• negative allergy tests, including negative immediate skin tests
• no family allergy history
• normal or low IgE levels
• asthma onset in adulthood
• chronic asthma.

Possibly caused by infection, intrinsic asthma usually strikes older patients and may resist treatment.

Note: Intrinsic and extrinsic asthma can't always be differentiated; for this reason, many experts no longer use these terms.

wheezing, tightness in the chest, and cough with thick or clear sputum. The patient may have a suffocating feeling. During a severe attack, he may be unable to speak more than a few words without pausing for breath.

When examining such a patient, you'll find tachypnea (although respiratory rate's frequently normal), audible wheezing, obvious use of accessory respiration muscles, rapid pulse, profuse perspiration, hyperresonant lung fields, and diminished breath sounds with wheezes and rhonchi. Cyanosis, confu-

sion, and lethargy indicate the onset of life-threatening status asthmaticus and respiratory failure.

Diagnosis

Studies that may be ordered to confirm asthma include chest X-ray, pulmonary function tests (PFTs), serum IgE and eosinophil counts, and arterial blood gas (ABG) analysis.

• PFTs reveal signs of obstructive airway disease, including decreased forced expiratory volume in 1 second (FEV_1), decreased FEV_1 to forced vital capacity ratio, low normal or decreased vital capacity, and increased total lung capacity and functional residual capacity. However, PFT results may be normal between attacks. Even when the asthma attack appears under control, spirometric values (FEV_1 and forced expiratory flow between 25% and 75% of vital capacity) remain abnormal. Residual volume remains abnormal for the longest period—up to 3 weeks after the attack.

• Serum IgE level may rise from an allergic reaction.

• Complete blood count with differential shows increased eosinophil count.

• ABG analysis serves as an essential guide for proper treatment of the asthmatic patient. It commonly shows hypocapnia and mild hypoxia in patients with mild to moderate asthma; hypercapnia and profound hypoxia in patients with severe asthma. Typically, the patient has decreased PaO_2 and $PaCO_2$ levels. However, in patients with severe asthma, the $PaCO_2$ level may be normal or above normal, indicating severe bronchial obstruction. Thus, consider frequent ABG analysis mandatory.

• Chest X-ray may show hyperinflation, with areas of focal atelectasis (mucus plugs).

If the patient has asthma symptoms but no history of allergy, he may need to undergo skin testing for specific allergens and, later, inhalation bronchial challenge testing to evaluate the clinical significance of allergens identified by skin testing.

Before testing for asthma, other causes of airway obstruction and wheezing must be ruled out. In children, such causes include cystic fibrosis; aspiration; congenital anomaly; benign or cancerous tumors of the bronchi, thyroid gland, thymus, or mediastinum; and acute viral bronchitis. In adults, such causes include obstructive pulmonary disease and congestive heart failure.

Treatment and clinical considerations

Consider prevention—identification and avoidance of precipitating factors such as allergens or irritants—the best treatment for asthma. Because such stimuli usually can't be removed entirely, desensitization to specific antigens may be helpful but rarely proves totally effective or long-lasting.

Drug therapy for asthma, which usually includes a bronchodilator, is most effective when begun soon after the symptom onset. Drugs used include rapid-acting epinephrine; terbutaline; aminophylline; theophylline and theophylline-containing oral preparations; corticosteroids; oral sympathomimetics; aerosolized sympathomimetics, such as isoproterenol or albuterol; and cromolyn sodium to treat allergy-induced asthma.

ABG analysis helps determine the severity of the asthma attack as well as the patient's response to treatment.

During an acute asthma attack:
• First, maintain respiratory function and relieve bronchoconstriction, while allowing mucus plug expulsion.
• If the attack resulted from exercise, you can try to control it by having the patient sit down and rest and use diaphragmatic and pursed-lip breathing to help recover from shortness of breath.
• Find out if the patient has a metered-dose inhaler or home nebulizer and whether he has used it. The asthmatic patient should have access to a beta-

How Status Asthmaticus Progresses

Obstructed airways hamper gas exchange and increase airway resistance, leading to labored breathing.

Patient hyperventilates, which decreases $PaCO_2$ levels. (PaO_2 levels also decrease secondary to the disorder.) Decreased PaO_2 levels further decrease $PaCO_2$ levels. Respiratory alkalosis develops.

Patient tires from hypoxia and labored breathing; respiratory rate drops to a normal level.

$PaCO_2$ increases to a higher-than-baseline level; respiratory rate remains normal. (Asthma patients usually have low $PaCO_2$ levels.)

Patient hypoventilates from exhaustion.

Respiratory acidosis sets in as PaO_2 level continues to drop and $PaCO_2$ level increases.

Unless treated, patient develops acute respiratory failure.

adrenergic metered-dose inhaler (such as albuterol or metaproterenol) or home nebulizer at all times. But warn him not to take more than two or three whiffs every 4 hours. If he needs the treatment again in less than 4 hours, give it and call the doctor for further instructions.

How to Treat Status Asthmaticus

Unless treated promptly and correctly, status asthmaticus may lead to fatal respiratory failure. The patient with increasingly severe asthma who doesn't respond to drug therapy is usually admitted to the intensive care unit for the following care:

• As ordered, give corticosteroids, epinephrine, and I.V. aminophylline. For children, I.V. isoproterenol may be used.

• Check ABG measurements frequently to assess respiratory status, particularly after ventilator therapy or a change in oxygen concentration.

• Administer oxygen, as ordered (the patient will be hypoxemic), and, if necessary, assist with endotracheal intubation and mechanical ventilation (when he has an elevated $PaCO_2$ level).

• Administer I.V. fluids, as ordered, according to the patient's clinical status and age. Increase fluids, barring contraindications, to mobilize thick secretions. (Dehydration's likely because of inadequate fluid intake and increased insensible fluid losses.)

• Position the patient for frequent chest X-rays.

(Overuse of a metered-dose inhaler or nebulizer can progressively decrease the patient's response to the inhaled drug until the drug has no effect. Extended overuse can even lead to cardiac arrest and death in rare cases.)

• The patient may be terrified from shortness of breath, so reassure him that you'll help him. Then place him in semi-Fowler's position, encourage him to use diaphragmatic and pursed-lip breathing, and urge him to relax as much as possible.

• Consider status asthmaticus unrelieved by epinephrine a medical emergency.

• Administer oxygen by nasal cannula, as ordered, to ease breathing and increase arterial oxygen saturation. Adjust oxygen concentration according to the patient's vital functions and ABG measurements.

• Administer drugs and I.V. fluids, as ordered. Continue epinephrine and administer aminophylline I.V. as a loading dose, followed by I.V. drip. Draw blood to determine the aminophylline level before administering this drug if the patient takes it at home. (*Caution:* Elderly patients with hepatic or cardiac insufficiency or those taking erythromycin have an increased risk of aminophylline toxicity. Children and those who smoke or who are receiving barbiturates have increased aminophylline metabolism and require a larger dose.) Monitor the drip rate and, when possible, use an I.V. infusion pump. Simultaneously, you may give a loading dose of corticosteroids I.V. or I.M. Combat dehydration by giving I.V. fluids, as ordered, until the patient can tolerate oral fluids, which help loosen secretions.

During long-term care:

• Supervise the patient's drug regimen. Make sure he knows how to use aerosolized bronchodilator drugs properly. If the patient's receiving an aminophylline bronchodilator, monitor his blood drug levels, because oral absorption of aminophylline can be erratic. With long-term steroid therapy, watch for cushingoid side effects. Minimize these by giving alternate-day doses or administering orally inhalable steroid beclomethasone. Because of their respiratory depressant effect, sedatives and narcotics aren't recommended.

To prevent recurring asthma attacks:

• Instruct the patient to breathe deeply, expectorate secretions accumulated overnight, and allow time for medications to work. He can best loosen secretions by coughing correctly—inhaling fully and gently, then bending

over with arms crossed over the abdomen before coughing—and by drinking 3 qt (2.8 liters) of liquid daily. Also caution the patient and his family to avoid known allergens, irritating fumes, aerosol spray, smoke, and automobile exhaust. Refer the patient to community resource groups, such as the American Lung Association and the Asthma and Allergy Foundation.
• To prevent exercise-induced bronchospasm, advise an asthmatic adult or child to use an oral bronchodilator for 30 to 60 minutes or an inhaled bronchodilator for 15 to 20 minutes before exercising. Cromolyn sodium can also be used; have the patient inhale the medication no more than 1 hour before exercising.

Acute bronchitis

Description
Acute bronchitis is an inflammation of the tracheobronchial tree, usually associated with respiratory infection. Acute bronchitis most commonly occurs during the winter when the incidence of respiratory infections rises. Young children and elderly patients (particularly those with underlying chronic obstructive pulmonary disease [COPD]) stand the greatest chance for developing bronchitis. Attacks may become more severe with exposure to such pulmonary irritants as cigarette smoke or air pollutants.

Epidemiologic research suggests that acute respiratory infections play an important role in the pathogenesis of COPD. Pulmonary function studies in previously healthy adults with acute infection from certain viruses (such as respiratory syncytial virus) show prolonged abnormalities in airway resistance and reactivity.

Causes
• Common cold viruses (most commonly, rhinovirus and influenza)
• Bacterial infection

Pathophysiology
With acute bronchitis, mucous membranes of the tracheobronchial tree become hyperemic and edematous. Bronchial secretions increase.

Signs and symptoms
Common cold symptoms, such as sore throat, may precede bronchitis by a few days. Signs and symptoms may include cough, which typically begins during the initial cold, persists, and then produces purulent sputum, and burning and substernal pain with breathing and coughing.

Chest auscultation may reveal rhonchi and wheezing. No signs of chest consolidation occur unless the patient has pneumonia. Low-grade fever may be present.

Diagnosis
Diagnosis usually rests on signs and symptoms. Sputum may be cultured to determine if bacterial infection's a causative or complicating factor. Chest X-ray may show accentuated bronchial markings without significant infiltrates.

Treatment and clinical considerations
Acute bronchitis caused by bacterial rather than viral agents calls for antibiotics. Bronchodilators may be used if the patient has bronchospasms. Adequate hydration's critical to prevent bronchial secretion drying. A humidifier may also help. Cough suppressants, such as dextromethorphan, may be ordered. Aspirin or acetaminophen and bed rest can help reduce fever and malaise. (*Note:* Don't administer aspirin to a child.)

Encourage high-risk patients, such as elderly patients with underlying COPD, to receive an annual influenza vaccine and to avoid persons with colds and other infections.

If the patient smokes, encourage him to stop smoking or refer him to a smoking cessation program.

Chronic obstructive pulmonary disease
(Chronic obstructive lung disease)

Description
Chronic obstructive pulmonary disease (COPD) refers to a group of respiratory disorders characterized by persistent obstruction of bronchial airflow. Most COPD patients have a combination of chronic bronchitis, emphysema, and asthma. Emphysema alone usually occurs only with alpha$_1$-antitrypsin deficiency.

The most common chronic lung disease, COPD affects an estimated 17 million Americans and has a rising incidence. It affects more men than women, probably because until recently men were heavier smokers.

COPD causes varying degrees of dyspnea, wheezing, and productive coughing. Because victims don't get enough oxygen and have to work so hard at breathing, they tire easily.

However, COPD doesn't always produce signs and symptoms and, in many patients, causes only minimal disability. The disease tends to worsen with time and can cause complications. (See *Complications of COPD.*)

Causes
COPD usually results from some combination of:
• chronic bronchitis
• pulmonary emphysema
• bronchial asthma.
(See *Chronic Obstructive Pulmonary Disease,* pages 154 to 157, and *Predisposing Factors to COPD,* page 158.)

Pathophysiology
In a healthy patient, the breathing process continually moves enough air in and out of the lungs to meet metabolic needs. Anything that changes the airway's size reduces the lungs' ability to provide enough air. An airway obstruction—for example, from a foreign object or COPD—hinders alveolar ventilation. A foreign object usually can be removed. COPD, on the other hand, causes chronic and irreversible problems. Underinflated alveoli beyond the obstruction can't provide enough oxygen to the blood that perfuses them and can't rid the blood of carbon dioxide. As a result, these patients suffer chronic hypoxemia, hypoxia, and hypercapnia.

The chronic airway obstruction occurring in COPD mainly affects expiration, a passive process that depends on the lungs' elastic recoil. Because inspiratory muscles can pull air past most obstructions, air can enter but can't leave as easily. Instead, it's trapped in alveoli, severely limiting inspiration of oxygen-rich air.

To force air past the obstruction, the body uses abdominal and auxiliary thoracic muscles. However, this slows expiration, causing a classic COPD sign: reduced forced expiratory flow. The patient retains carbon dioxide and hypercapnia ensues. Compromised inspiration compounds hypoxia.

COPD creates a paradox: While the breathing process provides oxygen, accessory inspiratory and expiratory muscles consume more than their normal oxygen needs, depleting the patient's oxygen supply.

Besides overworking respiratory muscles, COPD strains the heart's right side, which serves pulmonary circulation. The heart compensates for hypoxemia by pumping faster to deliver more blood to the lungs and by pumping harder to push blood through constricted capillaries. As a result, the heart's right side hypertrophies (cor pulmonale). Another compensatory mechanism—polycythemia—develops to enrich the blood's oxygen supply.

Signs and symptoms
The typical patient, a long-term cigarette smoker, has no symptoms until

middle age, when his capacity for exercise or strenuous work gradually declines and he develops a productive cough. Subtle at first, these signs become more pronounced as the patient ages and the disease progresses. Eventually, the patient develops dyspnea on minimal exertion, frequent respiratory infections, intermittent or continuous hypoxemia, and grossly abnormal pulmonary function test results. In its advanced form, COPD may cause thoracic deformities, overwhelming disability, cor pulmonale, severe respiratory failure, and death.

Diagnosis

The following tests may be ordered for a COPD patient:

• *Arterial blood gas (ABG) analysis:* The COPD patient may suffer from hypoxemia, especially when his condition's acute. With mild to moderate COPD, expect a normal $PaCO_2$ level because central chemoreceptors in the anterior medulla respond to a $PaCO_2$ elevation by increasing ventilation. With moderate to severe COPD (especially chronic bronchitis), the patient can't sustain the increased work of breathing, and his $PaCO_2$ level increases. In response, the body retains bicarbonate to maintain normal pH.

• *Other blood tests:* Elevated hematocrit and hemoglobin levels and red blood cell counts occur in a COPD patient with polycythemia.

• *Sputum cultures:* Acute COPD episodes suggest an infection. Sputum cultures help the doctor choose an appropriate antibiotic. Always arrange for culturing of green or yellow sputum.

• *Chest X-ray:* A chest X-ray of a COPD patient with chest hyperinflation may look black. It may also show a flattened diaphragm, partially obscuring the costophrenic angles, and an increased retrosternal space.

• *Pulmonary function tests:* Expect decreases in vital capacity, forced expiratory volume in 1 second (FEV_1) peak flow, and FEV_1/FVC ratio in a COPD

Complications of COPD

Chronic obstructive pulmonary disease (COPD) can cause the following complications:

• Pulmonary hypertension (high blood pressure in the pulmonary vessels) develops because the blood (which typically has a thicker consistency and increased volume from polycythemia) must move through or around constricted vessels.

• Cor pulmonale (pulmonary heart disease) may follow hypertension, as the heart's right side pumps increasingly thicker blood against a rising pressure gradient. Chronic hypoxia reduces the heart's oxygen supply, which is needed to fight hypertension. Check for neck-vein distention during inhalation, edema in the arms and legs, and dyspnea on exertion. EKGs and chest X-rays show the heart's enlarged right side.

• Peptic ulcer can also stem from COPD, although researchers don't know why.

---

patient. Functional residual capacity, residual volume, and total lung capacity may increase from reduced elastic lung recoil, especially in a patient with chronic bronchitis or emphysema.

Treatment and clinical considerations

Treatment goals include relieving symptoms and preventing complications. Because most COPD patients receive outpatient treatment, they need comprehensive teaching to help them comply with therapy and understand the nature of this chronic, progressive disease. Encourage them to enroll in available pulmonary rehabilitation programs, such as the Better Breathing Club of the American Lung Association.

Pulmonary medications, such as beta adrenergics, methylxanthines, corticosteroids, antibiotics, expectorants, anticholinergics, and other

Chronic Obstructive Pulmonary Disease

Disease	Causes and pathophysiology	Clinical features
Emphysema • Abnormal irreversible enlargement of air spaces distal to terminal bronchioles caused by destruction of alveolar walls, resulting in decreased elastic recoil properties of lungs • Most common cause of death from respiratory disease in the United States	• Cigarette smoking, deficiency of alpha$_1$-antitrypsin • Recurrent inflammation associated with release of proteolytic enzymes from cells in lungs causes bronchiolar and alveolar wall damage and, ultimately, destruction. Loss of lung supporting structure results in decreased elastic recoil and airway collapse on expiration. Destruction of alveolar walls decreases surface area for gas exchange.	• Insidious onset, with dyspnea the predominant symptom • Other signs and symptoms of long-term disease: chronic cough; anorexia; weight loss; malaise; barrel chest; use of accessory respiratory muscles; prolonged expiratory period with grunting, pursed-lip breathing, and tachypnea; peripheral cyanosis; and digital clubbing • Complications include recurrent respiratory tract infections, cor pulmonale, and respiratory failure.
Chronic bronchitis • Excessive mucus production with productive cough for at least 3 months per year for 2 successive years • Only a minority of patients with the clinical syndrome of chronic bronchitis develop significant airway obstruction.	• Severity of disease related to amount and duration of smoking: respiratory infection exacerbates symptoms. • Hypertrophy and hyperplasia of bronchial mucous glands, increased goblet cells, damage to cilia, squamous metaplasia of columnar epithelium, and chronic leukocytic and lymphocytic infiltration of bronchial walls; widespread inflammation, distortion, airway narrowing, and mucus within the airways produce resistance in small airways and cause severe ventilation-perfusion imbalance.	• Insidious onset, with productive cough and exertional dyspnea the predominant symptoms • Other signs and symptoms: colds associated with increased sputum production and worsening dyspnea that take progressively longer to resolve; copious sputum (gray, white, or yellow); weight gain from edema; cyanosis; tachypnea; wheezing; prolonged expiratory time; use of accessory respiratory muscles

Confirming diagnostic measures	Management
• *Physical examination:* hyperresonance on percussion, decreased breath sounds, expiratory prolongation, quiet heart sounds • *Chest X-ray:* in advanced disease, flattened diaphragm, reduced vascular markings at lung periphery, overaeration of lungs, vertical heart, enlarged anteroposterior chest diameter, large retrosternal air space • *Pulmonary function tests:* increased residual volume, total lung capacity, and compliance; decreased vital capacity, diffusing capacity, and expiratory flow • *Arterial blood gas measurements:* reduced PaO_2 with normal $PaCO_2$ level until late in disease • *EKG:* tall, symmetric P waves in leads II, III, and AVF; vertical QRS axis; signs of right ventricular hypertrophy late in disease • *RBC count:* increased hemoglobin late in disease when persistent severe hypoxia is present	• Bronchodilators, such as aminophylline, to promote mucociliary clearance • Antibiotics to treat respiratory infection; flu vaccine to prevent influenza; and Pneumovax to prevent pneumococcal pneumonia • Adequate fluid intake and, in selected patients, chest physiotherapy to mobilize secretions • O_2 at low-flow settings to treat hypoxia • Avoidance of smoking and air pollutants
• *Physical examination:* rhonchi and wheezes on auscultation, expiratory elongation, neck vein distention, pedal edema • *Chest X-ray:* may show hyperinflation and increased bronchovascular markings • *Pulmonary function tests:* increased residual volume, decreased vital capacity and forced expiratory flow, normal static compliance and diffusing capacity • *Arterial blood gas measurements:* decreased PaO_2 level, normal or increased $PaCO_2$ level • *Sputum:* contains many organisms and neutrophils • *EKG:* may show atrial dysrhythmias; peaked P waves in leads II, III, and AVF; and, occasionally, right ventricular hypertrophy	• Antibiotics for infections • Avoidance of smoking and air pollutants • Bronchodilators to relieve bronchospasm and facilitate mucociliary clearance • Adequate fluid intake and chest physiotherapy to mobilize secretions • Ultrasonic or mechanical nebulizer treatments to loosen secretions and aid in mobilization • Occasionally, patients respond to corticosteroids. • Diuretics for edema • Oxygen for hypoxia

(continued)

Chronic Obstructive Pulmonary Disease   *(continued)*

Disease	Causes and pathophysiology	Clinical features
Asthma • Increased bronchial reactivity to various stimuli, which produces episodic bronchospasm and airway obstruction • Asthma with onset in adulthood: typically without distinct allergies; asthma with onset in childhood: typically associated with definite allergens. Status asthmaticus is an acute asthma attack with severe bronchospasm that fails to clear with bronchodilator therapy. • Prognosis: More than half of asthmatic children become asymptomatic as adults; more than half of asthmatics with onset after age 15 have persistent disease, with occasional severe attacks.	• Possible mechanisms include allergy (family tendency, seasonal occurrence); allergic reaction results in release of mast cell vasoactive and bronchospastic mediators. • Upper airway infection, exercise, anxiety, and rarely, coughing or laughing can precipitate an asthma attack. • Paroxysmal airway obstruction associated with nasal polyps may occur in response to aspirin or indomethacin ingestion. • Airway obstruction from spasms of bronchial smooth muscle narrows airways; inflammatory edema of the bronchial wall and inspissation of tenacious mucoid secretions are also important, particularly in status asthmaticus.	• History of intermittent attacks of dyspnea and wheezing • Mild wheezing progresses to severe dyspnea, audible wheezing, chest tightness (a feeling of being unable to breathe), and cough productive of thick mucus. • Other signs: prolonged expiration, intercostal and supraclavicular retraction on inspiration, use of accessory respiratory muscles, flaring nostrils, tachypnea, tachycardia, perspiration, and flushing; patients commonly have symptoms of eczema and allergic rhinitis (hay fever). • Status asthmaticus, unless treated promptly, can progress to respiratory failure.

drugs, may be used to control the underlying disease. Other interventions include administering oxygen therapy, mobilizing secretions, improving breathing techniques, stopping smoking, improving physical fitness, conserving energy, ensuring good nutrition, and relieving depression and anxiety.

Administering medications

• *Beta adrenergics:* Bronchodilators (including beta adrenergics [sympathomimetics] and methylxanthine derivatives) top the list of drugs most commonly used to treat COPD. Classified as beta$_1$ and beta$_2$, beta adrenergics mimic sympathetic nervous system activity. Beta$_1$ drugs, such as epinephrine, increase heart rate and contractility and stimulate coronary vasodilation and bronchodilation. Beta$_2$ drugs dilate bronchial passages and veins and relax smooth muscles. Most bronchodilators affect both the heart and lungs. However, some (for example, albuterol and metaproterenol sulfate) act mainly on the respiratory system. Isoproterenol hydrochloride mainly affects the cardiovascular system.

Confirming diagnostic measures	Management
• *Physical examination:* usually normal between attacks; auscultation shows rhonchi and wheezing throughout lung fields on expiration and, at times, inspiration; absent or diminished breath sounds during severe obstruction. Loud bilateral wheezes may be grossly audible; chest is hyperinflated. • *Chest X-ray:* hyperinflated lungs with air trapping during attack; normal during remission • *Sputum:* presence of Curschmann's spirals (casts of airways), Charcot-Leyden crystals, and eosinophils • *Pulmonary function tests:* during attacks, decreased forced expiratory flows that improve significantly after inhaled bronchodilator; increased residual volume and, occasionally, total lung capacity; may be normal between attacks • *Arterial blood gas measurements:* decreased Pao_2 level; decreased, normal, or increased $Paco_2$ level (in severe attack) • *EKG:* sinus tachycardia during an attack; severe attack may produce signs of cor pulmonale (right axis deviation, peaked P wave) that resolve after the attack • *Skin tests:* may identify allergens	• Aerosol-containing beta-adrenergic agents, such as metaproterenol or albuterol; also, oral beta-adrenergic agents (terbutaline) and oral methylxanthines (aminophylline). Occasionally, patients require inhaled, oral, or I.V. corticosteroids. • *Emergency treatment:* O_2 therapy, corticosteroids, and bronchodilators, such as subcutaneous epinephrine, I.V. aminophylline, and inhaled agents, such as isoproterenol • Monitor for deteriorating respiratory status and note sputum characteristics; provide adequate fluid intake and oxygen, as ordered. • *Prevention:* Tell the patient to avoid possible allergens and to use antihistamines, decongestants, inhalation of cromolyn, and oral or aerosol bronchodilators, as ordered. Explain the effects of stress and anxiety on asthma and frequent association with exercise (particularly running) and cold air.

Because beta-adrenergic abuse (especially with inhalers) can be a major clinical problem, teach your patient not to overuse these medications. Also teach him to use and clean inhalers correctly. Always have him give a return demonstration after your initial instructions and then periodically after treatment begins.

• *Methylxanthines:* Aminophylline and theophylline relieve smooth muscle spasms of the respiratory tract. Remind the patient taking these drugs to decrease his consumption of caffeine-containing beverages, including coffee, tea, or colas. Too much caffeine can interact with theophylline and cause jitteriness and toxicity. Also, monitor the patient's serum theophylline levels. Instruct the patient taking theophylline to take his medication on time. Skipping doses or stopping the drug can cause symptoms to reappear.

• *Corticosteroids:* These drugs help relieve inflammation. Warn the patient never to discontinue corticosteroids abruptly to avoid adrenal crisis, a life-threatening disorder. Also explain that these drugs can cause serious adverse effects, including Cushing's syndrome,

Predisposing Factors to COPD

- Cigarette smoking
- Recurrent or chronic respiratory infections
- Allergies
- Familial and hereditary factors (such as alpha$_1$-antitrypsin deficiency)
- Chronic exposure to lung irritants or air pollution
- Advanced age
- Male sex

Smoking—by far the most important predisposing factor—impairs ciliary action and macrophage function and causes airway inflammation, increased mucus production, destruction of alveolar septae, and peribronchiolar fibrosis. Early inflammatory changes may reverse if the patient stops smoking before extensive lung destruction occurs.

weight gain, osteoporosis, diabetes, peptic ulcers, masking of infections, and psychosis.

Beclomethasone, a steroid taken orally via metered-dose inhaler, causes fewer adverse systemic effects than oral corticosteroids. The doctor may order beclomethasone for a patient who is tapering off or has stopped oral steroids.

If your patient uses a beta-adrenergic spray, such as metaproterenol, in addition to beclomethasone, tell him to use the beta adrenergic first, to wait 15 minutes, then to use beclomethasone. The beta adrenergic will open the airway, allowing better beclomethasone distribution.

• *Antibiotics:* These drugs help treat a COPD patient's acute bacterial infection and control infectious bronchiectasis.

• *Expectorants:* Expectorants usually don't liquefy mucus effectively. Drinking plenty of fluids usually eliminates the patient's need for expectorants. (However, increased fluid intake

may be contraindicated by a cardiac problem or other disorder.)

• *Anticholinergics:* When stimulated, the cholinergic nervous system constricts bronchial airways. Anticholinergic drugs, such as atropine sulfate, counteract this effect, relaxing smooth muscles and dilating bronchial tubes.

• *Other medications:* Advise all COPD patients to avoid sedatives, sleeping pills, and narcotics, which can cause respiratory depression. (Morphine's especially risky for a COPD patient, and its use isn't advocated for these patients. Besides depressing respiration, morphine increases histamine release, which constricts airways.)

Administering oxygen therapy

A COPD patient usually needs oxygen therapy during acute episodes and possibly for routine home care also. The doctor usually orders low-flow oxygen via nasal cannula for a patient with a PaO$_2$ level less than 55 mm Hg or with cor pulmonale.

Use caution when administering oxygen to a COPD patient; too much may eliminate his breathing stimulus. In a healthy person, an increased PaCO$_2$ level stimulates breathing. (See *The Hypoxic Drive* on page 244 in Chapter 11.)

But because the COPD patient retains CO$_2$, he doesn't respond to a PaCO$_2$ increase. Instead, hypoxia stimulates his breathing—a phenomenon called hypoxic drive. A COPD patient who receives too much oxygen may stop breathing.

Stopping smoking

The more a COPD patient smokes, the faster his condition deteriorates. Encourage him to quit; if necessary, refer him to a stop-smoking clinic.

Improving breathing techniques

The COPD patient breathes ineffectively, using his upper chest and accessory muscles too much and his diaphragm too little. Teach him how to breathe with his diaphragm. He'll probably need several training sessions to master the technique. (However, a patient with severe disease or a flattened diaphragm may never properly incorporate diaphragmatic breathing into his normal breathing pattern.) See Chapter 10 for information on proper deep-breathing methods.

Mobilizing secretions
Postural drainage, chest percussion, and vibration help the COPD patient remove secretions. Teach him and his family how to perform these techniques at home. See Chapter 10 for more information on these techniques.

Improving physical fitness
Many COPD patients experience dyspnea on exertion and may avoid activity whenever possible. However, a sedentary life-style decreases physical fitness so that eventually any activity becomes intolerable.

To help your patient break the in-activity cycle, encourage him to set short-term goals to gradually increase his activity level. Instruct him to walk regularly, for instance, but not to the point that he tires or feels extremely short of breath.

Coordinating the patient's activities with his respiratory cycle will also help him increase his activity level. For example, have him use this pattern when climbing stairs: Exhale when climbing a stair or two, then inhale while resting. When walking, he should take two steps while inhaling and four while exhaling. (Of course, these patterns may not work for everyone. Help your patient find what works best for him.) Be sure to check with your hospital's physical therapy department before increasing your patient's activity level, and include this department in patient teaching.

Conserving energy
Teach your patient the following energy-conserving strategies to help him carry out activities of daily living without taxing his respiratory system:
• Sit for as many activities as possible—sitting requires less energy than

standing. While showering, sit on a bathtub seat; while shaving, sit in front of the sink.
• Alternate easy and hard tasks instead of trying to do several hard tasks in a row.
• Organize the home logically, placing frequently used items within easy reach. If necessary, consult an occupational therapist for more energy-conserving techniques.

Ensuring good nutrition
Encourage your patient to eat nutritious, well-balanced meals. If he has a dietary problem, consult a nutritionist. To help ensure adequate nutrition and prevent his condition from worsening, also suggest the following:
• Eat six small daily meals instead of three large meals. A large meal can lead to abdominal distention, which interferes with diaphragm movement.
• Avoid gas-forming foods, such as broccoli, cauliflower, and onions, and carbonated beverages, which may also distend the abdomen.
• Rest for 30 minutes before eating to avoid tiring during a meal.
• Lose weight if necessary; obesity restricts lung movements.
• Take breathing treatments, such as postural drainage, at least 1 hour before eating so secretions won't interfere with the meal.
• Practice good mouth care before meals so secretions won't dull the appetite.
• If the patient is receiving oxygen via nasal cannula, he should wear the cannula while eating to maintain adequate oxygenation.

Relieving depression and anxiety
A COPD patient may become depressed about his disease and the physical limitations it imposes. Encourage him to express his feelings. If he's also anxious, suggest relaxation exercises or biofeedback. If these measures don't help, consider referring him to individual counseling or a support group. The doctor may order psychothera-

Bronchiectasis

In this chronic lung disorder, repeated episodes of acute bronchial infection with heavy, productive coughing alternate with periods of chronic infection and mild coughing. The disease's chief physiologic characteristics include destruction and dilation of the airways' inner lining.

Like chronic bronchitis, bronchiectasis causes violent coughing, dyspnea, and heavy sputum production. However, in bronchiectasis, sputum stagnates in dilated bronchi. When finally expectorated, it usually smells foul and separates into three distinct layers: a cloudy top layer; a central layer of clear saliva; and a bottom layer of heavy, thick, purulent matter. Hemoptysis also suggests bronchiectasis rather than chronic bronchitis.

A routine chest X-ray of a bronchiectasis patient may show lung scarring, atelectasis, and fluid accumulation. To confirm the diagnosis, the doctor will order bronchography, which outlines bronchial walls so that an X-ray can then reveal affected areas.

Treatment aims to control any respiratory infection; remove irritants; and loosen and drain secretions with aerosols, percussion, and postural drainage.

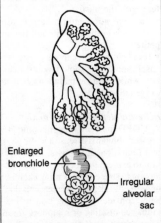

Enlarged bronchiole

Irregular alveolar sac

peutic drugs to reduce anxiety, but only in a low dosage that won't cause respiratory depression. (See *Bronchiectasis.*)

Cystic fibrosis
(Mucoviscidosis)

Description
Cystic fibrosis (CF) is a generalized dysfunction of the exocrine glands. An incurable chronic progressive disease, it affects multiple organ systems in varying degrees of severity. It's the most common fatal genetic disease among white children. CF shortens the patient's life span; the median survival age is 26 years. Approximately 25% of CF patients are adults (age 18 and older).

Cause
CF is inherited as an autosomal recessive trait.

Pathophysiology
The underlying biochemical defect probably reflects a protein or enzyme alteration. (Cystic fibrosis accounts for almost all cases of pancreatic enzyme deficiency in children.)

Immediate causes of CF symptoms include increased viscosity of bronchial, pancreatic, and other mucous gland secretions and subsequent obstruction of glandular ducts.

Researchers now theorize that CF results from an abnormality in chloride transport across the cell membrane. This leads to dehydration and mucosal thickening in the respiratory and intestinal tracts. This theory explains the elevated sweat chloride levels typical in this disorder.

Signs and symptoms
Clinical effects of CF may become apparent soon after birth or may take years to develop. They include major aberrations in sweat gland, respiratory, and gastrointestinal (GI) func-

tions. Sweat gland dysfunction ranks as the most consistent abnormality. Increased sodium and chloride concentrations in the sweat lead to hyponatremia and hypochloremia and may eventually induce fatal shock and cardiac dysrhythmias, especially in hot weather, when sweating's profuse.

Respiratory symptoms reflect disabling obstructive changes in the lungs: wheezy respirations; a dry, nonproductive, paroxysmal cough progressing to a moist cough that produces tenacious yellow-green sputum; dyspnea; and tachypnea. These changes stem from accumulation of thick, tenacious secretions in the bronchioles and alveoli and eventually lead to severe atelectasis and bronchiectasis. Consequently, children with advanced CF typically have a barrel chest, cyanosis, and clubbed fingers and toes. They suffer recurring bronchitis and pneumonia and may have associated nasal polyps and sinusitis. Pneumonia or atelectasis usually causes death.

The GI effects of CF occur mainly in the intestines, pancreas, and liver. Among the earliest symptoms is meconium ileus. Because the newborn with CF doesn't excrete meconium—a dark green mucilaginous material found in the intestine at birth—he develops signs and symptoms of intestinal obstruction, such as abdominal distention, vomiting, constipation, rectal prolapse, dehydration, and electrolyte imbalance. Eventually, pancreatic duct obstruction and resulting deficiency of trypsin, amylase, and lipase prevent conversion and absorption of fat and protein in the GI tract. Undigested food is then excreted in characteristically frequent, bulky, foul-smelling, pale stools with a high fat content. This malabsorption causes other abnormalities: poor weight gain and growth, ravenous appetite, distended abdomen, thin extremities, and sallow skin with poor turgor. Inability to absorb fats causes deficiency of fat-soluble vitamins (A, D, E, and K), leading to clotting problems, retarded bone growth, and delayed sexual development. Males may experience azoospermia; females may have delayed menarche or secondary amenorrhea. Rectal prolapse, secondary to malnutrition and wasting of perirectal supporting tissues, typically complicates CF in infants and children with these signs and symptoms.

In the pancreas, fibrotic tissue, multiple cysts, thick mucus, and, eventually, fat replace the acini—small, saclike swellings normally found in this gland. This results in signs and symptoms of pancreatic insufficiency: insufficient insulin production, abnormal glucose tolerance, and glycosuria. These findings usually occur in the older CF patient. Biliary obstruction and fibrosis may prolong neonatal jaundice. In some patients, cirrhosis and portal hypertension may lead to esophageal varices, hematemesis episodes, and, occasionally, hepatomegaly.

Diagnosis

Elevated electrolyte (sodium and chloride) concentrations in sweat in a patient with pulmonary disease or pancreatic insufficiency confirm CF. The sweat test (stimulation of sweat glands, collection of sweat samples, and laboratory analysis) shows that the sweat volume remains normal but its weight increases from higher chloride and sodium concentration. (Sweat's normal sodium concentration is less than 40 mEq/liter; in cystic fibrosis, it rises above 60 mEq/liter.) Although sodium and chloride concentrations normally rise with age, any value greater than 50, even in an adult, strongly suggests CF and calls for repeated testing. Recently, a new screening test has been developed for cystic fibrosis. (See *Cystic Fibrosis: Neonatal Screening Test*, page 162, for more information.)

Examination of duodenal contents for pancreatic enzymes, and stools for trypsin or a 72-hour stool collection for fecal fat content can confirm pan-

Cystic Fibrosis: Neonatal Screening Test

This test, still largely investigational, measures serum immunoreactive trypsinogen (IRT) in neonates to screen for cystic fibrosis (CF).

Unlike most neonatal screening tests that detect inborn errors of metabolism, the IRT test identifies pancreatic disease manifestations. Although this test may not detect CF in neonates without pancreatic involvement (about 15% of the total affected), its results have been encouraging. In studies of the test's effectiveness, infants who tested positive on initial screening were tested again. If they tested positive on the second screening, they were referred for a diagnostic sweat test. Based on those results, researchers estimated the predictive value of a positive IRT test (specificity) with two-tiered screening at 75%; specificity based only on initial screening ranges from 15% to 22%. The predictive value of a *negative* test result (sensitivity) hasn't yet been determined.

The test requires a blood sample obtained via heel stick. The test's purpose, procedure, and limitations must be discussed with the parents, especially because of the relatively high risk of false-positive results on initial screening. Also, parents must be told that if the child tests positive, additional studies must be done to confirm the diagnosis.

Normal and suspect IRT levels are based on percentiles derived from reference neonate populations. Currently, the 99.8 percentile (an IRT concentration of 140 ng/dl) means a positive result on the first screening; the 99.5 percentile (120 ng/dl) means a positive result on the second screening.

No other reliable CF screening methods exist. Although researchers believe the CF gene's located on chromosome 7, they haven't identified the specific gene, and available genetic markers can't be used for wide-scale screening of the general population. Carrier detection and prenatal diagnosis can be done for families who have a living child with CF, provided both biological parents are available for testing. No carrier testing or prenatal diagnosis now exists for the general public. However, scientists believe that the CF gene will soon be identified, making widespread carrier testing and prenatal diagnosis available in large genetic centers.

creatic insufficiency; trypsin's absent in over 80% of children with CF. Chest X-rays, pulmonary function tests, and arterial blood gas determinations assess the patient's pulmonary status. Sputum culture's usually positive for *Staphylococcus aureus, Pseudomonas aeruginosa,* or *Pseudomonas cepacia.* Family history may show siblings or other relatives with CF.

Treatment and clinical considerations

Because CF has no cure, treatment aims to help the child lead a life that's as normal as possible. Teach the child's family about the disease and its complications, and refer them for genetic counseling. The emphasis of treatment depends on the organ systems involved.

• To combat sweat electrolyte losses, treatment measures include replacing sodium losses during hot weather and avoiding strenuous activity to prevent dehydration. Providing an air-conditioned environment also proves helpful, particularly to infants.

• To offset pancreatic enzyme deficiencies, treatment measures include administering oral pancreatic enzymes with meals and snacks. Such supplements improve absorption and digestion and satisfy hunger within a reasonable calorie intake. Ensure a diet that's moderate in fat but high in protein and calories; include supplements of water-miscible, fat-soluble vitamins (A, D, E, and K) if laboratory analysis identifies a deficiency of any of these vitamins.

• Measures to treat pulmonary dysfunction include physical therapy, postural drainage, and breathing exercises several times daily, to aid removal of secretions from lungs. Aerosol therapy includes intermittent nebulizer treatments before postural drainage, to loosen secretions and dilate bronchi. Home care is critical for the CF patient; make sure to teach caregivers these techniques.

• Oxygen therapy may be used in advanced stages.

• Heart-lung transplants may be needed for some patients.

Treatment of pulmonary infection requires:

• loosening and removal of mucopurulent secretions, using an intermittent nebulizer and postural drainage to relieve obstruction

• aggressive use of sputum-sensitive, specific antimicrobials (usually with acute pulmonary infections, because prophylactic use of these drugs causes resistant bacterial strains)

Throughout this illness:

• thoroughly explain all treatment measures, and teach the patient and his family about his disease.

• provide much-needed emotional support. Be flexible about care and visiting hours to allow continuation of schooling and friendships. Because many CF patients now reach adulthood, they must plan for higher education, employment, and marriage. Most men with CF are sterile; some women experience decreased fertility. A few women with mild CF have given birth to healthy children, although some others have experienced significant health deterioration and have delivered premature infants.

For further information on the disease and support groups, refer the patient and his family to the Cystic Fibrosis Foundation and the closest CF treatment center.

Selected References

Emergency Care Handbook. Springhouse, Pa.: Springhouse Corp., 1986.

Glauser, F.L., ed. *Signs and Symptoms in Pulmonary Medicine.* Philadelphia: J.B. Lippincott Co., 1983.

"The Growing Problem of Lung Disease: 1984-1985." American Lung Association Annual Report.

Hahn, K. "Slow-Teaching the COPD Patient," *Nursing87* (17)4:34-41, April 1987.

Higgins, M. "Epidemiology of COPD: State of the Art," *Chest* 85(6): 3S-8S, June 1984.

Mandell, G., et al., eds. *Principles and Practice of Infectious Diseases,* 2nd ed. New York: John Wiley & Sons, 1985.

Nursing Yearbook87. Nurse's Reference Library. Springhouse, Pa.: Springhouse Corp., 1986.

Professional Guide to Diseases, 2nd ed. Springhouse, Pa.: Springhouse Corp., 1987.

Rakel, R. *Textbook of Family Practice,* 3rd ed. Philadelphia: W.B. Saunders Co., 1984.

Respiratory Problems. NurseReview Series. Springhouse, Pa.: Springhouse Corp., 1986.

Shapiro, B.A., et al. *Clinical Applications of Respiratory Care,* 3rd ed. Chicago: Year Book Medical Pubs., Inc., 1985.

Wade, J.F. *Comprehensive Respiratory Care: Physiology and Technique,* 3rd ed. St. Louis: C.V. Mosby Co., 1982.

6 PULMONARY VASCULAR DISORDERS

Introduction

Pulmonary vascular disorders rank among the most serious complications of cardiovascular or respiratory disease. These disorders include pulmonary hypertension, pulmonary edema, and pulmonary embolism.

Pulmonary hypertension occurs in primary and secondary forms. Primary pulmonary hypertension is the only pulmonary vascular disorder that can't be attributed to preexisting cardiovascular or respiratory disease. Secondary pulmonary hypertension may result from congenital or acquired cardiovascular disease as well as from obstructive or restrictive respiratory disease. Pulmonary edema usually stems from cardiac disease; pulmonary embolism, from thrombi formation originating in the venous system; however, nonthrombotic emboli can also occur.

Untreated, these disorders cause severe lung damage that can drastically impair or threaten a patient's life-style. (See *Pulmonary Vascular Disorders and Cor Pulmonale: Clinical Findings in Acute Episodes,* pages 166 and 167.) To promote prompt treatment that helps prevent irreversible complications, you must be able to identify patients at risk for developing these disorders. (See *Pulmonary Vascular Disorders: Complications.*) To minimize permanent respiratory damage, you must know how to evaluate the effectiveness of prescribed therapy when caring for a patient with a known pulmonary vascular disorder. You also must know how to recognize significant and potentially life-threatening changes in the patient's condition.

Pulmonary circulation vs. bronchial circulation

Two main pulmonary arteries originating from the heart's right side supply blood to the alveolar-capillary membrane for gas exchange. Blood reaches the pulmonary trunk from the heart's right ventricle. The trunk branches into the right and left pulmonary arteries, which continue to subdivide as they follow the bronchial airways through the lungs. Eventually, pulmonary arteries branch into microscopic structures called arterioles and venules, which enter the lung lobules and form capillary beds around the alveoli.

Gas exchange occurs at the alveolar-capillary membrane, where the pulmonary capillary and alveolus meet. Oxygenated blood then travels to the left atrium via the pulmonary veins.

Two main bronchial arteries serve as the main sources of bronchial circulation. They descend from the aorta and its branches, supplying oxygen-rich blood to the conducting airways and pleurae. Because they're part of the systemic circulation, they play no part in blood oxygenation.

Compensatory mechanisms

All pulmonary vascular disorders increase pulmonary vascular resistance; however, the pathophysiology of these disorders varies with the underlying cardiovascular or respiratory disease.

To propel blood through a healthy pulmonary vascular system requires only about 10 mm Hg of pressure—roughly 10% of the average systemic intravascular pressure. In pulmonary vascular disorders, however, pressure within the pulmonary circulation must be great enough to overcome pulmonary vascular resistance to ensure adequate lung perfusion for gas exchange. To compensate for this resistance, the body reacts with two mechanisms: tachycardia and tachypnea.

Tachycardia

Although tachycardia may help propel oxygenated blood through a resistant pulmonary vascular system, it may reduce cardiac output because of the concomitant decrease in ventricular filling pressure. As a result, blood flow to the coronary arteries decreases; together with the heart's increased work load, this can cause chest pain.

If pulmonary vascular resistance becomes chronic, the right ventricle's inability to adequately expel its contents against high pulmonary vascular pressure during systole may eventually lead to right ventricular failure. Blood then accumulates in the venous system, causing jugular vein distention and liver engorgement. As right ventricular failure progresses, systemic venous pressure and hydrostatic pressure in peripheral veins rise. Peripheral edema results.

Tachypnea

This second mechanism, coupled with increased depth of respirations, attempts to compensate for decreased oxygenation. The body tries to take in more oxygen while expelling excess carbon dioxide. In chronic conditions, however, persistent tachypnea may result in overcompensation. Then, too much carbon dioxide's expelled, causing respiratory alkalosis.

Pulmonary Vascular Disorders: Complications

If untreated, pulmonary vascular disorders can lead to any of the following complications:

Pulmonary hypertension
- Decreased pulmonary blood flow
- Right ventricular overload
- Right ventricular hypertrophy, possibly leading to cor pulmonale
- Impaired gas exchange
- Increased dead space

Pulmonary embolism
- Pulmonary infarction
- Emboli extension, blocking additional vessels
- Hepatic congestion and necrosis
- Pulmonary abscess
- Shock and adult respiratory distress syndrome
- Massive atelectasis
- Venous overload (evidenced by jugular vein distention, pedal edema)
- Ventilation/perfusion mismatch
- Death (with massive embolism)

Pulmonary edema
- Impaired gas exchange
- Intrapulmonary shunt
- Atelectasis secondary to surfactant depletion
- Adult respiratory distress syndrome
- Respiratory failure

Medical management

Effective treatment of a pulmonary vascular disorder can begin only after its cause has been identified. This requires correlation of diagnostic test results with history and physical findings. Careful analysis of all subjective and objective data may also reveal the disease's extent and identify significant events in the patient's life that may have led to disease development. A typical diagnostic workup for a patient with a suspected pul-

Pulmonary Vascular Disorders and Cor Pulmonale: Clinical Findings in Acute Episodes

Body system or area	Pulmonary hypertension	Pulmonary edema
Respiratory system	• Tachycardia • Cyanosis* • Decreased breath sounds (with loud tubular sounds) • Decreased diaphragmatic excursion and respiration depth	• Dyspnea • Orthopnea • Cyanosis* • Crepitant crackles • Dullness on percussion • Possible wheezing
Cardiovascular system	• Tachycardia • Displaced point of maximal impulse (beyond the midclavicular line) • Possible neck vein distention • Widely split S_2, S_3, or S_4 • Systolic ejection murmur	• Tachycardia • Neck vein distention • Gallop rhythm • Pulsus alternans
Neurologic system	• Restlessness, agitation • Decreased level of consciousness • Confusion, memory loss	• Restlessness, agitation • Decreased level of consciousness • Confusion, memory loss
Abdomen	• Liver enlargement or tenderness	• Liver enlargement or tenderness • Possible use of abdominal muscles

* Development of cyanosis varies depending on the patient's hemoglobin level.

monary vascular disorder includes chest X-rays, lung scan, arterial blood gas analysis, electrocardiography, complete blood cell count, sputum analysis, pulmonary function tests, and pulmonary angiography.

Pulmonary hypertension

Description
In adults, resting systolic pulmonary artery pressure above 30 mm Hg and mean pulmonary artery pressure above 18 mm Hg indicate pulmonary hypertension. The disorder may be primary (rare) or secondary (far more common). Primary or idiopathic pulmonary hypertension occurs most commonly in women between ages 20 and 40. Usually fatal within 3 to 4 years, it has the highest mortality among pregnant women. It's the only pulmonary vascular disorder that can't be attributed to preexisting cardiovascular or respiratory disease.

Secondary pulmonary hypertension results from existing cardiac or pulmonary disease. Prognosis depends on the severity of the underlying disorder.

Causes
Primary pulmonary hypertension
Although the cause remains unknown, a hereditary defect appears likely be-

Pulmonary vascular obstruction	Cor pulmonale
• Tachypnea • Cyanosis* • Decreased diaphragmatic excursion and respiration depth • Crackles at lung bases • Pleural friction rub	• Tachypnea • Shortness of breath with mild exertion • Cyanosis* • Possible crackles at lung bases
• Tachycardia • Widely split S_2, possible S_3 or S_4 • Normal or bounding pulses (may be weaker in legs)	• Tachycardia • Displaced point of maximal impulse (beyond the midclavicular line) • Gallop rhythm • Neck vein distention • Lower extremity and presacral edema
• Restlessness • Decreased level of consciousness • Confusion, memory loss	• Restlessness • Decreased level of consciousness • Confusion, memory loss
• Possible use of abdominal muscles	• Liver enlargement or tenderness

cause this disorder tends to occur within families.

Secondary pulmonary hypertension
Usually, this disorder is secondary to hypoxemia from an underlying disease process, including:
• chronic hypoxemia from chronic obstructive pulmonary disease (most common cause in the United States), sarcoidosis, diffuse interstitial pneumonia, cancer metastases, and scleroderma; other disorders that cause chronic hypoxemia without lung tissue damage include obesity and kyphoscoliosis
• vascular obstruction from pulmonary embolism, vasculitis, and disorders that cause obstructions of small or large pulmonary veins, such as left atrial myxoma, idiopathic veno-occlusive disease, fibrosing mediastinitis, and mediastinal neoplasm
• chest-wall abnormalities, such as thoracic cage deformities
• primary cardiac disease, which may be congenital or acquired. This includes congenital defects that cause left-to-right blood shunting, such as patent ductus arteriosus and atrial or ventricular septal defect. Acquired cardiac disease includes rheumatic valvular disease and mitral stenosis, which increases pulmonary venous pressure by restricting blood flow leaving the heart.

Pathophysiology

Primary pulmonary hypertension

This disorder has a unique pathology. The pulmonary arteries' intimal lining thickens for no apparent reason. This narrows arterial diameter and impairs distensibility, increasing pulmonary vascular resistance. Primary pulmonary hypertension usually causes no symptoms until lung damage becomes severe. This disorder may not be found until autopsy.

Secondary pulmonary hypertension

Various pathologic processes can lead to this disorder—for example, preexisting cardiovascular disease (congenital or acquired). Acyanotic congenital cardiac defects, such as patent ductus arteriosus and atrial and ventricular septal defects, allow left-to-right blood shunting into the pulmonary artery. As a result, blood reroutes through the lungs twice; the additional blood flow can cause pulmonary hypertension. If severe enough and accompanied by sufficiently increased pulmonary vascular resistance, the shunts can decrease and even reverse.

In acquired cardiac disease, left ventricular failure diminishes the flow of oxygenated blood from the lungs. As a result, pulmonary vascular resistance increases, along with right ventricular pressure.

Secondary pulmonary hypertension resulting from obstructive or restrictive respiratory disease may destroy alveoli, causing the lungs to shunt incoming blood to the remaining healthy alveoli. As these alveoli decrease in number, pulmonary vascular resistance rises as more and more blood shunts to a progressively smaller lung area. (See *Pulmonary Hypertension: Tracking the Destructive Cycle*.) Hypoxemia resulting from this ventilation/perfusion mismatch also causes pulmonary vasoconstriction, further increasing pulmonary vascular resistance. If the underlying respiratory defect is chronic, the overwhelming work load on the right ventricle eventually causes it to dilate and hypertrophy, resulting in cor pulmonale. (See *Understanding Cor Pulmonale*, page 170.)

Signs and symptoms

Most patients complain of increasing dyspnea on exertion, weakness, syncope, and fatigability. Many also show signs of right-sided heart failure, including peripheral edema, ascites, neck vein distention, and hepatomegaly. Auscultation reveals abnormalities associated with the underlying disorder. Tachycardia commonly occurs; the point of maximal impulse may be displaced beyond the midclavicular line. Other clinical effects vary according to the underlying disorder.

Diagnosis

Characteristic diagnostic findings include the following:
- *Arterial blood gas (ABG) measurements:* hypoxemia (decreased PaO_2 level)
- *EKG:* right axis deviation and tall or peaked P waves in inferior leads with right ventricular hypertrophy
- *Cardiac catheterization:* increased pulmonary artery pressures (PAPs)—pulmonary systolic pressure above 30 mm Hg; pulmonary capillary wedge pressure (PCWP) usually remains normal but increases if the underlying cause is left atrial myxoma, mitral stenosis, or left ventricular failure. These pressures can also be determined at the bedside using Swan-Ganz catheterization.
- *Pulmonary angiography:* filling defects in pulmonary vessels, such as those that develop in patients with pulmonary emboli
- *Pulmonary function tests:* in underlying obstructive disease, possible decreased flow rates and increased residual volume; in underlying restrictive disease, possible decrease in total lung capacity.

Pulmonary Hypertension: Tracking the Destructive Cycle

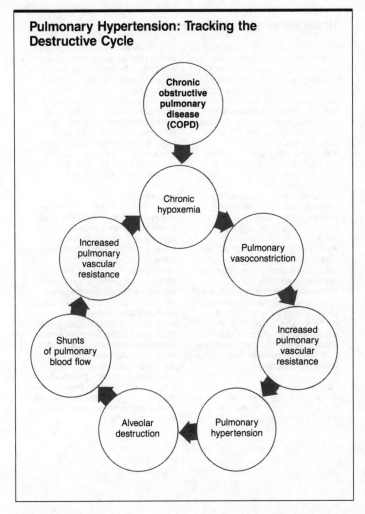

Treatment and clinical considerations

Treatment usually includes oxygen therapy to decrease hypoxemia and resulting increased pulmonary vascular resistance. For patients with right ventricular failure, treatment also includes fluid restriction, digitalis to increase cardiac output, and diuretics to decrease intravascular volume and extravascular fluid accumulation. The most definitive treatment is combined heart/lung transplant. Correction of the underlying cause is another important treatment goal.

Care measures include keen observation and careful monitoring as well as skilled supportive care.

• Administer oxygen therapy, as ordered, and observe the patient's re-

Understanding Cor Pulmonale

Cor pulmonale, or right ventricular hypertrophy, occurs as the end stage of chronic disorders that effect lung function or structure. Although this disorder carries a poor prognosis, treatment aims to reduce hypoxia, increase exercise tolerance, and, when possible, correct the underlying causes. These causes include:
• pulmonary diseases that affect the airways (such as chronic obstructive pulmonary disease and bronchial asthma)
• disorders affecting pulmonary parenchyma (such as sarcoidosis, pulmonary fibrosis, pneumoconiosis, periarteritis nodosa, and tuberculosis)
• vascular diseases (such as vasculitis, pulmonary emboli, or external vascular obstruction caused by tumor or aneurysm)
• chest-wall abnormalities, including such thoracic cage deformities as kyphoscoliosis and pectus excavatum
• other external factors occurring in obese patients, in those living in high altitudes, and in those with neuromuscular disorders (such as muscular dystrophy and poliomyelitis).

Pathophysiology

In cor pulmonale, pulmonary hypertension increases cardiac work load. To compensate, the right ventricle hypertrophies to force blood through the lungs. However, this compensatory mechanism begins to fail and larger amounts of blood remain in the right ventricle at the end of diastole, causing dilatation. In response to hypoxia, the bone marrow produces more red blood cells, resulting in polycythemia. Blood viscosity increases, further aggravating pulmonary hypertension, increasing the right ventricle's work load, and causing failure.

Assessment

Diagnosis rests mainly on the patient's history and the physical findings supported by diagnostic tests. During the physical examination, you'll find displacement of the point of maximal impulse, indicating right ventricular enlargement. You'll hear a gallop rhythm, a loud pulmonic sound, and, with tricuspid insufficiency, a pansystolic murmur at the left sternal border. You'll also detect distended neck veins; dependent edema; tachycardia; an enlarged, tender liver from venous pooling; and a weak pulse and hypotension from decreased cardiac output. Diagnostic tests, such as an echocardiogram, EKG, and chest X-ray, show right ventricular hypertrophy. The complete blood count shows an elevated hematocrit value, reflecting erythrocytosis.

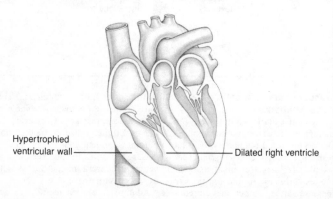

Hypertrophied ventricular wall —   — Dilated right ventricle

sponse. Report any signs of increasing dyspnea so that the doctor can adjust treatment accordingly.

• Monitor ABG measurements for hypoxemia, hypercapnia or hypocapnia, and acidosis or alkalosis. Immediately report any change in level of consciousness.

• When caring for a patient with right-sided heart failure, especially one who's receiving diuretics, record weight daily, carefully measure fluid intake and output, and explain all medications and dietary restrictions. Check for increasing neck vein distention, which may indicate fluid overload. Provide special skin care for dependent edema.

• Monitor vital signs, especially blood pressure and heart rate. Watch for hypotension and tachycardia. If the patient has a pulmonary artery catheter, check PAP and PCWP, as ordered, and report any changes.

• Before discharge, help the patient adjust to the limitations imposed by this disorder. Advise against overexertion and suggest frequent rest periods between activities. Refer the patient to the social services department if he needs special equipment, such as oxygen equipment, for home use. Make sure he understands his prescribed diet and medications.

Pulmonary embolism and infarction

Description

A common pulmonary complication in hospitalized patients, pulmonary embolism (PE) is an obstruction of the pulmonary arterial bed by a dislodged thrombus or foreign substance. It strikes an estimated 6 million adults each year in the United States, resulting in 100,000 deaths. Typically, though, it resolves within 2 weeks.

Pulmonary infarction (tissue death) occurs in 10% to 30% of pulmonary embolism patients. Although pulmo-

nary infarction may be so mild as to be asymptomatic, massive pulmonary embolism, defined as occlusion of 50% or more of the pulmonary arterial circulation, can cause lethal hemodynamic changes, suddenly or within a few hours. Embolism of medium-sized vessels may cause pulmonary infarction, which also can be rapidly fatal. (See *Who's at Risk for Pulmonary Embolism?*, page 173.)

Causes

The causes of PE include dislodged thrombi, most commonly originating in deep leg veins, typically from thrombophlebitis. Less common sources include the pelvic veins, renal veins, hepatic vein, right heart, upper extremities, and tricuspid or pulmonic valves. (Thrombi may embolize spontaneously during clot dissolution or may be dislodged during trauma, sudden muscle action, or a change in peripheral blood flow.)

Rarely, PE may stem from nonthrombic emboli such as fat emboli (may occur after long bone fracture), septic emboli (from I.V. injection of drugs intended for oral administration), amniotic emboli, and air emboli.

Pulmonary infarction may evolve from PE, especially in patients with chronic cardiac or pulmonary disease.

Pathophysiology

Pulmonary embolism occurs when a mass lodges in a pulmonary artery branch, partially or completely obstructing it. The mass can be bone, air, fat, amniotic fluid, a thrombus (blood clot), or a foreign object, such as a needle or catheter part.

If a thrombus (caused by trauma, sudden muscle action, or intravascular pressure changes) occludes the vein, it may loosen or fragmentize. Once dislodged, the thrombus floats to the heart's right side and enters the lung through the pulmonary artery. The thrombus—now called an embolus—may dissolve, continue to fragmentize, or grow. If it's small enough to dissolve or fragmentize before symptoms develop, phagocytes will digest the remains. On the other hand, if the embolus enlarges, it may clog most or all pulmonary vessels and cause death.

Once an embolism develops, platelets and red and white blood cells in the clot release vasoactive substances, including serotonin, histamine, prostaglandin, and thromboxane. These substances constrict bronchial passages, decreasing lung volume and compliance.

Hypoxemia also arises in PE, resulting from ventilation/perfusion ($\dot{V}/\dot{Q}$) mismatch. Dead space increases markedly. When an embolus blocks the vessel, some alveoli can't be adequately perfused but can be normally ventilated. Consequently, adjacent alveoli become overperfused as the body redistributes blood to nonembolized vessels.

Intrapulmonary shunting also occurs during PE. Because the pulmonary artery's occluded, alveoli can't produce enough surfactant to maintain alveolar integrity. As a result, alveoli collapse and atelectasis develops. As pulmonary artery pressure (PAP) increases, preexisting pulmonary arteriovenous anastomoses open. Finally, increasing PAPs (which damage endothelial cells and increase capillary permeability) cause postembolic edema.

In a patient with a normal cardiopulmonary history, occlusions of less than 50% rarely cause hemodynamic problems because the normal lung has patent but unperfused capillaries. As pulmonary artery pressure increases, these capillaries maintain pulmonary vascular circulation.

Expect a patient with recurrent or massive PE (occlusion greater than 50%) to develop pulmonary hypertension—a result of increased vascular resistance. The pressure needed to move a given volume of blood through the lungs significantly increases with arterial occlusion. Chronic multiple

small PEs can also cause cor pulmonale. (See *Understanding Cor Pulmonale*, page 170.)

Right atrial pressure, right ventricular pressure, and PAP also increase. Initially, the volume of blood that enters the left ventricle from the pulmonary circulation decreases. To maintain cardiac output, the right ventricle contracts with a greater-than-normal force. However, the heart can't maintain this increased effort indefinitely, and ventricular strain and right-sided heart failure develop.

PE may precipitate pulmonary hemorrhage and pulmonary infarction. Hemorrhaging causes congestion that may lead to hemoptysis. Pulmonary infarction occurs in a small percentage of PE patients, even when the embolus totally obstructs the pulmonary artery. Because the lung's parenchyma has three oxygen sources—alveolar air, bronchial circulation, and pulmonary circulation—infarction can usually be circumvented. However, it may occur in patients with underlying heart disease and left ventricular failure. In most cases, parenchymal hemorrhaging and necrosis result. Eventually, cavitation or scarring develop in the infarcted area. But death can also occur from pulmonary infarction. In this case, the occlusion's usually total and the patient dies immediately.

If total occlusion does occur, one of two defense mechanisms may correct the problem. The first mechanism—resolution—restores normal vascular flow by dissolving the embolus. The second mechanism—organization—incorporates the damaged area into the affected vessel's lining.

Signs and symptoms

Total occlusion of the main pulmonary artery rapidly proves fatal; smaller or fragmented emboli produce symptoms that vary with emboli size, number, and location. Usually, the first symptom of PE is dyspnea, which may be accompanied by anginal or pleuritic chest pain. Other clinical features in-

Who's at Risk for Pulmonary Embolism?

Hospitalized patients risk developing pulmonary embolism (PE) for many reasons. For example, the anesthestic used during surgery can injure lung vessels. Surgery itself or prolonged bed rest can promote venous stasis, which compounds the risk.

Conditions that promote venous stasis include:
• prolonged bed rest or immobilization
• obesity
• advanced age (over 40)
• burns
• postpartum
• orthopedic casts.

Conditions that can cause venous injury include:
• surgery, particularly on the legs, pelvis, abdomen, or thorax
• leg or pelvic fractures or injuries

• I.V. drug abuse
• I.V. therapy.

Conditions that increase blood coagulability include:
• cancer
• use of high-estrogen oral contraceptives.

Disorders that put patient at higher risk of developing PE include:
• lung disease, especially chronic types
• heart disease
• infection
• diabetes mellitus
• history of thromboembolism, thrombophlebitis, or vascular insufficiency
• polycythemia
• long-bone fracture
• manipulation/disconnection of central line.

clude tachycardia, productive cough (sputum may be blood-tinged), low-grade fever, and pleural effusion. Less common signs include massive hemoptysis, chest splinting, leg edema, and, with a large embolus, cyanosis, syncope, and distended neck veins.

In addition, PE may cause pleural friction rub and signs of circulatory collapse (such as weak, rapid pulse and hypotension) and hypoxia (such as restlessness).

In pulmonary infarction, sharp pleuritic chest pain accompanied by fever or hemoptysis can occur if the patient has progressive dyspnea. Listen for pleural friction rub on auscultation.

Diagnosis

Patient history typically reveals predisposing conditions for PE.
• Chest X-ray usually is inconclusive in the immediate postembolism period (1 to 2 hours). However, it may help by ruling out other pulmonary diseases and showing atelectatic areas, elevated diaphragm and pleural effusion, prominent pulmonary artery, and, occasionally, the characteristic wedge-shaped infiltrate suggestive of PE.
• Lung scintigraphy may show uneven densities on the lung perfusion and ventilation scans, strongly suggesting PE. However, results may be inconclusive. Schedule these tests within 48 hours of symptom onset to increase their accuracy.
• Pulmonary angiography, the most definitive test, requires a skilled angiographer and radiologic equipment; it also poses some risk to the patient. Even so, it's usually used if facilities are immediately available. Two findings indicate PE: a pulmonary vessel filling defect and an abrupt vessel ending.

Pulmonary angiography proves especially important when accurate diagnosis must be made quickly, such as for patients considered for vena caval interruption, embolectomy, or fibrinolytic therapy, or when anticoagulant therapy is contraindicated.

• EKG is inconclusive but helps distinguish pulmonary embolism from myocardial infarction. In extensive embolism, EKG may show right axis deviation; right bundle branch block; tall peaked P waves; depressed ST segments; inverted T waves (reflecting right heart strain), and supraventricular tachydysrhythmias.

• Auscultation occasionally reveals a right ventricular S_3 gallop and increased intensity of a pulmonic S_2 component. Also, crackles and a pleural rub may occur at the embolism site.

• Arterial blood gas (ABG) measurements typically show decreased PaO_2 and $PaCO_2$ levels (although these don't always occur).

If the patient has pleural effusion, thoracentesis may rule out empyema, which indicates pneumonia.

• Magnetic resonance imaging may be helpful. This diagnostic test is based on the interaction of body organs and tissues with a magnetic field and radiofrequency pulses. In normal blood vessels, the radio signal doesn't transmit, creating a black image. In occluded vessels, signal intensity increases, either from the embolus itself or from a blood flow change.

Treatment

Treatment aims to maintain adequate cardiopulmonary function during resolution of the obstruction and to prevent recurrence of embolic episodes. It consists of oxygen therapy, as needed, and anticoagulation with heparin to inhibit new thrombus formation. (Heparin doesn't dissolve existing clots but can prevent new clots from forming.) Depending on specific conditions, other drugs may be ordered.

Drug therapy
Heparin. An anticoagulant typically given in suspected PE, heparin combines with thrombin to prevent the formation of fibrin, the major blood clot component.

Administer heparin by continuous I.V. infusion or intermittent I.V. bolus injection, as ordered. Monitor activated partial thromboplastin time (APTT) to maintain a level 1½ to 2 times the control level. Heparin therapy usually lasts 7 to 10 days.

Although associated with few complications, heparin may cause bleeding—a result of its anticoagulant effect and the thrombocytopenia it induces. Avoid administering antiplatelet drugs, such as aspirin and dipyridamole (Persantine), while the patient's on heparin therapy. Protamine sulfate will neutralize heparin's effects if bleeding occurs.

Sodium warfarin (Coumadin). The doctor may order long-term oral anticoagulant therapy (3 to 6 months) if the patient's at risk for recurrent thromboembolism. Warfarin acts by depleting the body's clotting factors. Usually, you'll give heparin concomitantly with warfarin for 3 to 4 days (before switching to warfarin alone) to allow for vitamin K depletion.

Warfarin's dosage depends on the patient's prothrombin time (PT), which the drug should maintain at twice his normal level. Check PT daily when therapy starts, then weekly for a month, and monthly thereafter.

Like heparin, warfarin can cause bleeding. If bleeding occurs, administer vitamin K, as ordered. Vitamin K takes approximately 4 hours to reverse warfarin's action. If bleeding is serious, your patient may need fresh frozen plasma to stabilize his PT.

Thrombolytic agent. Hemodynamically unstable patients or those with severely compromised respiratory status (resulting from PE) may require thrombolytic therapy with streptokinase or urokinase. Use of these agents is becoming increasingly common.

Initially, thrombolytic agents dissolve clots within 12 to 24 hours. Seven days later, these drugs lyse clots to the same degree as heparin therapy alone.

Obtained from the group C beta-hemolytic streptococci, streptokinase forms an activator complex with plasminogen, converting uncomplexed plasminogen to plasmin. Urokinase, obtained from renal cells, directly converts plasminogen to plasmin.

Your patient's coagulation profile will guide thrombolytic therapy. Before starting therapy, check his baseline complete blood count, platelet count, PT, partial thromboplastin time (PTT), and thrombin time. Then, as ordered, administer both streptokinase and urokinase in an initial loading dose followed by either streptokinase, given for 24 hours, or urokinase, given for 12 hours. Every 4 hours during treatment, check the patient's PTT and thrombin times, which should be maintained at 2 to 5 times normal (streptokinase) or 1½ to 5 times normal (urokinase).

When thrombolytic therapy stops, initiate I.V. heparin therapy, as ordered, when thrombin time or PTT falls below twice baseline. Then manage heparin and long-term anticoagulation as if the patient never received thrombolytic agents.

Bleeding, a common side effect, occurs because streptokinase and urokinase lyse not just the PE but also clots formed as a hemostatic defense mechanism. If bleeding occurs with thrombolytic treatment, stop the drug and administer fresh frozen plasma, cryoprecipitate, and fibrinogen, as ordered.

Dihydroergotamine mesylate/heparin sodium (Embolex). Recently approved for the treatment of PE, this combination drug constricts veins, counteracts venous stasis, and promotes venous return from the legs. By inactivating thrombin and preventing fibrinogen's conversion to fibrin, it also inhibits hypercoagulation.

As ordered, administer the drug 2 hours postoperatively; then give every 12 hours for 5 to 7 days by subcutaneous injection in the abdominal fat pads above the iliac crest.

Embolex may cause hemorrhaging, mild pain, local irritation, ecchymosis,

or hematoma at the injection site. Be sure to monitor the patient's PT and APTT.

Surgical interventions
Vena caval interruption. Venous interruption is indicated when:
• heparin therapy is contraindicated or fails
• multiple, small PEs causing cor pulmonale and pulmonary hypertension develop
• pulmonary embolectomy is performed
• PEs lead to septic emboli
• the patient couldn't tolerate another PE.

Doctors once used plication, clipping, and ligation of the inferior vena cava to interrupt venous flow. Today they rarely perform these procedures because of the high mortality. Instead, they use a catheterization technique, guided by a fluoroscope, to insert a Mobin-Uddin or Kim-Ray-Greenfield filter through the jugular or femoral vein (see *Embolism Surgery*, page 176). This procedure requires only local anesthesia, a key factor in its low mortality.

Although vena caval interruption prevents recurrent PE, it doesn't treat existing emboli. The patient will need heparin therapy 12 hours after filter placement and long-term anticoagulation treatment for deep-vein thrombosis.
Surgical embolectomy. A surgical procedure that extracts the embolus, embolectomy is usually reserved for patients with:
• massive PE causing shock
• systolic blood pressure less than 90 mm Hg
• urine output less than 20 ml/hour
• PaO$_2$ level below 60 mm Hg after 1 hour of unsuccessful PE management.

The patient's usually placed on cardiopulmonary bypass during open surgical embolectomy. Because the procedure's so extensive and used only as a last resort, be prepared to give comprehensive care to the patient if he survives surgery.

Embolism Surgery

These illustrations show two surgical interventions to prevent recurrent pulmonary embolism. In the filter method, a Mobin-Uddin or Kim-Ray-Greenfield filter, inserted through the jugular or femoral vein, traps emboli while allowing blood to flow to the lungs. In the ligation method, the surgeon ties off the vena cava to stop emboli from migrating to the lungs.

Filter Method

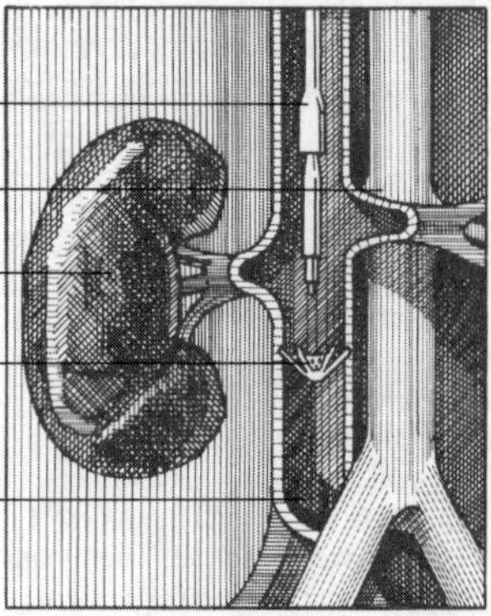

Applicator stylet unscrewed from filter and about to be withdrawn

Aorta

Kidney

Filter in place with spokes imbedded in vena caval walls

Inferior vena cava

Ligation method

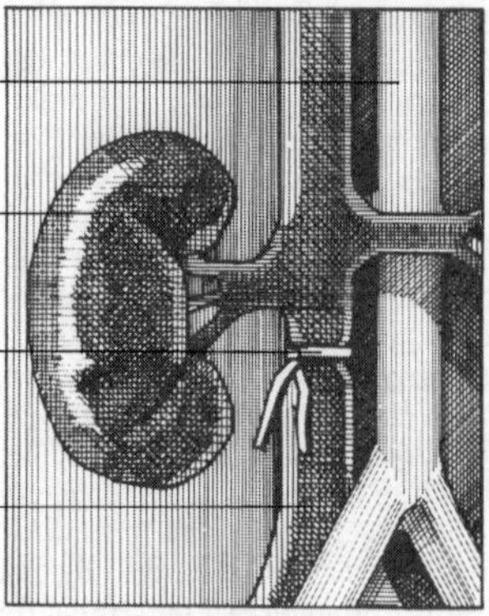

Aorta

Kidney

Ligation

Inferior vena cava

Transvenous catheter embolectomy, a promising alternative to surgical embolectomy, involves only local anesthesia. The surgeon inserts a catheter with a cup device into the femoral vein. Using fluoroscopy, he guides the catheter to the embolus, then applies suction to the cup, using an attached syringe. If the cup's in the right position, a vacuum will develop, suctioning the clot. The patient's PAPs drop immediately whereas his PaO_2 level and cardiac output increase.

If the patient suffers cardiopulmonary arrest during transvenous catheter embolectomy, the doctor will perform open surgical embolectomy.

Other interventions

If your patient's hypoxemic or dyspneic, you may administer supplemental oxygen. Monitor serial ABG measurements for improvement during oxygenation. Encourage coughing, deep breathing, and incentive spirometry to help keep the alveoli inflated. Give sedatives and analgesics as ordered.

To prevent venous stasis, elevate the patient's legs 6″ to 8″ if he's been on bed rest for 24 hours or more. If he's bedridden, make sure he wears thromboembolic stockings to divert venous flow to large veins, or wrap his legs with an Ace bandage. Help him exercise his legs, both actively and passively. Encourage early ambulation.

Intermittent calf compression decreases the risk of deep-vein thrombosis and PE, especially in orthopedic patients. A cuff applied to the leg automatically inflates at 1-minute intervals, increasing venous blood flow and fibrinolysis. *Important:* Because patients on bed rest are at risk for thrombus development in the lower extremities, never massage the legs of these patients. This may result in thrombus dislodgment.

Continuous passive motion devices help prevent thrombosis after surgery by improving venous blood flow.

Clinical considerations

• As ordered, give oxygen by nasal cannula or mask. Check ABG measurements if the patient develops new emboli or worsening dyspnea. Be prepared to help with endotracheal intubation with assisted ventilation if breathing's severely compromised.

• Administer heparin, as ordered. Monitor coagulation studies, particularly the patient's PT and APTT. Report values greater than 1½ to 2 times normal. Watch closely for nosebleeds, petechiae, and other signs of abnormal bleeding; check stools for occult blood. Tell the patient to prevent bleeding by using an electric razor instead of a safety razor, to brush his teeth with a soft toothbrush, and to avoid injections whenever possible.

• After the patient's stable, encourage him to move about often and assist with isometric and range-of-motion exercises. Check pedal pulses, temperature, and foot color to detect venostasis. *Never* vigorously massage the patient's legs. Offer diversional activities to promote rest and relieve restlessness.

• Have the patient ambulate as soon as possible after surgery to prevent venostasis.

• Maintain adequate nutrition and fluid balance to promote healing.

• Report frequent pleuritic chest pain; the doctor may order analgesics. Encourage incentive spirometry to assist in deep breathing. Provide tissues and a bag, for easy disposal of expectorated material.

• Warn the patient not to cross his legs because this promotes thrombus formation.

• To relieve anxiety, explain all procedures and treatments. Encourage the patient's family to participate in his care.

• Most patients need an oral anticoagulant (warfarin) for 4 to 6 months after PE. Advise these patients to watch for signs of bleeding (bloody stools, blood in urine, large ecchymoses), to take prescribed medication exactly as ordered, and to avoid taking any additional medication (even for headaches or colds) or changing medication doses without consulting the doctor. Stress the importance of avoiding aspirin or over-the-counter products containing aspirin. Tell patients to inform dentists and other health-care providers that they're receiving anticoagulant therapy. Stress the importance of follow-up laboratory tests (such as PT) to monitor anticoagulant therapy effects.

• Consider prevention of PE a crucial responsibility when planning care for the patient at risk for PE. For example, be sure to encourage early ambulation in high-risk patients. With close medical supervision, low-dose heparin may be useful prophylactically.

Pulmonary edema

Description
Pulmonary edema refers to fluid accumulation in extravascular lung spaces. In cardiogenic pulmonary edema, fluid accumulation results from elevated pulmonary venous and capillary hydrostatic pressures. A common complication of cardiac disorders, pulmonary edema can occur as a chronic condition or can develop quickly and rapidly cause death.

Causes
Pulmonary edema usually results from left ventricular failure caused by arteriosclerotic, hypertensive, cardiomyopathic, or valvular cardiac disease. Pulmonary edema from decreased colloid osmotic pressure occurs with burns, severe malnutrition, and hepatic disease. (See *Pulmonary Edema: Predisposing Factors.*)

Pathophysiology
Two mechanisms can result in pulmonary edema: increased pulmonary capillary hydrostatic pressure and decreased colloid osmotic pressure. Under normal circumstances, the two pressures remain in balance. When this balance changes, pulmonary edema may result.

In the first mechanism, the compromised left ventricle requires increased filling pressures to maintain adequate output; these pressures are transmitted to the left atrium, pulmonary veins, and pulmonary capillary bed. This increased pulmonary capillary hydrostatic force promotes transudation of intravascular fluids into the pulmonary interstitium, resulting in pulmonary edema; it also decreases lung compliance and interferes with gas exchange. In the second

mechanism, decreased colloid osmotic pressure, the natural pulling force that keeps fluids intravascular, is lost—nothing opposes the hydrostatic force. Thus, fluid can flow freely into the interstitium and alveoli, resulting in pulmonary edema.

Signs and symptoms
Early evidence of pulmonary edema reflects interstitial fluid accumulation and diminished lung compliance: dyspnea on exertion, paroxysmal nocturnal dyspnea, orthopnea, and coughing. Other clinical features include tachycardia, tachypnea, dependent crackles, and a diastolic (S_3) gallop. With severe pulmonary edema, alveoli and bronchioles may fill with fluid and intensify early symptoms. Respiration becomes labored and rapid, with more diffuse crackles and coughing productive of frothy pink-tinged or bloody sputum. Tachycardia increases and dysrhythmias may occur. Skin becomes cold, clammy, diaphoretic, and cyanotic. Blood pressure drops and pulse becomes thready as cardiac output falls.

Signs and symptoms of severe heart failure with pulmonary edema may also include a decreased level of consciousness and confusion as gas exchange becomes increasingly impaired. When pulmonary edema results from decreased colloid osmotic pressure, the respiratory signs and symptoms described earlier occur. Concomitant symptoms arise less commonly but include generalized edema secondary to leaky capillaries.

Diagnosis
Clinical features of pulmonary edema permit a working diagnosis. Arterial blood gas (ABG) measurements usually show hypoxia; the $PaCO_2$ level varies. Profound respiratory alkalosis or acidosis may occur. When cardiac output drops, metabolic acidosis occurs from anaerobic metabolism and lactic acid buildup. Chest X-ray shows diffuse haziness of lung fields and, often,

cardiomegaly and pleural effusions. Pulmonary artery catheterization helps identify left ventricular failure by showing elevated pulmonary capillary wedge pressures (PCWPs). This helps rule out adult respiratory distress syndrome, because PCWP usually remains normal in this disorder.

Treatment and clinical considerations

Treatment of pulmonary edema aims to reduce extravascular fluid, improve gas exchange and myocardial function, and, if possible, correct the underlying pathologic process. Administration of high oxygen concentrations improves oxygen delivery to tissues and may help manage acid-base disturbances. Mechanical ventilation with positive end-expiratory pressure helps decrease alveolar fluid/volume ratio (the positive pressure may help push fluid back across the alveolar-capillary membrane). A bronchodilator, such as aminophylline, may relieve bronchospasm and enhance myocardial contractility. Diuretics, such as furosemide and ethacrynic acid, promote diuresis, thereby helping to mobilize extravascular fluid.

Treatment of myocardial dysfunction includes digitalis or pressor agents to increase cardiac contractility, antiarrhythmics (particularly for dysrhythmias associated with decreased cardiac output), and occasionally arterial vasodilators, such as nitroprusside, which decrease peripheral vascular resistance and thereby reduce left ventricular work load. Other treatment measures include morphine to relieve anxiety and dyspnea and to dilate the systemic venous bed. Rotating tourniquets may be used as an emergency measure to reduce venous return to the heart from the extremities.

• Carefully monitor the high-risk patient for early signs of pulmonary edema, especially tachypnea, tachycardia, and abnormal breath sounds. Report any abnormalities. Check for peripheral edema, which may indicate fluid accumulation in pulmonary tissue.

Pulmonary Edema: Predisposing Factors

The following factors may predispose the patient to pulmonary edema:
• infusion of excessive volumes of I.V. fluids
• decreased serum colloid osmotic pressure as a result of nephrosis, protein-losing enteropathy, extensive burns, hepatic disease, or nutritional deficiency
• impaired lung lymphatic drainage from Hodgkin's disease or obliterative lymphangitis after radiation
• mitral stenosis and left atrial myxoma, which impair left atrial emptying
• pulmonary veno-occlusive disease.

• Administer oxygen, as ordered.
• Monitor vital signs every 15 to 30 minutes while administering nitroprusside in dextrose 5% in water by I.V. drip. Protect it from light by wrapping the bottle or bag with aluminum foil. Discard unused nitroprusside solution after 4 hours. Watch for dysrhythmias if the patient's receiving digitalis, and check for marked respiratory depression if he's receiving morphine.
• Assess the patient's condition frequently, and record his response to treatment. Monitor ABG measurements, oral and I.V. fluid intake, urinary output, and, if he has a pulmonary artery catheter, pulmonary end diastolic and wedge pressures. Check the cardiac monitor often, and report changes immediately.
• Record the sequence and time of rotating tourniquets.
• In a calm voice, reassure the patient, who will be frightened by respiratory impairment. Be sure to explain all procedures. Provide emotional support to his family, too. (See also *Pulmonary Edema: A Crisis Situation,* pages 180 and 181.)

Pulmonary Edema: A Crisis Situation

The situation
John Wilson, age 72, arrives at your emergency department (ED) at 3 a.m., complaining of shortness of breath and a cough that has worsened during the night. He's producing frothy, pink-tinged sputum and appears restless and apprehensive. A frequent visitor to the ED, Mr. Wilson has congestive heart failure, and he's known to be noncompliant with his drug therapy. Your physical findings include cool, clammy skin; peripheral edema; and distended neck veins. Auscultation reveals crackles, wheezes, a heart rate of 146, and an S_3 gallop.

The problem
A patient with congestive heart failure is exhibiting classic signs and symptoms of pulmonary edema.

The worst case
Fluid continues to leak into the lung parenchyma and alveoli and progresses into the larger airways, leading to respiratory arrest. Subsequent dysrhythmias and heart failure lead to cardiogenic shock or cardiac arrest.

The best case
Administration of oxygen and medication relieves the patient's distress. His noncompliance with drug therapy is explored, and new strategies are developed and implemented to encourage compliance, which should help prevent future episodes of pulmonary edema.

The assessment
You observe a patient whose medical history and current signs and symptoms (cough; orthopnea; paroxysmal nocturnal dyspnea; crackles; wheezes; frothy, pink-tinged secretions; gallop rhythm; tachycardia; apprehension; and cool, clammy skin) indicate pulmonary edema of cardiac origin.

Immediate actions
Stay with Mr. Wilson and summon the ED doctor. Quickly review the goals in treating pulmonary edema: decreasing hypoxemia and improving ventilation, retarding venous return and improving cardiac output; and providing mental and physical relaxation.

Place Mr. Wilson in a high Fowler's position with his legs dangling over the side of the bed; this will decrease preload. Administer 30% to 60% oxygen by face mask and start an infusion of dextrose 5% in water at a keep-vein-open rate. Place him on a cardiac monitor and take a 12-lead EKG; look for acute cardiac changes. Also, draw an arterial blood gas sample to determine the level of hypoxemia and associated metabolic acidemia.

As you do these procedures, explain to Mr. Wilson that they'll help ease his distress. Remember, he may feel that the face mask is suffocating him and try to remove it. Because only a face mask can deliver the high oxygen concentration he needs, you'll have to constantly reassure him to reduce his anxiety. If he still can't tolerate the mask, intubation may be needed.

Administer morphine I.V. as ordered; this will cause venodilation and venous pooling, decreasing venous return and myocardial irritability. The drug's euphoric effect will also reduce the patient's anxiety, decreasing catecholamine release. Be prepared to give increased doses, but keep monitoring the patient for signs and symptoms of respiratory depression, and have a narcotic antagonist available.

The doctor will probably order furosemide (Lasix, Novosemide, SK-Furosemide, Uritol), a rapid-acting diuretic, to decrease circulating volume and help eliminate excess fluid. Obtain the patient's baseline vital signs before giving the drug

Pulmonary Edema: A Crisis Situation *(continued)*

and especially note any signs or symptoms of hypotension. Insert an indwelling catheter so that you can measure urine output.

Next, have the respiratory therapist give Mr. Wilson an intermittent positive-pressure breathing treatment, as ordered. This will force fluids from the airways into pulmonary vasculature and expand alveolar spaces. Also, positive pressure in the intrathoracic cavity decreases venous return. Stay alert, though—decreased venous return may cause further deterioration in the patient's condition.

As ordered, administer digoxin (which slows the heart rate and improves cardiac output) and aminophylline (which also improves cardiac output as well as relieves bronchospasm). With both drugs, monitor the patient closely; digoxin toxicity can develop if the patient has hypokalemia, and aminophylline may produce severe ventricular dysrhythmias.

Later actions
Although Mr. Wilson's anxiety should decrease as his breathing becomes easier, continue to give him emotional support. He'll probably be fatigued, so allow him to rest as much as possible.

Try to determine the cause of this pulmonary edema episode. When Mr. Wilson's ready, talk to him about his recent activities. Has he changed his exercise or dietary patterns? Has he recently consumed foods or beverages high in sodium?

Review his medication regimen, and determine why he has trouble complying with it. Work with him and his doctor to establish a regimen that he can agree to follow. Consider your goal creating a care plan that will keep Mr. Wilson healthy and fit his life-style.

Thorough patient teaching, supported by home care if necessary, should make him a less familiar face in the ED.

Selected References

Assessment. Nurse's Reference Library. Springhouse, Pa.: Springhouse Corp., 1983.

*Emergency Care Handbook.*Springhouse, Pa.: Springhouse Corp., 1986.

Luce, J.M., et al. *Intensive Respiratory Care.* Philadelphia: W.B. Saunders Co., 1984.

Professional Guide to Diseases, 2nd ed. Nurse's Reference Library. Springhouse, Pa.: Springhouse Corp., 1987.

Respiratory Disorders. Nurse's Clinical Library. Springhouse, Pa.: Springhouse Corp., 1984.

Respiratory Emergencies. NursingNow Series. Springhouse, Pa.: Springhouse Corp., 1984.

Respiratory Problems. NurseReview Series. Springhouse, Pa.: Springhouse Corp., 1986.

Shapiro, B.A., et al. *Clinical Applications of Respiratory Care,* 3rd ed. Chicago: Year Book Medical Pubs., Inc., 1985.

Wollschlager, C.M., et al. "Secondary Pulmonary Hypertension: Clinical Features," *Heart & Lung* 15(4):336-40, July 1986.

7 ACUTE INHALATION DISORDERS

Introduction

A normal person breathes approximately 12 million cubic centimeters of air per day. During this process, the pulmonary system uses its sophisticated ability to filter impurities before they reach the tracheobronchial tree. The atmospheric character changes constantly; as we continue to pollute the air with numerous chemicals, the lungs respond by further rallying their protective mechanisms. However, in such situations as smoke inhalation and near-drowning, these defense mechanisms are overwhelmed. Toxic materials enter the tracheobronchial tree and can cause severe lung damage. The patient may initially be asymptomatic but quickly deteriorate over the next 48 hours. Astute physical assessment is crucial; a detailed history also is important to determine the length and severity of exposure to the offending element.

Near-drowning and smoke inhalation may lead to an acute inflammatory response in the lung parenchyma. The inflammatory response may also result from various other agents: illicit and therapeutic drugs, radiation therapy, environmental exposure, and aspiration. Although aspiration of many substances can occur, aspiration of gastric acid contents ranks as the leading cause of chemical pneumonitis. Persons who suffer gastric aspiration typically have a decreased level of consciousness, which interferes with defense mechanisms—the swallow, gag, and cough reflexes. Gastric aspiration poses a danger because it's associated with a high incidence of adult respiratory distress syndrome (ARDS), which has a high mortality.

Aspiration pneumonitis, near-drowning, and smoke inhalation can lead to severe lung damage without overt clinical signs. The degree of lung damage may be deceiving. Such patients require careful assessment, early intervention, and supportive care. Treatment goals include minimizing lung injury, promoting oxygenation, and preventing fibrosis formation secondary to pneumonitis.

Near-drowning

Description
In the United States, drowning claims nearly 8,000 lives annually. Children under age 4 account for nearly half of these deaths. Near-drowning refers to surviving—at least temporarily—the physiologic effects of hypoxemia and acidosis that result from submersion in fluid. No statistics are available for near-drownings.

Near-drowning occurs in three forms. In *wet drowning,* by far the most common form, the victim swallows or aspirates water while submerged. In response, he holds his breath, which increases his $PaCO_2$ level. After a certain point, however, increased $PaCO_2$ levels stimulate the brain's respiratory center, forcing the victim to breathe.

However, as the victim breathes, he swallows or aspirates greater quantities of water, causing him to vomit and perhaps aspirate some vomitus. He then loses consciousness, convulses, and aspirates more water. Asphyxia or secondary changes from fluid aspiration occur. Hypercapnea, hypoxia, and metabolic acidosis present the main problems.

In *dry drowning*, the first aspiration causes laryngospasm, which blocks the trachea and prevents further aspiration. The victim asphyxiates, becomes hypoxic, and loses consciousness. Hypoxia's the main problem. The dry-drowning victim has a better chance of surviving.

A third drowning type, *secondary drowning*, can occur several minutes or even several days after the accident if respiratory distress (for example, aspiration pneumonia or pulmonary edema) recurs. Near-drowning is a common cause of adult respiratory distress syndrome (ARDS).

Causes
Near-drowning results from an inability to swim or, in swimmers, commonly from panic, a boating accident, a medical emergency (such as a heart attack), a blow to the head while in the water, spinal cord injury, hypothermia, heavy alcohol consumption before swimming, or a suicide attempt.

Pathophysiology
Asphyxia results in hypoxemia and hypercapnia, causing tissue hypoxia, anaerobic metabolism, metabolic and respiratory acidosis, unconsciousness, convulsions, and dysrhythmias that lead to cardiac arrest and death, unless the victim's successfully resuscitated.

The brain responds to hypoxemia by shifting water and sodium from surrounding blood vessels into brain cells. The resulting cerebral edema and increased intracranial pressure can lead to permanent brain damage in a resuscitated victim. In addition, renal failure may result from acute tubular necrosis

caused by prolonged hypoxia and hypotension, and disseminated intravascular coagulation may occur from release of certain activators of the extrinsic clotting and fibrinolytic systems from the victim's damaged lungs.

Research shows that fresh water and salt water have different damaging effects on the body's fluid volume and electrolyte balance. (See *Freshwater and Saltwater Aspiration: Two Routes to Hypoxia,* page 184.)

Signs and symptoms
Immediately after a near-drowning, your first priority is to check the victim for the following signs and symptoms of asphyxia and pulmonary edema:
• rapidly worsening dyspnea
• apnea
• wheezing, crackles, and rhonchi
• productive cough with pink, frothy sputum
• substernal chest pain that worsens with breathing
• tachycardia
• tachypnea
• vomiting
• abdominal distention
• cyanosis
• confusion
• lethargy
• irritability
• restlessness
• unconsciousness
• seizure
• coma
• elevated body temperature (However, if the accident occurred in cold water, the patient's temperature may be abnormally low.)
• respiratory or cardiac arrest.

Diagnosis
Diagnosis requires a history of near-drowning along with characteristic features and auscultation of crackles and rhonchi. Supportive tests include:
• *Arterial blood gas (ABG) measurements:* decreased oxygen content, low

Freshwater and Saltwater Aspiration: Two Routes to Hypoxia

Although the cause of death in drowning—and the ultimate danger in near-drowning—is hypoxia, the type of fluid aspirated determines how hypoxia develops. Fresh water, hypotonic compared to blood, rapidly penetrates the pulmonary capillary membrane. Large amounts of lung surfactant are either lost or altered, causing alveolar collapse, intrapulmonary shunting, and hypoxia.

Salt water, hypertonic compared to blood, disrupts osmotic pressure, forcing fluid into the alveoli. Pulmonary edema, intrapulmonary shunting, and hypoxia result.

Freshwater aspiration

When a hypotonic fluid, such as fresh water, enters the alveolus, it can chemically alter the capillary membrane and destroy pulmonary surfactant. Intrapulmonary shunting, atelectasis, and hypoxia result. The fresh water also passes through the alveolar membrane and causes hemodilution, as shown in the illustration at right. This sudden circulatory overload is thought to cause freshwater pulmonary edema. In rare cases, ventricular fibrillation and death result.

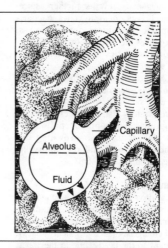

Saltwater aspiration

Salt water's hypertonicity draws fluid from the pulmonary capillary bed into the pulmonary interstitium and the alveoli (see the illustration at right). Consequently, the lung parenchyma undergoes damage. Fluid floods the alveoli, leading to intrapulmonary shunting and hypoxia.

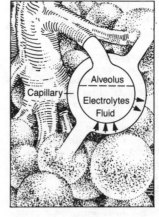

Understanding the Mammalian Diving Reflex

A drowning victim is rushed into the ED. Despite the CPR done at the scene and during transport, he has no detectable pulse, heartbeat, or breathing, he's cyanotic, and his pupils are fully dilated. He's dead. Or is he?

Don't give up your resuscitation efforts yet—he may still be alive. Why? Because, in a small percentage of apparently drowned persons, a protective mechanism—known as the *mammalian diving reflex*—is triggered. People submerged as long as 38 minutes have been resuscitated with little or no brain damage because of this reflex.

As you know, such aquatic mammals as whales and seals can remain underwater for long periods. They can do this because, when they submerge, blood is diverted from their extremities and concen-

trated in circulation to their heart, lungs, and brain. Their heart rate and brain metabolism also slow considerably, reducing these animals' need for oxygen and protecting their vital signs.

The same reflex can operate in humans. It doesn't occur in all drowning victims, however, because several factors must operate simultaneously to trigger it. These include:
• water temperature—the water must be 70° F. (21.1° C.) or colder; the colder the water, the more pronounced the reflex.
• age—young victims have a more easily stimulated diving reflex.
• facial immersion—the mechanism of the diving reflex is vagal stimulation with peripheral vasoconstriction, so the victim's face must be suddenly immersed in cold water to trigger the reflex.

HCO_3^-, and low pH; leukocytosis may occur.
• *Chest X-ray:* may be normal or show perihilar pulmonary edema, generalized pulmonary edema, or alveolar infiltrates. Chest X-ray changes occur within 12 hours and usually resolve within 10 days after the insult, if ARDS does not occur.
• *EKG:* supraventricular tachycardia, occasional premature contractions, and nonspecific ST segment and T wave abnormalities may occur.

Treatment and clinical considerations

Cardiopulmonary resuscitation (CPR) can begin as soon as the victim's head is above water. If a spinal injury is suspected, a board should be placed under the victim's head and back while he's still in the water.

When the victim arrives at the hospital, your first priority is to maintain an

open airway. Continue CPR, if necessary. Then take the following measures:
• Relieve hypoxia. Administer low-percentage oxygen until you can obtain ABG measurements. Then ventilate the patient, as ordered, using positive-pressure breathing with 100% oxygen or positive end-expiratory pressure. Suction the patient's airway frequently to remove secretions.
• Assess ABG values. Increased ventilation may be used to treat respiratory acidosis.
• Give medications, as ordered. Much controversy exists about the benefits of drug therapy for near-drowning victims. Such therapy may include sodium bicarbonate for metabolic acidosis, possible corticosteroids for cerebral edema, antibiotics to prevent infection, and bronchodilators to ease bronchospasms.
• If the patient has a distended abdomen, insert a nasogastric tube. (A

qualified practitioner should intubate an unconscious patient first.)

• Start I.V. lines, and insert an indwelling (Foley) catheter, as ordered.

• Remember, all near-drowning victims should be observed for 12 to 48 hours because of the chance of delayed drowning.

• Close assessment proves crucial. A patient who appears normal may deteriorate quickly, and one who appears critically ill may recover without sequelae.

• Observe for pulmonary complications and signs and symptoms of delayed drowning (confusion, substernal pain, adventitious breath sounds). Pulmonary artery catheterization may be useful in assessing cardiopulmonary status. Monitor vital signs, intake and output, and peripheral pulses. Check for skin perfusion and for signs of infection.

• Assess the patient for associated trauma, especially spinal cord injuries, internal injuries, and bone fractures.

• Patients who experience immersion hypothermia may develop serious cardiac dysrhythmias. Vasopressors and defibrillation prove ineffective until the victim's warmed. These patients may also experience hypoglycemia, especially if the accident resulted from alcohol intake.

• To facilitate breathing, raise the head of the bed slightly.

• To prevent near-drowning, advise swimmers to avoid drinking alcohol before swimming, to observe water safety measures, and to take a water safety course sponsored by the Red Cross, YMCA, or YWCA. (Also see *Understanding the Mammalian Diving Reflex*, page 185.)

Inhalation injuries

Description
Respiratory tract injury may accompany burn injuries and toxic chemical inhalation. Severe injuries may result from house fires or recreational accidents resulting in a fire. Kerosene heaters and wood or coal stoves also contribute to the increased incidence of inhalation injuries. The growing use of synthetic materials also raises the risk of a chemical accident leading to toxic lung injury—a dangerous respiratory disorder resulting from toxic chemical inhalation. Workers or bystanders may suffer toxic chemical and smoke inhalation from an accident, such as a fire at a chemical plant or an explosion at an oil refinery.

Toxic lung injury can occur within minutes after exposure to noxious chemicals contained in smoke or gas. Without proper treatment, this injury can lead to respiratory failure.

Causes
Respiratory tract injury can stem from inhalation of:
• steam
• superheated air
• smoke
• a toxic product of combustion, especially carbon monoxide
• a toxic chemical.
(See *Identifying Risk Factors for Toxic Inhalation Injuries*.)

Pathophysiology
The patient may sustain a thermal injury to his upper respiratory tract from excessive heat or steam, or damage to his lower respiratory tract from inhalation of a toxic product of combustion or toxic chemical. Or the patient may experience both thermal and toxic injuries together.

In a patient with a thermal inhalation injury, laryngeal edema—from increased capillary permeability in injured mucosal tissue—may rapidly cause airway obstruction. Damage to the lower airway occurs rarely and usually results from steam inhalation.

Identifying Risk Factors for Toxic Inhalation Injuries

Certain patients have a high risk of sustaining significant lung damage from inhaling a toxin. The following factors predispose a patient to serious lung damage:

• *Preexisting lung disease* that reduces ventilation, disturbs cell function, or destroys lung tissue; for example, tuberculosis, chronic obstructive pulmonary disease, or pleurisy. (Pulmonary edema is an exception. The excess fluid this condition produces helps mobilize harmful particles before they can irritate the alveolar wall.)

• *Cigarette smoking* paralyzes the mucociliary escalator—a system in which the cilia and a mucous blanket propel airway particles upward. This leads to bronchoconstriction and thick mucus buildup, which compromises the lungs' normal defense mechanisms by impairing macrophagic activity. Also, smoking increases carboxyhemoglobin levels.

• *Long-term exposure to toxic chemicals* can wear out the lungs' defense mechanisms. (Most lung diseases take years to develop.)

• *Exposure to high concentrations of toxic chemicals,* even over a short period, may overwhelm the lungs' defense mechanisms.

• *The size of a chemical's particles* determines where those particles lodge in the lungs. For example, particles 3 to 5 μ in diameter lodge in the alveoli and cause the greatest damage. Particles less than 1 μ in diameter (for example, those in smoke, fumes, or aerosols) cause less serious injury because they penetrate the alveolar walls and enter interstitial tissue.

In a patient with tracheobronchitis from smoke or fume inhalation, airway occlusion may be progressive. This occurs from bronchospasm, laryngeal edema, mucosal sloughing, and hypoxia. Chemical irritants also disrupt the alveolar capillary membrane in the lungs, allowing fluids and protein to accumulate and possibly cause noncardiogenic pulmonary edema or adult respiratory distress syndrome.

In a patient who's inhaled carbon monoxide, hypoxia occurs. (See *Carbon Monoxide Poisoning,* page 188, and *Gas Inhalation,* page 189.)

Signs and symptoms

Because a victim of an inhalation injury can deteriorate rapidly, consider recognition and intervention critically important. Clinical features may include singed nasal hairs, circumoral or orofacial burns, soot-stained sputum, coughing or hoarseness, anxiety, confusion, combativeness, possibly cyanosis, respiratory distress, and additional signs and symptoms related to the injury source. Crackles, rhonchi, and wheezes may occur initially but more commonly occur 24 to 36 hours after injury. (See *Inhalation Injuries from Some Toxic Products,* page 190.)

Remember, however, that signs and symptoms of inhalation injury may not appear for up to 48 hours after exposure. About 50% of victims are asymptomatic initially. Delaying treatment for such a period could have serious consequences.

Diagnosis

Suspect inhalation injury whenever the patient's history includes exposure to burning agents in an enclosed space or loss of consciousness accompanying burns. The major diagnostic tests include:

• *Arterial blood gas (ABG) measurements:* may show hypoxemia, hyper-

Carbon Monoxide Poisoning

Pathophysiology

Carbon monoxide poisoning, one of the most common poisoning types, accompanies smoke inhalation injuries. It ranks as the leading cause of death from fires.

A colorless, odorless gas, carbon monoxide results from incomplete burning of organic substances, such as gasoline, coal products, tobacco, and building materials. You'll see carbon monoxide poisoning most commonly in burn victims with smoke inhalation and in persons who've tried to commit suicide by inhaling automobile exhaust fumes. Anyone who inhales air containing a high level of carbon monoxide risks cardiopulmonary failure, CNS damage, and death. Here's why: Once it's inhaled, carbon monoxide crosses the alveolocapillary membrane, which provides the means for gas exchange between alveolar air and capillary blood in the lungs. Because it has a high affinity for hemoglobin (nearly 240 times that of oxygen), carbon monoxide quickly binds to it, forming carboxyhemoglobin. This causes hypoxemia, because the hemoglobin can no longer carry oxygen, and it prevents oxygen release from unaltered hemoglobin to the tissues. Also, carbon monoxide binds with myoglobin in muscle cells and interferes with cellular respiration. Hypoxia and metabolic acidosis result.

Assessment

To assess the severity of carbon monoxide poisoning, the doctor will order blood tests to determine the patient's carboxyhemoglobin level. Signs and symptoms of carbon monoxide poisoning vary in severity, depending on the carboxyhemoglobin level. A level of 20% causes headache and mild dyspnea, whereas a level between 20% and 40% produces fatigue, irritability, diminished judgment, dimmed vision, and nausea.

With a carboxyhemoglobin level between 40% and 60%, the patient suffers confusion, convulsions, hallucinations, ataxia, collapse, and coma. His skin and mucous membranes typically turn cherry red.

Although arterial blood gas measurements reveal a normal PaO_2 level, oxygen release to peripheral tissues drops sharply when carboxyhemoglobin levels are high. Therefore, oxygen saturation decreases.

Management

The doctor will order 100% high-flow oxygen, which reduces the half-life of carboxyhemoglobin from 4 hours to 30 minutes. He may order blood transfusions or hyperbaric oxygen therapy, which provides 100% oxygen at high pressure in a controlled environment.

Besides administering oxygen, keep the patient on total bed rest for at least 48 hours, or as ordered. Also watch for signs and symptoms of reduced cardiac output or CNS impairment, which may not appear for 3 weeks.

capnea, respiratory or metabolic acidosis
• *Chest X-ray:* may initially be clear, but may show pulmonary edema or complete whiteout indicating adult respiratory distress syndrome (usually develops 4 to 7 days later)

• *Carboxyhemoglobin levels:* elevated in smoke inhalations caused by carbon monoxide poisoning (*Note:* Normally, this level ranges from 1% to 3%; in smokers, from 5% to 10%.)
• *Fiberoptic bronchoscopy:* may show mucosal damage. This serves as the best diagnostic tool because it pro-

vides direct visualization of upper and lower respiratory tract mucosa. (Can also be used to establish an airway and to lavage and suction the lungs.)
• *Lavage:* fluid can be sent for analysis
• *Xenon lung scan:* may show decreased secretion if lungs are damaged
• *Spirometry:* measures forced expiratory volume, peak flow, and forced vital capacity to detect airflow (may be performed at the bedside).

Treatment and clinical considerations

Priorities for the patient include providing adequate oxygenation and preventing progression to respiratory failure.
• Assess and maintain airway, breathing, and circulation. Initiate cardiopulmonary resuscitation if necessary.
• Administer low-percentage humidified oxygen until you can obtain ABG measurements.
• Assist with insertion of an endotracheal tube to improve breathing. Major indications for intubation include CNS depression, visible edema or mucosal injury of the upper airway, and circumferential neck burns.
• Prepare and assist with endotracheal tube insertion and with placing the patient on mechanical ventilation before airway obstruction can occur. (Tracheostomy is rarely performed because of the associated increased sepsis risk and high mortality.)
• For toxic inhalation injuries, administer bronchodilators, as ordered, to help maintain airway patency; give corticosteroids, if ordered, to help reduce tissue damage (although corticosteroid use is controversial); administer antibiotics, if ordered, based on culture results; insert a nasogastric tube, if ordered, to help remove ingested chemicals.
• Assess breath sounds frequently for wheezes, crackles, and rhonchi, and

---

Gas Inhalation

Responses to gas inhalation vary according to gas solubility. A person who's inhaled a water-soluble gas, such as ammonia, usually flees the area immediately because such a gas is extremely irritating to the upper airways. By fleeing, he reduces the risk of lung damage.

But if he's trapped in the contaminated area, he'll inhale a much greater gas volume. Consequently, the gas penetrates deeper into the respiratory system, causing potentially acute respiratory dysfunction.

Insoluble gases, such as nitrogen dioxide, cause only mild upper airway irritation. A person exposed to such a gas is more likely to inhale a greater volume before fleeing and thus suffer greater lung damage at the alveolar level.

---

suction carefully to avoid further tracheal damage. Also assess for decreased or tubular breath sounds.
• Anticipate pulmonary therapies, such as bronchoscopy, for lavage of secretions and diagnosis of damage extent; nebulizer treatments; coughing and deep breathing; and chest physiotherapy. (These procedures mobilize thick bronchial tree secretions.)
• If your patient's on a ventilator and requires positive end-expiratory pressure (PEEP) for oxygenation, closely assess him for pneumothorax. Inhaled chemicals may weaken the alveolar capillary membranes, making these patients especially vulnerable to barotrauma from PEEP.
• Watch for signs of pneumonia (fever, increased and purulent secretions, and respiratory distress); report such signs immediately and obtain cultures as necessary.
• Watch for complications from therapy, such as pneumothorax and gastric distention.

Inhalation Injuries from Some Toxic Products

Toxic product of combustion	Sources	Signs and symptoms
Hydrochloric acid	Burning products made of polyvinyl chloride, such as unbreakable bottles, electrical insulation, wall coverings, and car interiors	• Dyspnea • Burning pain in mucous membranes
Hydrocyanic acid	Burning products made of polyurethane or nylon, such as thermal insulation, wall coverings, seat cushions, carpeting, and mattress materials	• Light-headedness • Nausea • Dyspnea • Chest pain • Syncope
Styrene	Burning products made of styrene, such as piping, wall coverings, luggage, appliances, and plastic food and drink containers	• Conjunctivitis • Rhinorrhea • Burning pain in mucous membranes
Acrolein	Burning products made of acrylics, such as textiles, wood finishes, wall coverings, furniture, and piping	• Burning pain in mucous membranes • Light-headedness • Dyspnea
Ammonia	Burning products made of nylon, such as carpeting, clothing, and upholstery	• Conjunctivitis • Burning pain in mucous membranes • Laryngeal and pulmonary edema
Carbon monoxide	Burning of organic substances, such as gasoline, coal products, and building materials	• Headache • Light-headedness • Nausea and vomiting • Dyspnea • Visual disturbances • Seizures • Coma

Aspiration pneumonitis

Description

Aspiration means inhalation (usually of gastric contents) into the tracheobronchial tree and then into the lung parenchyma. Normally, the swallowing, gag, and cough reflexes protect the lung parenchyma from harm. In aspiration, however, one or all aspects of these protective mechanisms malfunction. *Pneumonitis* from aspiration refers to inflammation of lung tissue without development of infection. *Aspiration pneumonia* refers to aspiration pneumonitis plus an infection. The extent of pulmonary impairment depends on the type of material swallowed, aspirate volume and pH, frequency of aspiration, and the patient's baseline pulmonary status. A pH of 2.4 or less or aspirate volumes of 2 to 4 ml/kg (approximately 150 ml) cause the greatest lung damage. This section focuses mainly on gastric acid aspiration, because it's the most common type and has the highest mortality.

Causes

Aspiration of gastric acid contents is the most common cause of aspiration pneumonitis. (See *Gastric Aspiration: Risk Factors,* and *Chemical Pneumonitis,* page 194.)

Pathophysiology

Gastric aspiration results in edematous, hemorrhagic, inflamed alveoli. The trachea and bronchi become desquamated, and the mucociliary mechanism's destroyed. Alveolar infiltrates develop, acid destroys surfactant, and hyaline membranes form. Obstructive bronchiolitis occurs if food particles block bronchioles. After this initial chemical pneumonitis, pneumonia commonly develops secondary to lost defense mechanisms.

Signs and symptoms

Subtle aspiration typically causes no symptoms (many people aspirate in their sleep). In large aspiration, the patient coughs profusely if the cough reflex is intact. Over the next hour or so, tachypnea, dyspnea, bronchospasms, and tachycardia occur. Crackles, wheezes, and tubular breath sounds can be heard on auscultation.

Diagnosis

Gastric aspiration proves hard to diagnose unless vomiting was witnessed. However, suspect this disorder in any patient at risk.

Chest X-ray reveals infiltrates, which may be localized or diffuse. Usually, patients aspirate into the most dependent portions of the lung (posterior and inferior parts). Aspiration is usually greater on the right side be-

---

Gastric Aspiration: Risk Factors

Patients at highest risk for aspirating gastric contents include those with:
• an altered level of consciousness caused by:
—general anesthesia, especially in emergency and obstetrical cases that don't allow time for adequate gastric emptying
—CNS disturbances, such as seizures, strokes, and head trauma
—narcotics, sedatives, alcohol, and drug overdose
• gastrointestinal problems, such as achalasia, delayed gastric emptying, tracheoesophageal fistulas, gastric distention, diverticuli, gastroesophageal reflux, and tumors
• tube feedings
• placement of endotracheal or tracheostomy tube, incompetent glottis, and impaired mucociliary or lung defense mechanisms.

---

cause of the straighter position of the right mainstem bronchus. If infiltrates persist longer than 5 days, adult respiratory distress syndrome (ARDS) or pneumonia may be developing.

Arterial blood gas (ABG) measurements may show severe hypoxemia, which may be refractory to oxygen if ARDS is developing. The $PaCO_2$ level is initially below normal or normal if the patient can compensate, but increases as he decompensates.

In a patient with endotracheal or tracheal tubes who is receiving tube feedings, suctioning the endotracheal tube may detect gastric secretions or feeding solution. (Aspiration of feeding solution causes much less damage because the feeding has a higher pH than gastric contents.) To detect feeding-solution aspiration, you can use one of these methods:
• Use glucose oxidase reagent strips to detect glucose in bronchial secre-

Aspirated Feeding Solution

The situation
The patient in Room 247 suffered a cerebrovascular accident (CVA) 3 weeks ago. Although he's been unresponsive since then and his gag and swallowing reflexes remain depressed, his condition's otherwise stable. He'll be transferred to an extended care facility when a room is available.

Because the patient's family would not consent to a gastrostomy for placement of a feeding tube, the patient's being fed through a nasogastric tube. He's receiving a continuous feeding at a rate of 100 ml/hour, regulated by a Kangaroo pump.

When you enter the patient's room to take noon vital signs, you hear a loud gurgling sound. You immediately see that 4″ to 6″ of the feeding tube has slid out of his nose. The patient's diaphoretic, pale, and dusky.

The problem
The patient's feeding tube has come out of his stomach. He has aspirated the feeding solution and is choking.

The worst case
The patient's airway becomes completely occluded and he goes into respiratory arrest. Cardiac arrest will most likely follow.

The best case
You suction the patient's airway and he resumes breathing normally.

The assessment
The patient has aspirated feeding solution and is in respiratory distress. His pallor, duskiness, and diaphoresis—along with increased pulse (140), increased respiratory rate (34), and decreased blood pressure (110/70)—indicate impaired gas exchange. Don't even try to assess his breath sounds because the noise from his upper airway is so loud that it'll be transmitted through his lung fields.

Immediate actions
Call for help, and remove the feeding tube. (Don't replace it—that would waste time, and you could inadvertently place it in the trachea.) Next, lower the head of the bed and place the patient on his left side. Because the left bronchus is less vertical than the right, this position reduces the risk of the feeding solution moving further down into his lungs. (If the CVA has affected his left side, however, move him from this position as soon as it's safe to do so.)

Now suction his mouth and pharynx. If a tonsil (Yankauer) suction catheter is readily available, use that. Otherwise, use a regular suc-

tions. Because normal sputum has no glucose, a positive result indicates tube feeding contents in secretions. (However, a false-negative result may occur if secretions contain blood.)

• Add food coloring to tube feedings to later identify feeding contents in tracheal secretions. Red and blue food coloring will cause a false-positive Hematest of stools and should be avoided. (See *Aspirated Feeding Solution*.)

Treatment and clinical considerations
A patent airway must be established by suctioning, use of bronchodilators, and chest physiotherapy. Bronchoscopy may be needed to remove large particles. Hypoxemia may be corrected via supplemental oxygen; ABG values must be closely monitored for hypoxemia that's refractory to increasing oxygen amounts. This may herald the onset of ARDS. Chest X-rays must be closely monitored for pneumonia and vital signs checked frequently for

tion catheter. (The rigid tonsil catheter is better because it can slide easily into the patient's pharynx. Be careful not to accidentally gag the patient, or he may vomit more.)

Begin administering oxygen through a mask. Be sure to have a manual resuscitation bag ready to use if the patient stops breathing.

After suctioning the patient's upper airway and starting oxygen administration, reassess his condition. Is he breathing more easily? Has his color improved? If so, he probably aspirated the solution only into his pharynx and upper trachea. But if his condition's unchanged, the solution has most likely entered his lungs.

If suctioning the upper airway doesn't improve the patient's condition, page his doctor. Prepare to call for a portable chest X-ray and to draw a sample for arterial blood gas (ABG) analysis, as ordered. The patient will also need deep tracheal suctioning.

After tracheal suctioning, continue to administer oxygen and monitor the patient's vital signs. Be prepared to call a code; he may still become bradycardic or severely hypotensive, or he may stop breathing.

If his condition remains unchanged, or if ABG analysis shows severe hypoxemia or hypercapnia, he'll need to be intubated. Set up

the supplies and drugs, according to hospital procedures, and assist as needed.

Later actions

If the patient's transferred to the intensive care unit, inform the nurses there of his condition. He'll need to be closely watched for signs of pneumonia and ARDS during the next 48 hours. Be sure to notify his family of the transfer.

Now determine how the nasogastric tube came out. Was it anchored properly? Was its placement checked frequently? Did it come loose when the patient was repositioned? Also, was the patient placed on his unaffected side with the head of the bed elevated to reduce the risk of aspiration?

Review your response to the situation. Did you know what to do? Was the suction apparatus available and did it work? Were the supplies you needed right at hand? If a tonsil catheter wasn't stocked on the crash cart, suggest that it be included.

Finally, call for a team meeting to find out why the family wouldn't consent to placement of a gastrostomy tube. Perhaps they rejected the idea because they weren't fully informed. See whether better communication could have changed their minds—and prevented the incident.

evidence of shock. The doctor may order steroids; however, their use remains controversial.

Start antibiotics, if ordered, based on culture results. Bronchodilators may be used to treat bronchospasms. Closely monitor intake and output—these patients have a high risk for developing intravascular volume depletion and ARDS.

• Prevention is essential. Closely observe any patient at risk for aspiration

pneumonitis. Assess gag, cough, and swallowing reflexes.

• Patients with a decreased level of consciousness have the greatest risk of developing aspiration pneumonitis. Place these patients in a lateral position with the head of the bed elevated 30 degrees at all times.

• Closely assess a patient with abdominal distention and intervene appropriately. Assess his diet for gas-producing foods. The patient may need a nasogastric tube or food and fluid

Chemical Pneumonitis

The initial inflammatory response, chemical pneumonitis, may occur alone or with other responses to acute lung injury. Chemical pneumonitis commonly leads to pneumonia if untreated. After this inflammatory response occurs, reparative lung tissue develops in the form of pulmonary fibrosis. (Pulmonary fibrosis is the *chronic* response to injury; pneumonitis is the *acute* response. Although the two disorders often occur together, they're not synonymous.)

Chemicals that may cause pneumonitis include inhaled toxins, such as smoke or industrial agents in the work environment; inhaled gastric secretions; other fluids; and hydrocarbons, such as gasoline, paint thinners, and kerosene. Radiation therapy, chemotherapy, and such drugs as procainamide, hydralazine, nitrofurantoin, heroin, and amiodarone also can cause chemical pneumonitis. Signs and symptoms vary, and long-term effects depend on the amount of pulmonary fibrosis and damage to the lungs' protective mechanisms. Degrees of restrictive disease may occur.

---

withheld. As ordered and needed, administer metaclopramide to increase gastric emptying.

• If your patient has a nasogastric (NG) tube, be sure to check its patency and functioning frequently. Small-bore NG tubes should be used for feeding, because they can be passed into the duodenum and cause less interference with lower esophageal sphincter funtioning; large-bore tubes interfere with functioning of the lower esophageal sphincter and may result in aspiration. Cimetidine and antacids may be used to increase gastric secretion pH, thereby decreasing the destructive action of any aspirated gastric acids.

• To monitor your patient's tolerance of tube feedings, frequently check for residual; normally, this should be less than 100 ml or half the volume of the previous feeding. Assess the patient for fullness, distention, and cramping, and adjust the rate and concentration of tube feedings accordingly. Coughing, belching, and vomiting may displace the feeding tube. The tube may slip into the lung without initiating a cough or gag reflex. Because its position can't be absolutely verified by auscultation or aspiration of secretions alone, speak to the doctor, who may order a chest X-ray to verify tube position.

• If a patient has aspirated, help to identify and correct complications, such as refractory hypoxemia, decreased compliance, hypovolemia, and ARDS, as soon as possible.

Selected References

Baker, W., and Smith, S. "Pulmonary Aspiration and Tube Feedings: Nursing Implications," *Focus on Critical Care* 11(2):25-7, April 1984.

Dantzker, D.R., ed. *Cardiopulmonary Critical Care*. Orlando, Fla.: Grune and Stratton, 1986.

Emergency Care Handbook. Springhouse, Pa.: Springhouse Corp., 1986.

Glassroth, J., et al. "The Impact of Substance Abuse on the Respiratory System," *Chest* 91(4):596-602, April 1987.

Halpern, et al. "Propoxyphene and Acetaminophen Mixture (Darvocet)—Related Radiation-Induced Pneumonitis," *Archives in Internal Medicine* 145(8):1509-10, August 1985.

Israel-Biet, D., et al. "Bronchoalveolar Lavage in Amiodarone Pneumonitis: Cellular Abnormalities and Their Relevance to Pathogenesis," *Chest* 91(2):214-21, February 1987.

Kinni, M., and Strout, M. "Aspiration Pneumonitis: Predisposing Conditions and Prevention," *Journal of Oral and Maxillofacial Surgery* 44(5):378-84, May 1986.

Metheny, N., et al. "Aspiration Pneumonia in Patients Fed through Nasoenteral Tubes," *Heart & Lung* 15(3):256-61, May 1986.

Moseley, P., et al. "Lung Parenchymal Injury Induced by Bleomycin," *American Review of Respiratory Disease* 130(6):1082-86, December 1984.

Parrillo, J., *Current Therapy in Critical Care Medicine.* St. Louis: C.V. Mosby Co.,1986.

Professional Guide to Diseases, 2nd ed. Springhouse, Pa.: Springhouse Corp., 1987.

Respiratory Emergencies. NursingNow series. Springhouse, Pa.: Springhouse Corp., 1984.

Shapiro, B.A., et al. *Clinical Applications of Respiratory Care,* 3rd ed. Chicago: Year Book Medical Pubs., Inc., 1985.

St. Clair, E., et al. "Pneumonitis Complicating Low-Dose Methotrexate Therapy in Rheumatoid Arthritis," *Archives of Internal Medicine* 145(11):2035-38, November 1985.

Treolar, D., and Stechmiller, J. "Pulmonary Aspiration in Tube-Fed Patients with Artificial Airways," *Heart & Lung* 13(6):667-71, November 1984.

Van Barneveld, P., et al. "Predictive Factors for Bleomycin-Induced Pneumonitis," *American Review of Respiratory Disease* 130(6):1078-81, December 1984.

RESPIRATORY COMPLICATIONS OF NEUROLOGIC DISORDERS

Introduction

Normal respiration requires both a functioning respiratory system and an intact nervous system.

The central nervous system (CNS) is a major regulator of respiration. Central control mechanisms in the medulla and pons govern the automatic rhythm of inspiration and expiration. (Voluntary control of respiration originates in the brain's cortex.) Central control mechanisms receive impulses generated by chemoreceptors and proprioceptive receptors.

Chemoreceptors, thought to be centrally located in the medulla and peripherally in the bifurcation of the common carotid arteries, are especially sensitive to changes in $PaCO_2$. Because carbon dioxide is a strong stimulus for respiration, even minute changes in $PaCO_2$ can alter respirations. *Proprioceptive receptors* detect changes in lung tissues and airways and transmit these impulses via the vagus nerve to the respiratory control centers.

Next, these impulses must travel to the spinal cord. Here, the peripheral nervous system takes over. Peripheral motor nerves originating in cervical and thoracic cord areas transmit impulses over myoneural junctions to respiratory muscles. The impulse transmitted down the phrenic nerve to the diaphragm is the most important one. The main respiratory muscle, the diaphragm, moves downward in the chest with contractions, creating more space in the thorax, decreasing intra-

thoracic pressure, and drawing air from the atmosphere (inspiration). With expiration, a passive process, impulses at the diaphragm stop and the diaphragm relaxes.

When any part of this system is disrupted, respiratory dysfunction can occur. Two major problems that can affect the brain are brain injuries and conditions that decrease chemoreceptor sensitivity. Such injuries to the brain as trauma, tumors, and edema can cause increased intracranial pressure. This, in turn, may put pressure on central chemoreceptors and central respiratory control centers, thereby altering respiratory patterns.

Drug use ranks as the most common cause of decreased chemoreceptor sensitivity to carbon dioxide. For example, narcotics, barbiturates, and tranquilizers can decrease respirations by dulling chemoreceptor sensitivity.

Respiratory impulses reaching the spinal cord may be interrupted by spinal cord injuries. The most critical injuries are those which transect the cord, especially above C5 or C6. The phrenic nerve is vulnerable in higher injuries, and death may be almost instantaneous from complete interruption of respiration. With injuries below C5 or C6, the phrenic nerve's preserved, but the diaphragm may be the only functioning respiratory muscle, and respiratory reserve will be significantly limited. In this case, spinal cord injury causes muscle weakness, much like certain musculoskeletal diseases.

Neuromuscular disturbances can interfere with respiration through a different pathophysiologic process—but the end result is the same—respiratory muscles that can't contract powerfully. Myasthenia gravis affects the myoneural junction; amyotrophic lateral sclerosis affects motor neurons.

Muscular diseases can affect respiration, too. In these disorders, impulses may be transmitted normally to the respiratory muscles but the muscles can't respond. Although such muscular disorders as muscular dystrophy aren't neurologic in origin, they can cause diaphragmatic failure, resulting in similar problems.

Major respiratory problems secondary to neurologic impairment include loss of the ability to protect the airway and respiratory failure from disruption of respiratory muscles. Affected patients need close monitoring to detect these and other problems and to allow early intervention. Aggressive preventive care can sometimes eliminate the need for ventilator support. If respiratory failure does occur, the usual treatment is mechanical ventilation, which poses a challenge to the health care team. An unrelenting progressive neurologic or neuromuscular illness also presents an ethical question: Should mechanical ventilation be instituted if no hope of independent respiration exists? This issue should be addressed early in the course of a progressive neurologic illness with the patient, family, clergy, and other appropriate professionals. Because respiratory failure is fairly predictable in these patients, decisions about care shouldn't be delayed until an emergency arises.

Other treatment depends on the underlying pathophysiology. Care goals should be determined based on the course of the illness, the patient's needs, and community support systems. Sophisticated home-care devices, many of which have only recently become available, can greatly improve quality of life for the patient with respiratory failure caused by a neuromuscular disorder. Patients with polio were once doomed to a life in an iron lung machine with only a mirror to see the outside world. Today, portable ventilators and motorized wheelchairs allow some patients to maintain an active life-style despite severe handicaps.

Finally, sleep-related respiratory problems may stem from neurologic dysfunction. Diagnosing the cause of sleep apnea and providing appropriate treatment is also challenging.

Central nervous system disorders

Description
Central nervous system (CNS) disorders can lead to respiratory dysfunction when some aspect of neurologic control is disrupted. Careful assessment proves crucial to detect life-threatening complications, which can occur quickly. Prompt intervention may be needed to provide airway patency, adequate ventilation, and oxygenation.

Causes
• Increased intracranial pressure (ICP) from such conditions as head injury, brain tumor, intracranial abscess, hydrocephalus, and vascular disruption
• Direct injury to respiratory centers in the brainstem, such as from tumor or infarction
• Cerebral depression (unconsciousness) from such conditions as drug overdose, metabolic disturbance, trauma, or brain lesions

Pathophysiology
Increased ICP is a major cause of respiratory complications. Because the skull is rigid and inflexible, any brain swelling or space-occupying lesion will exert pressure on the brain and, if untreated, may affect the respiratory centers. This pressure can disrupt normal respiratory control. Direct injury to respiratory control centers also interferes with normal respiration.

Cerebral depression can directly affect respiratory patterns, resulting in hypoventilation with decreased respiratory rate and depth. It also can result in hypoventilation or aspiration because the patient can't clear secretions from his airway or mechanically maintain a patent airway. This can result in increased $PaCO_2$ and arterial hypoxemia, which can lead to further metabolic changes in the brain and the rest of the body.

Other respiratory complications of CNS disorders include adult respiratory distress syndrome (ARDS) and ventilation/perfusion ($\dot{V}/\dot{Q}$) mismatch caused by sympathetic stimulation from a severe head injury. (See Chapter 9 for more on ARDS.) Neurogenic pulmonary edema, an acute complication, probably occurs secondary to a massive sympathetic discharge following an abrupt ICP increase. Arterial blood gas (ABG) abnormalities resulting from these complications can create a vicious cycle that further compromises the brain, changing respiratory patterns and altering gas exchange.

Signs and symptoms
Respiratory signs and symptoms vary with the nature of the CNS disorder. A patient with CNS depression may experience impaired ability to cough, clear secretions, and inhale deeply. Auscultation may eventually reveal decreased ventilation in dependent areas. With mechanical insufficiency, shallow noisy respirations, accessory muscle use, and nasal flaring may occur. An alert patient may become increasingly restless, anxious, or confused. Marked inspiratory effort without air movement may result from complete airway obstruction—for example, soft tissue or foreign body obstructions in an unconscious patient. This condition calls for immediate life-support measures.

Abnormal respiratory patterns in a comatose patient may be the first sign of a respiratory complication. Careful assessment can help locate the injury level. (See *Abnormal Breathing Patterns Associated with Brain Injury.*)

Diagnosis
Diagnosis of the respiratory disorder usually occurs during diagnosis of the neurologic condition. ABG analysis helps determine the respiratory adequacy. The respiratory pattern may increase or decrease the $PaCO_2$ level. With hypoventilation, pH decreases and the $PaCO_2$ level increases, reflecting respiratory acidosis. With hyperventilation, pH increases and $PaCO_2$ decreases, reflecting respiratory alkalosis.

Treatment
First, make sure the patient can maintain a patent airway. If not, he'll need placement of an endotracheal tube or a tracheostomy.

Evaluate gas exchange with ABG measurements. Criteria for mechanical ventilation are usually more stringent for patients with head injuries or other brain disorders because carbon dioxide is a potent cerebral vasodilator. An increased $PaCO_2$ level increases blood flow, resulting in increased ICP. Patients with increased ICP will usually be iatrogenically hyperventilated to cause cerebral vasoconstriction in an attempt to lower ICP. The $PaCO_2$ shouldn't be maintained lower than approximately 25 mm Hg.

Hypoxemia can also cause increased cerebral blood flow, which may pose a danger to the patient. However, the constant threat of increasing ICP warrants extremely cautious treatment. Because suctioning causes tremendous spikes in ICP, the procedure should be minimized. To provide maximal protection in the patient with elevated ICP, the doctor may order sedation before suctioning and manual hyperventilation with 100% oxygen for 1 to 2 minutes just before suctioning. To minimize noxious stimulation, suctioning shouldn't be done in conjunc-

Abnormal Breathing Patterns Associated with Brain Injury

If your patient has a brain injury, his breathing will change as the injury affects certain vital brain areas. Use the chart below to review how abnormal breathing patterns indicate the location of brain injuries.

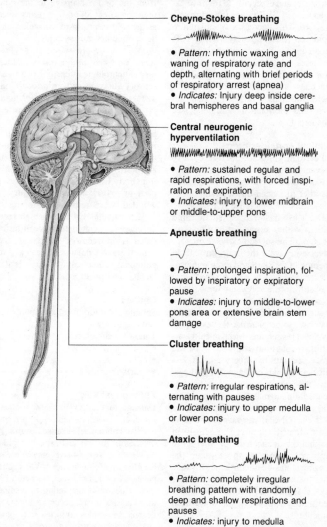

Cheyne-Stokes breathing

• *Pattern:* rhythmic waxing and waning of respiratory rate and depth, alternating with brief periods of respiratory arrest (apnea)
• *Indicates:* Injury deep inside cerebral hemispheres and basal ganglia

Central neurogenic hyperventilation

• *Pattern:* sustained regular and rapid respirations, with forced inspiration and expiration
• *Indicates:* injury to lower midbrain or middle-to-upper pons

Apneustic breathing

• *Pattern:* prolonged inspiration, followed by inspiratory or expiratory pause
• *Indicates:* injury to middle-to-lower pons area or extensive brain stem damage

Cluster breathing

• *Pattern:* irregular respirations, alternating with pauses
• *Indicates:* injury to upper medulla or lower pons

Ataxic breathing

• *Pattern:* completely irregular breathing pattern with randomly deep and shallow respirations and pauses
• *Indicates:* injury to medulla

tion with any other procedure and, when warranted, should be done for short periods.

Positive end-expiratory pressure (PEEP) is another therapeutic procedure with potential complications for the neurologic patient. Used to increase gas exchange, and especially to improve oxygenation, PEEP raises intrathoracic pressure. This decreases venous return from the head, possibly raising ICP. Protecting the brain by minimizing ICP increases while maintaining oxygenation adequate to maintain metabolic functions requires a delicate balance. For more information on airway management and mechanical ventilation, see Chapters 12 and 13.

Clinical considerations

• Perform good supportive care to prevent atelectasis and pneumonia.

• Never place a patient with a cerebral disorder in a head-down position, because this may increase ICP.

• Don't use nasotracheal suction in a patient with a suspected basilar skull fracture. The suction catheter may inadvertently enter the brain through an opening in the skull and nasal mucosa.

• A restless patient with a head injury may still need a computed tomography scan or X-rays. If he can't be sedated enough to lie still for the procedure, he may have to be pharmacologically paralyzed. This requires mechanical ventilation throughout the course of the procedure until the drug wears off. Extubation depends on diagnostic findings, any anticipated surgery, and the patient's ability to maintain a patent airway and gas exchange on his own.

If the CNS disturbance results in brain death, support the family in making the decision about whether to stop ventilatory support (once the prognosis has been confirmed). Make sure you know and follow hospital policy and legal criteria for discontinuing ventilatory support in the brain-dead patient.

Spinal cord injury

Description

Spinal cord injury (SCI) impairs the conduction of electrical impulses to or from the brain. Damage to the cord then can affect all body systems, such as the respiratory, cardiovascular, and autonomic nervous systems.

SCI can be classified in several ways. *Complete injury* refers to total loss of neurologic integrity (motor and sensory function and proprioception) distal to the injury site. *Incomplete injury* indicates partial or total preservation of movement, feeling, or proprioception. Complex by nature, incomplete injuries result in varying degrees of disability; some functions are destroyed while others are mildly impaired. Complete injury carries a poor prognosis; incomplete injury, a guarded but more positive prognosis.

SCI patients also have a high incidence of associated thoracic injuries (such as rib fractures, flail chest, and hemothorax or pneumothorax) and of pulmonary complications (such as atelactasis and pneumonia).

Causes

Spinal cord injury most commonly results from:

• motor vehicle accidents
• penetrating wounds
• falls
• sports injuries.

Pathophysiology

Damage to the cervical and thoracic spinal cord portions can result in respiratory compromise, because respiratory muscles are innervated by specific spinal nerves. (See *Spinal Cord Innervation of the Muscles of Respiration*.) When complete SCI occurs between C1 and T12, loss of nervous innervation to respiratory muscles always occurs to a varying degree. Incomplete injuries may have less effect on muscle groups if motor function is not completely affected;

Spinal Cord Innervation of the Muscles of Respiration

This lateral view of the spinal cord shows the level of origin for the nerves supplying the respiratory muscles. Function remains intact above the level of injury but is lost below it. Therefore, the higher the lesion, the more severe the respiratory dysfunction. Also note that complete transection above T1 causes quadriplegia; below, paraplegia.

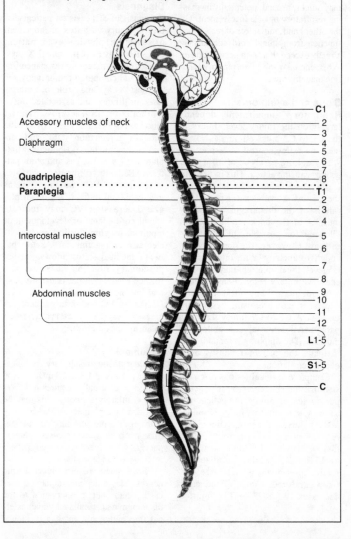

Accessory muscles of neck

Diaphragm

Quadriplegia

Paraplegia

Intercostal muscles

Abdominal muscles

C1
2
3
4
5
6
7
8
T1
2
3
4
5
6
7
8
9
10
11
12
L1-5
S1-5
C

however, if sensory function is spared and motor function in the upper thoracic or cervical regions is affected, significant respiratory compromise may result.

Spinal cord edema associated with SCI also has important implications. First, in the immediate post-injury period (several days) of an acute SCI, edema may worsen and the lesion level may quickly ascend, potentially increasing respiratory muscle involvement. On the other hand, initial loss of respiratory function from spinal cord edema may already exceed that from nerve damage. When edema resolves, respiratory function may improve.

Signs and symptoms

Respiratory impairment depends largely on the injury level. Injury to the C1 to C2 areas eliminates voluntary and reflex control of respiration, with resulting paralysis of all muscle groups causing apnea. This injury typically causes death instantly. Injury to the C3 to C4 levels causes partial paralysis of the diaphragm. Accessory muscles of the neck retain function, allowing for possible shallow respirations. However, the patient can't cough voluntarily. With injury to the C5 level, the diaphragm may be weakened. Voluntary respirations are usually adequate, but vital capacity decreases, compromising respiratory reserve. A C6 to C7 injury results in paralyzed intercostal and abdominal muscles. The diaphragm remains normal and the patient retains spontaneous ventilation.

Complete cervical lesions often destabilize the rib cage. You may detect paradoxical breathing; the patient may show rapid respiratory fatigue from the loss of muscle function. Diminished respiratory excursion prevents secretion expulsion. With injury at the T1 to T7 levels, breathing is diaphragmatic; intercostal muscles are partially paralyzed. Cough effectiveness decreases. With T7 to T12 injuries, impaired cough and abdominal muscle weakening occur.

The patient with SCI often sustains other traumatic injuries that may be life-threatening and that may present other significant signs and symptoms, such as flail chest with paradoxical chest wall movement.

Diagnosis

Diagnosis of SCI rests on patient history of injury with loss of movement or sensation, physical examination, and such tests as plain spinal X-rays, myelography, magnetic resonance imaging, and computed tomography.

Chest X-rays may rule out atelectasis, infiltrates, and associated pneumothorax or rib fractures. Arterial blood gas (ABG) analysis evaluates the patient's oxygenation status and carbon dioxide retention. Abdominal flat-plate X-rays assess gas and stool patterns. Bedside spirometry evaluates vital capacity (VC), which may be as low as 800 ml in C3 to C4 quadriplegia. Decreasing VC may indicate spinal cord edema or development of a pulmonary complication, such as atelectasis or pneumonia. As the patient's medical status allows, further pulmonary function tests are performed. Tidal volume is usually normal but may decrease in some cases. Decreased VC and a subsequent decrease in respiratory reserve can result in an increased $PaCO_2$ level.

Treatment

Consider treating respiratory complications a priority. A C1 to C3 quadriplegic who survives usually requires full, lifelong ventilatory support. This may be provided by a permanent tracheostomy with positive pressure mechanical ventilation or, in selected cases, phrenic pacing, which permits greater patient mobility and independence.

Phrenic pacing requires intact phrenic nerves. Electrodes are implanted over each phrenic nerve innervation to the diaphragm and stimulated via an external transmitter and antenna to induce respiration. Short-term stimulation is initiated with the expectation of multiple hours of pacing. Phrenic stimulators usually aren't implanted until several months to 1 year after injury, in case spontaneous respiration returns. All paced patients require stand-by ventilatory support in case of mechanical failure. (See *Phrenic Pacemaker*.) Also, ventilator-dependent quadriplegics may be able to use accessory muscles (sternocleidomastoid and scalene muscles), and glossopharyngeal breathing (air forced into the lungs by the mouth and throat) to provide short intervals of voluntary respiration. This method proves valuable in the event of short-term equipment failure. However, both glossopharyngeal and accessory-muscle breathing are exhausting and therefore not suitable for prolonged use.

Patients with C4 to C5 injury will require ventilatory support in the acute phase. However, these patients have a better chance of regaining spontaneous ventilation, avoiding the need for mechanical ventilation, at least during the day. Bronchial hygiene is important. Ventilatory assist devices, such as a rocking bed, may be used. (See *Rocking Bed*, page 204.)

Patients with SCI who can breathe spontaneously need initial and ongoing evaluation for respiratory reserve impairment and inefficient oxygenation.

When pulmonary hygiene is compromised or ABG measurements show deterioration, the patient must be intubated. Initially, an endotracheal tube is used to facilitate ventilation; however, if weaning is difficult or prolonged, a tracheostomy tube may be placed to prevent further vocal cord trauma and enhance secretion removal. In most cases, the tube's removed after the acute phase.

Patients with decreased respiratory reserve and weak muscle innervation may not generate a sufficiently strong cough and may therefore need suctioning assistance. In these cases, a

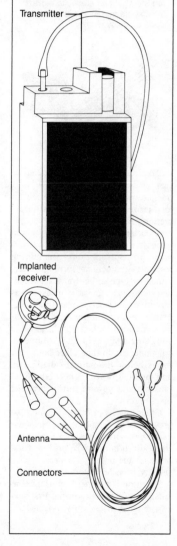

Phrenic Pacemaker

A phrenic pacemaker may be used to induce respiration in selected patients, such as those with high cervical cord injury or central alveolar hypoventilation.

Transmitter

Implanted receiver

Antenna

Connectors

Rocking Bed

A rocking bed offers an alternative to conventional mechanical ventilation for selected patients. Its slow, rocking movements improve ventilation by using the abdominal content's weight and gravity to move the diaphragm up on expiration and down on inspiration.

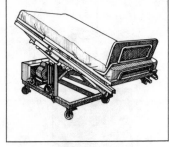

tracheostomy tube may be placed for long-term use to allow access for secretion removal.

A patient who can breathe spontaneously needs individualized treatment to optimize his remaining respiratory function. Turning (determined by type of bedframe and medical stability) and such measures as incentive spirometry, percussion, vibration, postural drainage, and breathing exercises may be helpful. Assistive coughing may help add volume to coughing. To do this, place both your hands below the patient's diaphragm and push upward. The abdominal pressure and upward thrust force the diaphragm up.

Other aspects of acute care focus on prevention of complications. Hemodynamic monitoring lines help manage I.V. fluid administration to prevent fluid overload and pulmonary edema. Occasionally, bronchodilators are necessary.

Nutrition is another important consideration, especially in the first several months after injury. Nasogastric feedings, gastrostomy feedings, or total parenteral nutrition should begin early.

Clinical considerations
• Make every effort to successfully wean the patient from the ventilator to increase his chances for survival and meaningful rehabilitation.
• Closely monitor the patient in the early post-injury period, even if he's breathing spontaneously. Spinal cord edema can quickly cause the lesion to ascend, requiring immediate ventilatory support.
• Teach the patient to recognize and report signs and symptoms of respiratory infection. Instruct him and his family to avoid crowds during heavy infection seasons. Encourage him to receive influenza and pneumonia vaccines.
• Encourage the patient to have a good understanding of his care needs and to teach others to perform necessary tasks.
• Teach the patient and family how to recognize equipment failure and emergency management.
• Encourage mobility and activity to minimize pulmonary complications.
• Provide psychological support and referrals to appropriate counseling to help the patient cope with the effects of his injury.

Neuromuscular disorders

Description
A neuromuscular disorder can cause life-threatening respiratory dysfunction. Its onset may be sudden, occurring within hours, or, in some cases, it may be slowly progressive. Prognosis also varies. Some disorders that temporarily weaken respiratory muscles may be potentially reversible, provided the patient receives careful assessment and aggressive respiratory treatment. In other cases, respiratory muscle involvement is permanent, and

respiratory failure can be the expected cause of death.

Causes
- Myasthenia gravis
- Amyotrophic lateral sclerosis (ALS)
- Poliomyelitis
- Guillain-Barré syndrome
- Duchenne's muscular dystrophy

Pathophysiology
Neuromuscular diseases can affect the motor neurons and the myoneural junction or may cause general nerve demyelination. In any case, if impulse transmission from the brain and along the phrenic nerve to the diaphragm is seriously impaired, respiratory failure can occur. Less severe impairment may result in decreased respiratory muscle function, with diminished respiratory reserve and decreased chest wall tone. This can result in retained secretions, decreased functional residual capacity, atelectasis, and respiratory tract infection. Genetically determined myopathies may cause respiratory problems from actual muscle degeneration.

Additionally, some neuromuscular disorders affect muscles supplied by cranial nerves. This can interfere with the gag, cough, and swallowing reflexes, resulting in inability to protect the airway. (For more specific information on neuromuscular disorders most likely to cause respiratory problems, see *Understanding Neuromuscular Disorders,* pages 206 and 207; for details on respiratory failure, see Chapter 9.)

Signs and symptoms
Neurologic signs and symptoms typically precede respiratory involvement, although the time frame varies considerably. In the patient with myasthenia gravis, the interval may be only minutes; in the patient with muscular dystrophy, it may be months. Patients with progressive respiratory weakness usually first notice shortness of breath

on exertion. Initially, this respiratory impairment may be wrongly attributed to fatigue from use of weakened muscles during exertion.

When respiratory muscles are markedly weakened, tidal volume decreases. Respiratory rate increases in an attempt to blow off carbon dioxide. Soon fatigue sets in. Eventually, the patient's cough becomes ineffective in clearing his airway. Respiratory failure follows shortly.

Diagnosis
Evaluating the respiratory status of a patient with neuromuscular disease is a priority. To ensure prompt intervention, frequently monitor vital capacity (VC), negative inspiratory force, respiratory rate, and arterial blood gas (ABG) measurements. (Frequency should be determined by progression of neurologic signs and symptoms and respiratory assessment results.)

Normally, VC ranges from 30 to 70 ml/kg. If it falls below 30 ml/kg, monitor the patient closely. If it falls below 15 ml/kg, the patient will need an artificial airway and, possibly, mechanical ventilation. (With inadequate VC, the patient can't take in a deep breath to cough and protect his airway, nor can he breathe deeply if respiratory demands increase.)

Inspiratory force is normally 50 to 100 cmH$_2$O. Closely monitor the patient if it falls below normal; anticipate artificial airway placement if it drops below 25 cmH$_2$O. (Decreasing negative inspiratory force has the same consequences as decreasing VC.)

Respiratory rate is normally 12 to 25 breaths/minute. Closely monitor the patient for fatigue if the rate starts to exceed normal limits. Unless complications exist, a respiratory rate above 35 breaths/minute indicates that tidal volume has decreased markedly; an increased respiratory rate reflects an attempt to maintain gas exchange. A rate this high, with other abnormal assessment findings, may warrant mechanical ventilation.

Understanding Neuromuscular Disorders

Condition	Pathophysiology	Clinical features
Myasthenia gravis	This disease results in impaired transmission of nerve impulses. It's thought to result from an autoimmune response causing autoantibody formation. These antibodies block and destroy acetylcholine receptor sites on the post-synaptic membrane. Muscle weakness and easy fatigability result from receptor site decrease.	The characteristic feature is muscle weakness, which increases with exertion and fatigue but improves with rest. Common signs and symptoms include ptosis, diplopia, and blurred vision. Difficulty swallowing, difficulty speaking, nasal speech, and facial muscle weakness occur with cranial nerve involvement. Respiratory muscle weakness may also occur with signs and symptoms of respiratory failure.
Guillain-Barré syndrome	This presumably is an autoimmune, postinfectious process striking spinal nerve roots as well as peripheral nerves. It results in inflammation, edema, and areas of segmental demyelination. Typically, the disease ascends the spinal cord, beginning with leg weakness and progressing quickly over a period of hours to several days. The point at which demyelination stops varies, but it may ascend up to and beyond the cervical level. Because both dorsal and ventral roots are involved, sensory and motor impairment may occur.	Typically, primary motor weakness or paralysis begins in the lower extremities and ascends upward at an unpredictable rate. Paresthesias and mild sensory loss, although less common, may accompany motor weakness. If respiratory muscles are involved, signs and symptoms of respiratory failure may occur. Other clinical features may include facial diplegia (possibly with opthalmoplegia), dysphagia, or dysarthria.
Amyotrophic lateral sclerosis	This rapidly progressing, fatal degenerative disease results in destruction of anterior gray horn cells (motor cells) and pyramidal tracts of the spinal cord. It can also attack the brain stem.	In early disease, weakness and spasticity in hands or arms occurs, along with fasciculations, muscle atrophy, and fatigue. When the disease is advanced, flaccid quadriplegia and respiratory muscle weakness occur along with dysphagia and dysarthria, with possible choking. Death usually results from respiratory failure.
Duchenne's muscular dystrophy	This myopathy is inherited as an x-linked recessive trait. It probably results	This muscular dystrophy initially involves the proximal pelvic girdle muscles. Eventually, muscle

Understanding Neuromuscular Disorders*(continued)*

Condition	Pathophysiology	Clinical features
Duchenne's muscular dystrophy *(continued)*	from abnormal cellular metabolism in muscle fibers, leading to muscular degeneration and wasting over a period of years.	atrophy and weakness immobilize the patient. In late disease, cardiac and respiratory muscles weaken. Death commonly results from sudden heart failure, respiratory failure, or infection.
Poliomyelitis	An acute communicable disease, poliomyelitis is caused by any of three polioviruses. Inflammation, scarring, and shrinking of the anterior horn and brain stem may occur.	In *paralytic poliomyelitis*, flaccid paralysis of muscles innervated by destroyed neurons causes prolonged immobility. The most dangerous type, *bulbar paralytic poliomyelitis*, results in facial weakness; dysphasia; difficulty chewing; inability to swallow or expel saliva; dyspnea; and abnormal respiratory rate, depth, and rhythm, which may lead to respiratory failure.

ABG measurements usually include an increased $PaCO_2$ level from reduced overall ventilation. When the patient can no longer compensate for decreasing tidal volume by increasing his respiratory rate, the $PaCO_2$ level rises, strongly suggesting the need for mechanical ventilation.

Treatment and clinical considerations

As respiratory compromise progresses along with the neurologic disorder, pulmonary hygiene becomes critical. Ensure adequate hydration to help maintain fluid secretions (unless contraindications rule out generous fluid intake). Teach the patient how to use an incentive spirometer to help focus his attention on deep breathing and to preserve vital capacity as long as muscle strength allows. If secretions collect and impair respirations, chest physiotherapy and suctioning should begin.

If assessment findings indicate impending respiratory failure and the neurologic diagnosis is clear, mechanical ventilation will be initiated.

• Patients with neuromuscular disease and potentially reversible respiratory failure may require long-term mechanical ventilation before adequate spontaneous ventilation resumes. Therefore, instead of intubating the patient and later performing a tracheotomy, the doctor may perform a tracheotomy initially. This protects the vocal cords from damage caused by the endotracheal tube, leaves the mouth free for mouth care, and keeps the patient's face free of tape.

• Wean the patient with intermittent mandatory ventilation to allow respiratory muscles gradual reconditioning. (See Chapter 13 for more information.)

• Remember that these patients may be weaned from ventilatory support and breathe on their own during the day but may hypoventilate at night. Therefore, provide nighttime ventilation until they regain muscle strength.

• Measure weaning parameters even if neurologic assessment findings haven't improved. Respiratory function may return first, and the sooner weaning begins, the sooner the patient can get off the ventilator.

• If the patient isn't likely to recover from a degenerative disease, discuss the issue of ventilatory support early in the course of treatment. ALS, for example, takes a relentless, progressive course, leaving the patient with an active mind but a totally unresponsive body. The patient may prefer death to prolonged ventilator dependency. Postponing the discussion may result in a hasty decision later, when respiratory failure occurs. Include any appropriate team members (such as a social worker or clergy member) in the discussion to provide support to the family, and allow the patient and his family time to make an informed decision.

• Home ventilation may be considered if the patient's clinical status is stable and his needs involve mainly ventilatory support and basic nursing care.

• Be sure to explain all procedures to the chronically ventilated patient. Totally dependent on others for all care, this patient may be extremely anxious, especially if caregivers perform procedures differently. If you must perform a procedure differently, be sure to explain why to the patient.

Sleep-related respiratory disorders

Description

Caused by disturbances in breathing, sleep-related respiratory disorders result in recurrent episodes of apnea, hypoventilation, or both. Apnea refers to cessation of airflow through the nose and mouth for longer than 10 seconds. The sleep apnea syndrome is characterized by more than 30 apneic episodes each night. Hypoventilation describes abnormally increased $PaCO_2$, which results from decreased respiratory depth or rate.

Causes

• Disruption of brainstem respiratory neurons, commonly associated with previous insult to the central nervous system

• Upper airway occlusion, commonly associated with adenotonsillar hypertrophy, lymphoma, acromegaly, goiter, and obesity. (See *Pickwickian Syndrome*.)

Pathophysiology

Four sleep-related abnormalities exist:
• central apnea
• obstructive apnea
• mixed apnea
• primary alveolar hypoventilation.

With *central apnea*, airflow through the nose, mouth, and lungs stops as respiratory muscle activity ceases secondary to neurologic dysfunction. If oxygen desaturation occurs, this may cause light sleep or arousal, thereby stimulating renewed respiratory efforts. Some researchers link central apnea with infantile apnea and sudden infant death syndrome. (See *SIDS Update*, page 210.)

With *obstructive apnea*, chest and abdominal wall muscles attempt to breathe, but no airflow occurs. The tongue or upper airway fatty tissue may occlude the airway. Also, certain physical characteristics combined with muscle relaxation during sleep increase upper airway resistance, which raises negative inspiratory pressures, causing oropharynx airway collapse. In most cases, oxygen desaturation arouses the person. Once awake, he can restore upper airway muscle tone and remove the obstruction. Without arousal, however, PaO_2 decreases and $PaCO_2$ levels increase. Eventually, abnormal blood gas levels or increased mechanical loads arouse the person and normal respiration resumes. But as soon as he falls asleep again, the cycle repeats itself.

Mixed apnea begins as a central breathing cessation. When breathing resumes, upper airway obstruction prevents airflow. Hypopnea is a decrease in both effort and flow that results in decreased tidal volume and desaturation.

Primary alveolar hypoventilation refers to a condition in which the lungs function normally but the breathing drive breaks down. Decreased alveolar ventilation results in CO_2 retention and may or may not occur while the person's awake. Hypoventilation usually worsens during sleep.

Persons with primary alveolar hypoventilation have normal pulmonary function test results. They can consciously alter their PaO_2 and $PaCO_2$ levels by increasing their respiratory rate and depth.

Signs and symptoms

Patients with sleep-related disorders may exhibit a range of daytime fatigue and lethargy, from mild sleepiness to severe hypersomnolence. For example, they may fall asleep while talking or even driving a car.

The patient may also experience decreased intellectual functioning, impotence, and personality changes that can lead to significant life-style changes. He may report impaired judgment and memory, especially in the morning. Or he may seek psychiatric or psychological counseling, to no avail. The negative results of these changes can create an altered self-image, leading to depression. Other signs and symptoms include headaches or confusion on awakening, morning nausea, and intermittent enuresis.

Many patients with obstructive sleep-related disorders have short, thick necks or large tongues and abnormally small lower jaws. Some have blocked or narrowed nasal passages from deviated nasal septums or adenotonsillar enlargements. Except for an elongated soft palate or redundant pharyngeal tissue, the pharynx usually appears normal. Such a patient may be obese, restless, and snore loudly, snort, and experience episodic apnea.

Pickwickian Syndrome

Pickwickian syndrome (also known as obese hypoventilation syndrome) derives its name from an obese character in Charles Dickens' novel *The Posthumous Papers of the Pickwick Club*. Like that character, obese persons may experience hypersomnolence during the daytime, a result of obstructive sleep apneas.

As muscle tone decreases in deep sleep, fatty soft tissue of the oropharynx can't resist the pull of inspiratory negative pressure. As a result, the oropharynx falls inward, blocking airflow. As oxygen desaturation increases, arousal to a lighter stage of sleep improves muscle tone. Also, the airway reopens. If this cycle continues uncorrected, the following conditions can develop: hypercapnia, polycythemia, periodic breathing, cor pulmonale, and right ventricular failure.

Because the patient may not be aware of his snoring or restlessness, his bed partner may need to supply the history. In addition, the patient may have systemic hypertension, which reverses when the obstruction's relieved.

Conversely, the central apneic patient may complain of insomnia and frequent awakenings. These patients (mean age 63) usually have normal or below-normal weights.

Patients with primary alveolar hypoventilation may also experience seizures or severe cardiac dysrhythmias during sleep, and may show signs and symptoms of right ventricular heart failure (cor pulmonale) and pulmonary hypertension.

Diagnosis

Appropriate medical intervention depends on diagnosing the specific sleep-related disorder and determining its effect on oxygen levels.

Polysomnography (sleep study) is warranted when the patient's history and

SIDS Update

Sudden infant death syndrome (SIDS) is the leading cause of death among infants aged 1 month to 1 year, with deaths occurring at a rate of 2 in every 1,000 live births. In the United States, 7,000 infants die of SIDS annually. Although SIDS has been described since ancient times, its causes are still obscure.

Formerly, SIDS was believed to be caused by accidental suffocation of infants during sleep or as a result of abuse. Diagnosis continues to be based on exclusion, but researchers believe that SIDS probably has more than one cause. They have uncovered the following information:

• Peak incidence occurs between age 2 and 4 months; incidence declines rapidly between 4 and 12 months. Sixty-one percent of SIDS victims have been boys.

• Infants die suddenly in their sleep, without warning, sound, or struggle.

• Incidence of SIDS is slightly higher in preterm infants, native Alaskan infants, disadvantaged Black infants, infants of mothers under age 20, and infants of multiple births. Incidence is 10 times higher in SIDS siblings; slightly higher in infants whose mothers smoke; and up to 10 times higher in infants whose mothers are narcotic addicts.

• Some SIDS-diagnosed infants show postmortem changes that indicate chronic hypoxia, hypoxemia, and large airway obstruction.

• *Clostridium botulinum* toxin has been linked to a few SIDS deaths.

• Infants commonly succumb to SIDS in the fall and winter. Many have a history of respiratory infection, suggesting viral infection as an etiology.

• Studies show conflicting data about abnormal hepatic or pancreatic processes in SIDS infants.

• The link between apneic episodes and SIDS is unclear. But about 60% of infants with near-miss respiratory events have second episodes of apnea; some succumb to SIDS.

When an infant dies of SIDS, assure parents that they were in no way responsible for the death. Answer questions about autopsy, and explain it as a benefit in achieving peace of mind as well as furthering knowledge of SIDS. Encourage parents to seek counseling about the risk of SIDS to siblings and their possible evaluation with cardiopneumogram and apnea monitoring. Parents can seek help from health care providers, clergy, and the National Sudden Infant Death Syndrome Foundation (1-800-221-SIDS).

Explain to parents of healthy infants who worry about SIDS that apnea/cardiac monitoring is generally recommended only for siblings of SIDS victims because of its high cost and often disruptive effects on family dynamics.

physical examination clearly indicate a sleep-related disorder. Whether the sleep study will be performed during a daytime nap or nighttime sleep depends on the degree of the patient's hypersomnolence and primary disease state. The primary factors evaluated in a standard sleep study include:

• sleep stages (including length of time in each stage, number of shifts from one stage to another, number of awakenings, and amount of awake time), using electroencephalography (EEG) and electro-oculography (EOG)

• cardiac rate and rhythm, using electrocardiography (EKG)

• oxygen saturation, using ear oximetry or transcutaneous monitoring.

• nose and mouth airflow using a thermistor, mask, and pneumotachygraph to quantitate volume moved

• inspiratory muscle activity, using devices that record chest and abdominal wall pressure changes.

If the patient's chest expands but air doesn't flow through his nose or mouth, suspect *obstructive apnea*. If you can't detect movement for more than 10 seconds, the patient has *central apnea*. When oxygen desaturation occurs, the sleep stage lightens or awakening occurs.

Another diagnostic test, capnography, measures exhaled CO_2 levels, using a mask to trap exhaled air.

Doctors rarely order invasive monitoring techniques, such as the esophageal balloon, which monitors transdiaphragmatic pressure swings that occur with obstruction, unless other diagnostic methods fail or require clarification.

The doctor may also ask the patient or his bed partner to keep a sleep diary to record sleep patterns, such as snoring, restlessness, and daytime somnolence. Also, a bedside tape recorder can document breath sounds that occur during sleep.

Treatment and clinical considerations

Treatment goals include correcting potentially life-threatening dysrhythmias and reversing depression, memory loss, and somnolence. Proper management requires an accurate diagnosis of the severity and cause of the sleep-related respiratory disorder.

For a patient with an obstructive disorder and dysrhythmias, a tracheotomy clears the airway. However, the risk of infection and patient reluctance may cause the doctor to forego this surgical technique. In addition, obese patients with neck sizes greater than 17″ may experience difficulty because the standard tracheostomy tube length is designed for smaller necks. Therefore, proper alignment with the airway may be difficult or the tracheostomy

tube may obstruct the airway, causing respiratory arrest. (Special-length tubes may be ordered for these patients.) If the patient's neck size decreases from a weight change, adjust the tube length or angle to the new tracheal wall depth. Improper tube fit will lead to excessive irritation and possible stenosis.

Nighttime oxygen administration to treat nocturnal hypoxemia raises baseline oxygen saturation, reducing the severity of apneas or hypopneas. Supplemental oxygen therapy also decreases the total amount of desaturation time, reducing the overall stress on the patient's cardiopulmonary system and averting potential pulmonary hypertension and right-sided heart failure.

Continuous positive airway pressure (CPAP) can provide a constant back pressure (greater than atmospheric pressure) to the upper airways of patients with obstructive sleep disorders. This helps maintain an open airway during inspiration when the usual negative pressure of inspiration would occlude it. As a result, CPAP can decrease or alleviate snoring associated with obstructive sleep apneas. (See *CPAP Mask,* page 245, in Chapter 11.)

Teach the patient and his family how to care for and maintain the CPAP system, especially the intake filter. A dirty filter can reduce airflow and cause the patient's inspiration pressure to drop below atmospheric pressure, negating the system's benefits.

Oxygen therapy for predominantly central apneas or primary alveolar hypoventilation usually isn't effective. However, a rocking bed or a negative pressure ventilator may offer assistance. For patients with mixed apnea, the doctor may perform a tracheotomy and order positive end-expiratory pressure ventilation. (Negative pressure ventilation could worsen the obstruction.)

Electrical diaphragm pacing is frequently used in patients with central alveolar hypoventilation to induce respiration. However, it can overstimulate the phrenic nerves and gradually decrease their responsiveness. You can decrease this risk by using the stimulator less than 8 hours per day and by alternating sides.

If the patient has a lesion, such as hypertrophied tonsils or adenoids, surgical intervention may be warranted. However, the doctor will carefully weigh risks against benefits.

Drug therapy may be helpful. The doctor will usually prescribe thyroid medications for hypothyroid patients with hypersomnolence.

Respiratory stimulants, such as progesterone, used in patients with central apnea and, to a lesser degree, obstructive apnea, decrease the number of apneic episodes and improve daytime ventilation.

Aminophylline, another respiratory stimulant, exerts a bronchodilatory effect when decreased airflow has been caused by bronchoconstriction during sleep (nocturnal asthma).

Protriptyline, a tricyclic antidepressant, treats central and obstructive apneas. By reducing the amount of REM sleep, it decreases the duration and frequency of apnea episodes. The usual protriptyline dose used for sleep apnea exceeds the normal dose prescribed for depression. Carefully monitor your patient for adverse effects, such as seizures, excitation, tremors, confusion, headache, nervousness, orthostatic hypotension, tachycardia, EKG changes, hypertension, blurred vision, tinnitus, mydriasis, constipation, dry mouth, and nausea.

Counsel obese patients in weight reduction techniques. Also, warn patients about the potential for injury if daytime hypersomnolence occurs, and assist them in planning to avoid hazardous activities.

Selected References

Martin, L. *Pulmonary Physiology in Clinical Practice: The Essentials for Patient Care and Evaluation.* St. Louis: C.V. Mosby Co., 1986.

Neurologic Disorders. Nurse's Clinical Library. Springhouse, Pa.: Springhouse Corp., 1984.

Raimond, J., and Taylor, J.W. *Neurological Emergencies: Effective Nursing Care.* Rockville, Md.: Aspen Systems Corp., 1985.

Respiratory Problems. NurseReview series. Springhouse, Pa.: Springhouse Corp., 1986.

Shapiro, B.A., et al. *Clinical Applications of Respiratory Care,* 3rd ed. Chicago: Year Book Medical Pubs., Inc., 1985.

Snyder, M., ed. *A Guide to Neurological and Neurosurgical Nursing.* New York: John Wiley & Sons, 1983.

Thompson, J.M., et al. *Clinical Nursing.* St. Louis: C.V. Mosby Co., 1985.

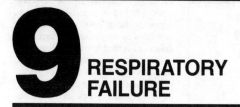

9 RESPIRATORY FAILURE

Introduction

Maintaining adequate respiration is essential to life: without the gas exchange that respiration provides, all body systems quickly fail. That's why respiratory failure demands early recognition and prompt treatment to improve the patient's chance of survival. To effectively intervene in respiratory failure, you must have a thorough knowledge of pathophysiology as well as current treatment methods.

Respiratory failure refers to a condition in which the lungs no longer efficiently exchange carbon dioxide and oxygen to keep pace with cellular metabolism. It may develop abruptly (acute respiratory failure) or insidiously (chronic respiratory failure). More a dysfunction than a disease, respiratory failure has many causes. A major cause of acute respiratory failure is chronic obstructive pulmonary disease. Adult respiratory distress syndrome also may quickly lead to acute respiratory failure.

Management of acute respiratory failure involves life-saving measures to correct hypoxemia, hypercapnia, and acidosis and to stabilize the patient's condition; diagnostic tests to confirm respiratory failure and identify its cause; and supportive therapy and care to treat the cause and prevent complications.

Acute respiratory failure

Description
With its myriad causes and variable clinical presentation, acute respiratory failure (ARF) defies easy definition. Basically, it occurs when the lungs no longer meet the body's metabolic needs. Arterial blood gas (ABG) levels usually provide clues to ARF. For most patients, a PaO_2 level of 50 mm Hg or below or a $PaCO_2$ level of 50 mm Hg or above indicates ARF. However, patients with chronic obstructive pulmonary disease (COPD) have chronically low PaO_2 levels and high $PaCO_2$ levels.

Therefore, a PaO_2 level that doesn't increase despite increased FIO_2 or an increased $PaCO_2$ level that results in a pH of 7.25 or lower suggests ARF. A pH of 7.25 is also significant because medications and enzymes don't function well in acidemia.

Causes
See *Acute Respiratory Failure: Reviewing Causes,* page 214, for a listing of major causes.

Pathophysiology
Four main mechanisms—alveolar hypoventilation, intrapulmonary shunting, ventilation/perfusion mismatch, and impaired diffusion across the respiratory membrane—can impair gas exchange in ARF. Regardless of the underlying mechanism, impaired gas

Acute Respiratory Failure: Reviewing Causes

VENTILATORY FAILURE
Brain
- Head trauma
- Cerebral hemorrhage
- Bulbar poliomyelitis
- Drug overdose
- Central alveolar hypoventilation syndrome

Neuromuscular
- Guillain-Barré syndrome
- Spinal cord trauma
- Polio
- Amyotrophic lateral sclerosis
- Myasthenia gravis
- Tetanus
- Drug blockade: kanamycin, polymyxin
- Botulism
- Organic phosphate insecticides
- Peripheral neuritis

Muscular-structural
- Muscular dystrophy
- Massive obesity
- Kyphoscoliosis
- Flail chest
- Rheumatoid spondylitis

GAS EXCHANGE FAILURE
Upper airways
- Sleep apnea
- Vocal cord paralysis
- Tracheal obstruction

Heart and vasculature
- Cardiogenic pulmonary edema
- Pulmonary embolism

Lower airways and alveoli
- Chronic obstructive pulmonary disease
- Asthma
- Cystic fibrosis
- Bronchiolitis
- Adult respiratory distress syndrome
- Interstitial lung disease
- Massive bilateral pneumonia

exchange ultimately affects the entire body. The hypoxemia and hypercapnia characteristic of ARF stimulate strong responses by the respiratory, cardiovascular, and central nervous systems.

Respiratory response. When the body senses hypoxemia or hypercapnia (or both), the brain's respiratory center responds by first increasing respiratory depth (tidal volume) and then increasing respiratory rate. These and other signs of labored breathing— flared nostrils, pursed-lip exhalation, and use of accessory breathing muscles—may signify ARF. As respiratory failure worsens, intercostal, supraclavicular, and suprasternal retractions may also occur. However, these signs don't always indicate ARF. For example, many COPD patients use pursed-lip breathing at all times. Also, patients with such ventilatory problems as Guillain-Barré syndrome and myasthenia gravis may suffer respiratory failure without obvious signs of labored breathing.

Cardiovascular response. Premature ventricular contractions (PVCs) are the most common cardiac ectopy related to hypoxia. The sympathetic nervous system usually compensates for an emergency, such as hypoxemia, by increasing the heart rate and constricting blood vessels. Besides helping to raise blood pressure and cardiac output, vasoconstriction makes the patient's skin cool, pale, and clammy.

This compensatory response can persist only for a limited time. When hypoxemia's severe enough and the compensatory response can no longer be maintained, blood pressure drops and coma may ensue.

Hypercapnia can have the opposite effect on smooth muscle lining of blood vessels, causing peripheral vasodilation. In this case, the skin becomes warm and flushed. If this opposing effect outweighs normal sympathetic vasoconstriction, blood pressure may drop, possibly leading to shock.

Central nervous system (CNS) response. Even a slight disruption in oxygen supply and carbon dioxide removal affects brain function and behavior. Hypoxia initially causes restlessness; the patient may use a pincerlike grasp to pick at items, such as bedclothes. This progresses to marked confusion and agitation and, finally, to coma. Headache is the primary sign of hypercapnia. It occurs as cerebral vessels dilate in an effort to increase the brain's blood supply. Lethargy, which may progress to somnolence, is another CNS sign. In addition, a high $PaCO_2$ level may cause confusion. If the $PaCO_2$ level continues to rise, the patient may have convulsions and lapse into a coma.

(See *Assessment Findings in Acute Respiratory Failure.*)

Signs and symptoms

Using your skills of inspection, palpation, percussion, and auscultation, examine the patient for signs of respiratory failure. Inspect the patient's chest for symmetry and degree of respiratory excursion. If you suspect chest trauma, stay alert for paradoxical movement and use of accessory muscles (perhaps the first clue that the patient's having difficulty breathing). Tachypnea usually signals impending respiratory failure. Also note whether the patient can speak and communicate with you. Inspect his lips and nailbeds for cyanosis, but remember, cyanosis isn't always a reliable indicator of hypoxemia. For example, blue nailbeds can result from local hypoperfusion and vasoconstriction.

Palpate your patient's chest for tenderness and for symmetrical chest movement; asymmetrical movement may suggest pneumothorax. If present, tactile fremitus decreases over an obstructed bronchi or pleural effusion but increases over consolidated lung tissue.

Assessment Findings in Acute Respiratory Failure

Respiratory response	Cardiovascular response	Central nervous system response
Increased $PaCO_2$		
• Decreasing tidal volume • Tachypnea	• Local vasodilation (flushing) • Decreased blood pressure (late response)	• Headache from cerebral vasodilation (cardinal sign) • Somnolence • Later convulsions, eventually coma
Decreased PaO_2		
• Tachypnea • Dyspnea	• Tachycardia • Ectopy (especially PVCs) • Initially, increased blood pressure from sympathetic response • Vasoconstriction as compensatory mechanisms fail • Bradycardia, vasodilation, and hypotension	• Initial restlessness, slight disorientation • Patient picks at sheet, gown, etc. • Anxiety progresses to frank disorientation, drowsiness, coma

With COPD patients, expect hyperresonance on percussion. Listen for a dull or flat percussion note if you suspect atelectasis, pneumonia, pleural effusion, or hemothorax.

COPD typically diminishes breath sounds; pneumothorax may silence them altogether, but you may hear sounds transmitted from other chest areas. In other cases of respiratory failure, you may hear adventitious breath sounds. For example, asthma may cause wheezes; bronchitis causes rhonchi. Suspect pulmonary edema or ARDS if you hear crackles.

Diagnosis

The following tests help confirm ARF:
• *ABG analysis.* This may show hypercapnia (with or without hypoxemia) and respiratory acidosis. ABG analysis is always performed whenever ARF is suspected. It's also indicated whenever PVCs occur in the absence of cardiac disease or indwelling cardiac catheters.
• *Chest X-ray.* This sometimes helps determine the underlying cause of ARF, such as pneumonia or flail chest. However, it's not diagnostic—pulmonary edema and ARDS can look alike on chest X-ray. Also, the chest X-ray is commonly inconsistent with the clinical picture. For instance, it may be normal with many causes of ventilatory failure, such as Guillain-Barré syndrome and poliomyelitis.
• *Sputum culture and sensitivity tests.* These isolate any causative infectious organism.
• *Bedside spirometry.* This can predict respiratory failure if vital capacity, tidal volume, inspiratory force, and other functional parameters decrease. (See *Respiratory Failure Criteria.*)
• *Serum electrolyte tests.* These may reveal electrolyte imbalances.
• *EKG.* This may detect dysrhythmias secondary to hypoxia.
• *Pulmonary artery catheterization.* This helps differentiate pulmonary and cardiovascular causes of respiratory failure and monitors hemodynamic pressures.

Treatment and clinical considerations

Unless promptly treated, ARF can precipitate respiratory and cardiac arrest. Major interventions for acute respiratory failure include intubation, mechanical ventilation, supplemental oxygen administration, and secretion removal. Intubation provides an adequate airway. Mechanical ventilation decreases the work of breathing, ventilates the lungs, and improves oxygenation. Positive end-expiratory pressure (PEEP) may be ordered during mechanical ventilation to improve gas exchange. PEEP maintains positive pressure at the end of expiration, preventing the airways and alveoli from collapsing between breaths. Oxygen is administered to achieve a PaO_2 level of 60 mm Hg. To prevent oxygen toxicity, expect to give the lowest FIO_2 level possible. If possible, teach the patient proper coughing techniques so that he can clear secretions effectively. As necessary, perform endotracheal suctioning and chest percussion and vibration. (See Chapters 10 through 13 for details on these procedures.)

Respiratory Failure Criteria

• Vital capacity < 15 ml/kg
• Tidal volume < 3 ml/kg
• Negative inspiratory force < -25 cmH_2O
• Respiratory rate > twice the normal rate
• Decreased PaO_2 level despite increased FIO_2
• Increased $PaCO_2$ level with pH < 7.25

Adult respiratory distress syndrome

Description
A form of pulmonary edema, adult respiratory distress syndrome (ARDS) can quickly lead to acute respiratory failure. Resulting from direct or indirect injury to the lungs, ARDS involves complex symptoms that lead to capillary leakage. These subtle symptoms make the disorder hard to recognize. And unless recognized early and treated promptly, ARDS can prove fatal within 48 hours of onset. Clinical features include dyspnea, hypoxemia, increased respiratory effort, reduced respiratory compliance, and diffuse infiltrates. Reduced respiratory compliance leads to an increased respiratory rate and increased respiratory effort. (See *Infant Respiratory Distress Syndrome [Hyaline Membrane Disease]: An Overview,* page 222.)

Causes
Common causes
• Trauma (most common). In most cases, ARDS strikes trauma victims, possibly because such complications as fat emboli, sepsis, shock, pulmonary contusions, head injury, and multiple transfusions increase the risk of developing microemboli.
• Aspiration of gastric contents
• Diffuse pneumonia (especially viral)
• Near-drowning
• Inhalation of noxious gases or smoke
• Anaphylaxis
• Oxygen toxicity
• Drug overdose (heroin, aspirin, and ethchlorvynol)
• Idiosyncratic drug reaction (to ampicillin and hydrochlorothiazide)

Less common causes
• Miliary tuberculosis
• Thrombotic thrombocytopenic purpura
• Leukemia
• Uremia

• Venous air embolism
• Pancreatitis
• Cardiopulmonary bypass
• Hemodialysis
Note: In critically ill patients, disseminated intravascular coagulation (DIC) may appear concomitantly in patients with ARDS. However, researchers don't know whether DIC causes ARDS or develops independently.

Pathophysiology
In healthy lung tissue, fluid—composed of water and low-molecular-weight substances—leaves the vascular bed and enters the interstitium, where it's absorbed by the lymphatic system. In ARDS, injury reduces normal blood flow to the lungs, allowing platelets to aggregate in the alveolar capillaries and permitting multiple microthrombi to form. These platelets also release substances (histamine, serotonin, and bradykinin) that inflame and damage the alveolar-capillary membrane, disrupting membrane permeability. These substances, especially histamine, increase capillary permeability, which allows fluid to shift into the interstitial space. As capillary permeability increases, large molecules (such as proteins, which normally remain within lung tissue cells) and more fluid leak into the interstitium, increasing interstitial osmotic pressure and causing pulmonary edema. (See *What Happens in ARDS,* page 218.)

Fluid in the alveoli and decreased blood flow damage alveolar surfactant and impair the cells' ability to produce more surfactant. Without adequate surfactant, alveoli collapse, impairing gas exchange.

Consequently, lung compliance drops and breathing becomes laborious. Although collapsed alveoli are still perfused, gas exchange doesn't occur because alveoli lack air. Consequently, pulmonary shunting occurs and unoxygenated blood enters arterial circulation. This atelectasis further impairs gas exchange and causes ventilation/perfusion ($\dot{V}/\dot{Q}$) mismatch.

What Happens in ARDS

ARDS enhances capillary membrane permeability. As a result, plasma and proteins leak from the capillaries into the interstitial spaces and alveoli, thereby reducing lung compliance and volume and inhibiting normal gas exchange.

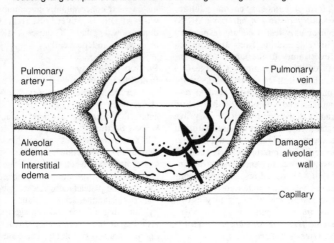

To compensate, the patient breathes faster. However, sufficient oxygen can't cross the alveolar-capillary membrane. Carbon dioxide, though, crosses more easily and is lost with every exhalation. PaO_2 and $PaCO_2$ levels then decrease.

Pulmonary edema worsens. Also, inflammation leads to fibrosis, which further impedes gas exchange. The resulting hypoxemia causes metabolic acidosis. Left untreated, hypoxemia and acidosis, along with a progressively increasing $PaCO_2$ level, can be fatal. (See *ARDS Pathogenesis.*)

Signs and symptoms and diagnosis
Phase 1
After the initial injury, tissue perfusion decreases and breath sounds may diminish. The chest X-ray appears clear or shows slight congestion. The patient experiences dyspnea on exertion and an increase in respiratory rate and depth. He remains alert, with high-normal respiratory and heart rates. Arterial blood gas (ABG) analysis shows a normal or slightly below-normal $PaCO_2$ level, averaging from 30 to 40 mm Hg.

Phase 2
The patient shows signs of subclinical respiratory distress. He uses his accessory muscles to breathe and appears anxious and restless. He experiences a dry cough with thick, frothy sputum and bloody, sticky secretions. His skin is cool, pale, and diaphoretic, and he may show signs of tachypnea, tachycardia, and elevated blood pressure. Auscultation may reveal basilar crackles. (At this point, these signs may be incorrectly attributed to other causes, such as multiple trauma.)

The chest X-ray may still appear normal during Phase 2. The patient's respiratory rate continues to increase. By this

ARDS Pathogenesis

```
Trauma, shock, and other causative factors
                    ↓
Pulmonary hypoperfusion and hypoxemia
                    ↓
Platelet aggregation in pulmonary capillaries
          ↓                          ↓
Mechanical obstruction        Release of vasoactive
from microvascular            substances from
thrombi                       disruption of platelets
                    ↓
Stagnation of blood and increased capillary
and bronchial permeability
                    ↓
Leakage of fluid and plasma protein
into tissues
                    ↓
Primary pulmonary edema
                    ↓
Decreased surfactant from damage of Type II
pneumocytes
                    ↓
Decreased pulmonary compliance
                    ↓
Atelectasis
          ↓                          ↓
Progressive hypoxemia         Hyperventilation
          ↓                          ↓
Hypercapnia                   Hypocapnia
          ↓
Acidosis
```

time, tidal volume decreases from decreased lung compliance. ABG analysis shows hypocapnia and hypoxia; administration of high oxygen concentrations doesn't relieve hypoxia. Watch for $\dot{V}/\dot{Q}$ mismatch or a respiratory quotient below 0.8, indicating pulmonary shunting. The $PaCO_2$ level usually ranges from 25 to 30 mm Hg.

Phase 3

The patient appears gravely ill. Expect severe dyspnea, tachypnea (more than 30 breaths/minute), and tachycardia with dysrhythmias (usually premature ventricular contractions). The patient visibly struggles for air. Other findings include pale, cyanotic skin; a wet cough; labile blood pressure; and decreased mentation. Auscultation reveals crackles and rhonchi. The patient must now be intubated and ventilated. Otherwise, he'll suffer continued hyperventilation, a decreased $PaCO_2$ level (from 20 to 35 mm Hg), a decreased PaO_2 level (from 50 to 60 mm Hg), pulmonary shunting ranging from 20% to 40%, and pulmonary edema (which appears on chest X-ray).

Phase 4

Now in acute respiratory failure, the patient has severe hypoxia. He lacks spontaneous respiration and lapses into a coma. (Ideally, the patient should have received treatment before Phase 4 to avoid many of the problems associated with this phase.) Other Phase 4 clinical manifestations include bradycardia with dysrhythmias; hypotension; and pale, cyanotic skin. Because the patient can't continue hyperventilating, his $PaCO_2$ level rises, indicating a marked reduction in functioning alveolar capillary units. Metabolic and respiratory acidosis develop. Pulmonary shunting approaches 50% to 60%. Chest X-ray shows a complete lung whiteout. When ARDS reaches this stage, the patient stands an increasing risk of fibrosis and pulmonary damage becomes life-threatening.

Other diagnostic tests

Besides ABG analysis and serial chest X-rays, diagnostic tests include pulmonary artery catheterization, which helps identify the cause of pulmonary edema by evaluating pulmonary capillary wedge pressure (PCWP). A measure of myocardial function, PCWP rules out cardiogenic pulmonary edema. (Normal PCWP ranges from 6 to 12 mm Hg; a pressure above 12 to 15 mm Hg indicates poor ventricular function. Always consider a PCWP reading of 12 mm Hg or less a hallmark of ARDS.) Pulmonary catheterization also allows for collection of pulmonary artery, mixed venous blood which shows decreased oxygen-saturation reflecting tissue hypoxia; measures pulmonary artery pressure as well as cardiac output by thermo-dilution techniques.

Besides cardiogenic pulmonary edema, differential diagnosis must rule out pulmonary vasculitis and diffuse pulmonary hemorrhage. To establish the etiology, laboratory work should include a sputum Gram stain with culture and sensitivity and blood cultures to detect infections; toxicology screening for drug ingestion; and a serum amylase determination when pancreatitis is possible.

Treatment and clinical considerations

Management of ARDS includes:
• increasing tissue oxygenation
• minimizing oxygen consumption
• preventing or treating complications.

To accomplish these goals, the doctor will select one or more of the following treatments.

Mechanical ventilation

This technique improves gas exchange between alveoli and pulmonary capillaries. By delivering tidal volume under positive pressure and using positive end-expiratory pressure (PEEP), ventilated alveoli can remain expanded, improving gas exchange and limiting the progression of atelectasis; however, hypoxemia may continue or worsen. Raising the FIO_2 level usually helps reverse hypoxemia; however, an FIO_2 of 0.5 or more for longer than 24 hours significantly increases the patient's risk of oxygen toxicity and pulmonary fibrosis. Because shunting's the real danger, PEEP will cause a greater improvement in PaO_2 than will increased FIO_2.

Two types of ventilators aid the ARDS patient. The volume-cycled ventilator ends inspiration after a preset volume. The high-frequency jet ventilator (HFJV) delivers small tidal volumes (up to 300 ml) at a respiratory rate of 60 to 100 breaths/minute. The HFJV introduces small bursts of gas into the airway through the extra lumen in the endotracheal tube. The small tidal volumes intensify in the patient's airway, forcing air into the alveoli. As a result, exhaled tidal volume exceeds the tidal volume delivered by the HFJV.

Unlike the volume-cycled ventilator, the HFJV doesn't cause the chest wall to rise and fall. Instead, it causes oscillations that carry air from large airways into the alveoli, where gas exchange occurs. (See Chapter 13 for details on mechanical ventilation.)

HFJV offers many advantages. The small tidal volumes it delivers allow lower peak airway pressures, which means lower mean intrathoracic pressures, even with administration of large amounts of PEEP. This significantly reduces the risk of barotrauma. Also with HFJV, spontaneous ventilation ceases at normal $PaCO_2$ levels, thus eliminating the need for increased sedation. Clinical trials show that HFJV distributes gas more effectively than conventional ventilation and usually doesn't reduce cardiac output, even with PEEP. Long-term effects of HFJV remain unknown. (*Note:* Whether your patient's on HFJV or conventional ventilation, be sure to maintain or increase humidification of inspired gas if secretions become thick and tenacious.)

PEEP

Normally, alveoli expand during inspiration and remain expanded throughout the respiratory cycle. But in ARDS, alveoli may not respond to ventilation by reexpanding. Or they may collapse at the end of expiration from surfactant abnormalities. When PEEP supplements mechanical ventilation, a constant pressure is exerted across the alveoli, preventing alveoli from collapsing and increasing the number and size of alveoli available for ventilation. Because alveoli remain expanded during expiration, functional residual volume (air remaining in the lungs after a normal expiration) increases. This results in an increased PaO_2 level with the same or even a lower FIO_2.

PEEP also redistributes alveolar fluid by pushing it to the alveolar wall. The reduced distance between capillaries and alveolar gas permits gases to diffuse across the alveolar membrane. Consequently, total lung volume increases and lung compliance improves.

Discontinuation of mechanical ventilation and PEEP causes immediate alveolar collapse. Hypoxemia may follow alveolar collapse within 1 minute. Once reinstated, PEEP increases the PaO_2 level. However, PEEP takes 20 to 30 minutes to become fully established and some collapsed alveoli may not reexpand.

Always use a PEEP adapter with a hand-held resuscitation bag or a special connector for the ventilator that allows suctioning during ventilation. If this is done, PEEP can be maintained, thereby decreasing the risk of alveolar collapse. This allows you to suction the patient, if necessary, while he's on the ventilator.

CPAP

The doctor may consider continuous positive airway pressure (CPAP) for hypoxemic patients who can breathe on their own. Based on the same principles as PEEP, CPAP continuously

Infant Respiratory Distress Syndrome (Hyaline Membrane Disease): An Overview

The most common cause of neonatal mortality, infant respiratory distress syndrome (IRDS) occurs in premature infants. Untreated, it proves fatal within 72 hours of birth in up to 14% of infants weighing less than 5.5 lb (2,500 g). Mild IRDS may subside after 3 days.

Like adult respiratory distress syndrome (ARDS), IRDS involves insufficient alveolar surfactant. In ARDS, this results from alveolar injury; in IRDS, from alveolar immaturity. Surfactant insufficiency results in widespread alveolar collapse, which causes atelectasis, which leads to inadequate alveolar ventilation with shunting of blood through collapsed lung areas, causing hypoxia, acidosis, and a progressively increasing $Paco_2$ level.

Signs and symptoms
• Rapid, shallow respirations developing within minutes or hours of birth
• Audible respiratory grunting
• Intercostal, subcostal, and sternal retractions
• Nasal flaring
• Possible hypotension, oliguria, and peripheral edema
• Apnea, bradycardia, and cyanosis (with severe disease)
• Pallor
• Frothy sputum
• Low body temperature

Diagnosis
• Chest X-ray is normal for the first 6 to 12 hours after birth in 50% of newborns with IRDS; it later shows a fine reticulonodular pattern.
• Arterial blood gas measurements reveal a decreased Pao_2 level with a normal, decreased, or increased $Paco_2$ level and a decreased pH (combined respiratory and metabolic acidosis).
• Amniocentesis to determine the lecithin/sphingomyelin (L/S) ratio is performed in women requiring a cesarean section before the 36th week of gestation, this test helps assess prenatal lung development and the risk of IRDS. An L/S ratio above 2 usually indicates fetal pulmonary maturity.

Treatment
• Oxygen administration via oxygen hood or mechanical ventilation
• Positive end-expiratory pressure (PEEP) with mechanical ventilation or continuous positive airway pressure (CPAP) ventilation via nose piece or endotracheal intubation in severe cases
• Radiant infant warmer or isolette for thermoregulation
• I.V. fluid administration to maintain fluid and electrolyte balance
• Tube feedings or I.V. hyperalimentation to maintain adequate nutrition, if the infant's too weak to eat

delivers oxygen via a tight-fitting mask or endotracheal tube. CPAP improves arterial oxygenation by increasing functional residual capacity and lung compliance.

When delivered through a mask, however, CPAP promotes gastric distention, vomiting, and aspiration. Furthermore, the mask is uncomfortable and predisposes the patient to skin excoriation. Also, regardless of the delivery method, the patient usually retains CO_2 as a result of fatigue. If this happens, the doctor may switch to mechanical ventilation with PEEP.

Drug therapy
When septic shock causes ARDS, the doctor may order high-dose steroids. (However, when other conditions cause ARDS, steroid therapy remains contro-

versial.) Steroids reduce inflammation and, in high doses, decrease white blood cell mobilization and chemotaxis. They also preserve vascular tone and endothelial cells, preventing the vascular permeability associated with ARDS. Steroids may work by stabilizing cell membranes and averting lysosomal enzyme release. Steroids also prevent complement activation. However, steroids can mask infection—a real risk with ARDS.

ARDS patients may also be given antiobiotics, based on the results of culture and sensitivity tests. Some doctors recommend prophylactic, broad-spectrum antibiotics from the onset of ARDS, reasoning that the extensive invasive procedures performed on these patients raise the risk of infection and that alveolar fluid provides an excellent medium for bacterial growth. However, although prophylactic antibiotics may inhibit bacterial colonization and reduce the chance of sepsis, they may also promote development of drug-resistant organisms, especially *Candida*.

Fluid management
Fluid management centers on maintaining a normal circulating blood volume. However, because of alveolar-capillary damage, overly aggressive treatment can increase fluid leakage into the interstitium. Because the ARDS patient has excessive alveolar fluid, you'll need to prevent fluid overload. For example, if hypotension develops, administer packed red blood cells and vasopressors, as ordered.

Fluid replacement is based on the patient's $PaCO_2$ level, blood pressure, PCWP reading, heart rate, and urine output. Administer colloid or crystalloid fluids, as ordered, to maintain normovolemia. Some health care professionals believe that colloids (which replace albumin and blood) restore oncotic and hydrostatic pressures in the vessels and interstitium, thereby decreasing capillary leakage. Others believe that ARDS stems from a discontinuity of the air-blood barrier (not from pressure changes) and that colloid therapy only increases the fluid shift from the vessels to the interstitium. Therefore, they support the use of crystalloid fluid replacement.

Administer I.V. fluids at the exact rates ordered. Report any changes in hemodynamic or clinical parameters immediately.

Diuretics also help in fluid management. Furosemide, a diuretic, may be ordered to restore the hydrostatic and oncotic pressure relationship and to remove lung fluid. Diuresis reduces intravascular volume, which decreases blood pressure—a potentially dangerous situation for the hypotensive patient. Such patients may require vasopressors or increased fluid intake to maintain blood pressure.

Monitor and assess your patient's response to diuretics frequently. Ventricular ectopy may signal hypokalemia.

When the patient no longer responds to diuretics, the doctor may choose hemodialysis or ultrafiltration to relieve pulmonary edema. Hemodialysis removes toxins and fluid via a semipermeable membrane and dialysate.

Ultrafiltration, which uses a dialysis circuit without dialysate, removes plasma volume by raising venous resistance to blood flow. It increases the oncotic pressure and may help repair the alveolar membrane.

Because both methods use heparin, observe your patient for bleeding. Obtain his dry weight to determine therapy effectiveness. Also, during and after hemodialysis or ultrafiltration, monitor vital signs frequently to determine if fluid removal has caused hypovolemia.

Pulmonary hygiene
Maintaining pulmonary hygiene aids patient recovery and helps prevent superimposed pulmonary infections, a leading cause of death in ARDS patients.

Before and after suctioning, sigh your patient, using a hand-held resuscitation bag with a PEEP valve and 100% oxygen. This offsets the PaO_2 decrease and $PaCO_2$ increase.

Alternatively, increase the FIO_2 level on the ventilator to 1.0 and deliver sighs by depressing the manual sigh button. Always remember to maintain PEEP and to decrease the FIO_2 level after suctioning.

Although humidifying the inspired air helps to thin secretions, parenteral hydration is the most effective way to liquefy secretions, which can be more easily removed by suctioning.

Frequent chest physiotherapy and postural drainage can help mobilize secretions from small, inaccessible airways into larger bronchioles for removal. Although you'll perform these techniques over the entire lung field, focus on the affected lobes (identified by auscultation and chest X-ray).

Nutrition
A carefully planned diet can prevent progressive respiratory muscle weakness and bolster the immune system to fight infection.

Ventilated patients consume approximately 2,500 to 3,000 calories daily. The septic patient needs 10,000 calories daily and will probably require I.V. hyperalimentation (IVH). IVH may increase CO_2 production because of the carbohydrate load. (See *Preventing ARDS.*)

Complications
Early diagnosis and aggressive treatment of ARDS and the associated hypoxemia help improve the patient's survival rate and longevity. However, these critically ill patients seem prone to multiorgan complications that increase the chance of death.

Some complications stem from mechanical ventilation. Many ARDS patients require airway pressures as high as 60 cmH_2O (average normal pressure is 20 to 30 cmH_2O). Concomitant PEEP puts the patient at risk for developing pulmonary barotrauma. Large volumes of air distend and sometimes rupture the alveoli, allowing air to travel along the blood vessels and into the mediastinum (pneumomediastinum), the tissues (subcutaneous emphysema), or the pleural space (pneumothorax).

ARDS and the high oxygen concentrations needed to reverse hypoxemia can lead directly to pulmonary fibrosis. As fibrous tissue replaces elastic lung tissue, the number of alveolar units available for gas exchange declines. The patient's ability to adequately ventilate his lungs without assistance may deteriorate, making weaning and extubation impossible. In addition, oxygen toxicity commonly occurs when the patient receives high oxygen levels (greater than 40%) for more than 24 hours.

Prolonged ventilation also can lead to complications associated with tracheal intubation, including tracheal stenosis, tracheal ulceration, tracheoesophageal fistula, and tracheomalacia. These complications occur most commonly when the pressure exerted by the cuff exceeds a capillary perfusion pressure of 15 mm Hg, thus creating an ischemic area within the tracheal mucosa. Most of these complications can be avoided or minimized if a tracheotomy is performed in patients requiring prolonged ventilation.

GI complications
Patients heavily sedated for long periods may develop paralytic ileus because GI motility decreases. Gastric distention, another possible complication, easily results when the patient swallows air that has leaked around the cuff.

GI hemorrhage, the most common and most serious GI complication, may arise from stress ulcers or other unidentified causes.

Renal complications
Sepsis, hypotension, and hypovolemia may predispose the patient to renal failure. Additionally, many drugs used to treat ARDS cause nephrotoxicity.

Cardiovascular complications
Dysrhythmias, the most common cardiovascular complication associated with ARDS, sometimes develop from hypoxemia and hypotension or from such interventions as diuresis. Also, because mechanical ventilation and PEEP restrict venous return, cardiac output temporarily drops.

Hematologic complications
ARDS may predispose your patient to thrombocytopenia and disseminated intravascular coagulation (DIC), which increase the risk of hemorrhage. Stay alert for signs and symptoms of these hematologic complications. If any develop, alert the doctor immediately. Prompt treatment may reduce mortality.

Infection
Superimposed bacterial pneumonias occur when sterile suctioning techniques fail or when the immune system is compromised. Many ARDS patients must undergo invasive procedures, ranging from placement of indwelling

Preventing ARDS

ARDS can't be prevented in any specific way because of its many causes, poorly understood pathophysiology, and lack of definitive clues. However, several interventions can lessen your patient's chance of developing ARDS; for example, use of blood filters for transfusions, nasogastric aspiration, and antiemetics (which prevent aspiration). Steroids and low levels of PEEP show promise for preventing ARDS in high-risk patients; however, these methods must withstand the test of time.

catheters to pulmonary arterial lines; each increases the infection risk. (Be sure to use sterile technique when caring for such patients.)

Malnutrition
Without proper nutrition, the body can't repair damaged tissue or fight infection. Malnutrition causes muscle weakness and loss of lean body mass. Weaning the malnourished patient from mechanical ventilation is virtually impossible.

Selected References
Burton, G.G., and Hodgkin, J.E., eds. *Respiratory Care: A Guide to Clinical Practice,* 2nd ed. Philadelphia: J.B. Lippincott Co., 1984.
Emergency Care Handbook. Springhouse, Pa.: Springhouse Corp., 1986.
Karnes, N. "Don't Let ARDS Catch You Off Guard," *Nursing87* 17(5):34-8, May 1985.
Luce, J.M., et al. *Intensive Respiratory Care.* Philadelphia: W.B. Saunders Co., 1984.
Respiratory Disorders. Nurse's Clinical Library. Springhouse, Pa.: Springhouse Corp., 1984.
Respiratory Emergencies. NursingNow series. Springhouse, Pa.: Springhouse Corp., 1984.
Respiratory Problems. Nurse Review series. Springhouse, Pa.: Springhouse Corp., 1986.
Zagelbaum, G.L., and Paré, J.A. *Manual of Acute Respiratory Care.* Boston: Little, Brown & Co., 1982.

10 CHEST PHYSICAL THERAPY AND HYPERINFLATION THERAPIES

Introduction

Initially developed and consistently used in England, chest physical therapy (CPT) techniques became popular in the United States during the polio epidemic. Patients immediately benefited from secretion clearance and muscle reeducation and strengthening. Since then, various CPT techniques have been effectively used for numerous pulmonary conditions. These techniques include effective coughing and deep-breathing exercises, postural drainage, percussion, and vibration. Besides postoperative use, indications for CPT include such acute conditions as pneumonia and atelectasis, and such chronic conditions as chronic obstructive pulmonary disease and neuromuscular diseases. Although CPT's effectiveness for some patients is controversial, this therapy continues to gain support among many pulmonary specialists. For example, percussion might be ordered for a patient experiencing an acute asthma attack who is retaining secretions and has bronchospasm. The desired effect of percussion is secretion removal; however, it can cause or intensify bronchospasm, which is a more serious problem.

Unlike many treatments, such as medication injection, CPT's success depends largely on the practitioner's skill and knowledge. Proper choice of techniques and their sequence can improve treatment outcome. For example, a dyspneic patient who retains secretions may be able to tolerate mod-ified postural drainage, percussion, and vibration if you have him perform relaxation and breathing techniques first. Patient motivation and involvement also promote effectiveness. To gain skill, consider training with a proficient practitioner.

Incentive spirometry, mainly used to prevent atelectasis, requires active patient participation. Intermittent positive-pressure breathing, once in widespread use, is rarely used today. (See *IPPB: Pros and Cons.*)

Deep breathing and coughing

Description
Coughing and deep breathing are usually performed together when used as a CPT treatment. The simplest pulmonary treatments, they can prevent as well as treat pulmonary problems when done correctly. One study found that patients who received more thorough instruction in proper coughing and deep-breathing techniques showed significantly fewer postoperative pulmonary complications than those with minimal instruction.

Deep breathing exercises increase normal respiratory volume to its maximal level. Other types of specific breathing exercises can also be used. Segmental breathing involves a conscious effort to breathe at greater depths in a localized area (usually the involved segment). Pursed-lip breathing improves alveolar ventilation by allowing more complete exhalation. This technique can increase tidal volume and decrease respiratory rate. With pursed-lip breathing, the patient creates back pressure by forcing air through pursed lips as he exhales. This allows airways to remain open. However, if the patient has chronic obstructive pulmonary disease (COPD), make sure he doesn't force expiration by contracting his abdominal muscles. This can collapse airways already damaged by disease and increase air trapping.

Deep diaphragmatic breathing, the most widely used technique, serves as the cornerstone of pulmonary treatments and relaxation techniques. In this technique, the diaphragm, the muscle responsible for 70% of the work of breathing, is used for maximal inspiration, improving basilar inflation and inferior segmental expansion. This technique decreases the respiratory rate and, as an added benefit, strengthens the diaphragm. Studies show that deep diaphragmatic breathing increases production of surfactant (the lipoprotein responsible for decreasing alveolar surface tension), which keeps the alveoli open. Therefore, deep diaphragmatic breathing can help prevent atelectasis.

Breathing exercises should always be followed by coughing to allow easier expectoration of secretions. Also, the deeper the preceding breath, the stronger the cough. Although coughing's a natural and spontaneous reflex, it can be improved upon through proper instruction.

The main contraindication for deep breathing and other breathing exercises is an *untreated* spontaneous or tension pneumothorax; breathing exercises will worsen these problems. After proper medical intervention, however, breathing exercises become a priority.

Coughing may also be harmful to patients with markedly elevated intracranial pressure, wound dehiscence, severe upper tracheal trauma, and untreated

IPPB: Pros and Cons

By delivering a mixture of air and oxygen to the lungs at a preset pressure, intermittent positive-pressure breathing (IPPB) treatments can:
• expand airways
• loosen secretions
• distend the tracheobronchial tree, lowering airflow resistance and reducing the work of breathing
• enhance distribution of inspired oxygen, improving ventilation/perfusion ratios.

As a rule, the doctor orders IPPB treatments for 10 to 20 minutes several times a day.

Despite the many *potential* benefits of IPPB therapy, many clinicians question its value. A patient who finds treatment frightening or painful (because of greater lung expansion) may decrease air delivery to the lungs by putting his tongue in front of the mouthpiece and letting the air fill his cheeks, instead of his lungs. This diminishes the volume of air available to inflate alveoli.

Other problems: IPPB easily inflates healthy alveoli but may have little effect on those with thickened or obstructed walls—the ones most difficult to inflate. Also, the patient can swallow air during treatments, causing gastric insufflation.

pneumothorax. (The patient with tracheal trauma will probably be intubated at some point and can then cough without added trauma to the upper trachea and larynx.)

Purpose
All breathing exercises
• Allow for maximal ventilation
• Prevent and treat atelectasis
• Increase alveolar ventilation
• Promote relaxation
• Decrease the respiratory rate
• Strengthen the diaphragm and other respiratory muscles.

Coughing
- Removes secretions
- Clears the airway
- Improves ventilation.

Procedure

All breathing exercises
- Explain the importance of the procedure to the patient.
- Make the room quiet and comfortable for maximal patient attention.
- Auscultate the lungs prior to treatment.

Deep diaphragmatic breathing
- Place the patient in semi-Fowler's position, with his knees and hips flexed to keep the abdominal muscles slack.
- Place your hand lightly on a point below the xiphoid process (to feel for diaphragmatic excursion).
- Instruct the patient to draw a full breath through his nose and try to pull the air toward your hand.
- Normally, you should feel the diaphragm descending—usually as a pressure against your fingers—about halfway into the inspiratory cycle.
- Encourage the patient to draw air in more and more deeply. The patient should feel the diaphragm stretching.
- Have the patient exhale through the mouth, then relax and allow the rib cage to settle down onto the lungs.
- After instruction, teach the patient how to palpate his own diaphragmatic movement so he can assess himself.
- If necessary, let the patient palpate your diaphragmatic movement to get an idea of what he should normally feel.
- Tell the patient to take 10 *deep* breaths each hour. Explain that 10 *deep* breaths are better than 50 shallow breaths.
- Check the patient's technique each time you see him until you're sure that he's exerting maximal effort and doing the exercise properly.
- Use this technique when instructing the patient in incentive spirometry.

- Auscultate the lungs after instruction and assess for improved breath sounds.
- Document patient teaching, the treatment, and any noticeable change in auscultation.

Segmental breathing
- Place the patient in the postural drainage position for segmental breathing to the involved lung segment. (See *Positioning Patients for Bronchial Drainage,* pages 230 and 231.) Alternatively, the patient can be in a sitting position.
- Place your hand over the lobe segment that you want to receive greater ventilation.
- Apply moderate pressure to this segment.
- Instruct the patient to pull the air into the region beneath your hand by breathing through his nose.
- As the patient begins to take a breath, give a quick stretch to the involved segment (apply intermittent pressure without limiting excursion). This provides tactile stimulation and helps increase localized inspiration. (As the patient practices this technique, you should feel increased rib movement on the involved side compared to the opposite side.)
- As excursion occurs, decrease the pressure over the lung segment to allow for full inspiration.
- When the patient's at end inspiration, release all pressure over the segment.
- As the patient exhales through his mouth, apply light pressure to the segment.
- Just before the patient takes his next breath, apply another quick stretch.
- Inform the patient to take about 10 breaths, with rests after every three breaths.
- After segmental breathing, auscultate the lung segment for improved breath sounds.
- Document patient teaching, the treatment, and any noticeable change in auscultation.

Pursed-lip breathing
• Place the patient in semi-Fowler's position, with his hips and knees flexed.
• Check the patient's respiratory rate.
• Instruct him to take a deep breath through his nose.
• Place your hand lightly on his abdomen. (In this technique, you'll focus more on exhalation than inhalation.)
• Tell the patient to purse his lips as he exhales to create a slight back pressure.
• Palpate the abdomen during exhalation to make sure the patient's not forcing air out through strong contraction of his abdominal muscles; this increases the work of breathing and causes distal airway closure in the end-stage COPD patient.
• Have the patient work toward a relaxed, rather than forced, exhalation that is twice as long as inspiration.
• Repeat pursed-lip breathing for 2 minutes. This will allow the patient to blow off CO_2 and decrease respiratory drive, thereby reducing a rapid respiratory rate.
• After the procedure, check the respiratory rate again.
• Document patient teaching, treatment, and any noticeable change in auscultation.

Coughing
• Explain the purpose of the procedure.
• Have tissues available.
• Place the patient in a sitting or semi-Fowler's position (sitting creates the highest intrathoracic pressures).
• Have the patient take a few deep diaphragmatic breaths.
• After the third breath, instruct him to cough twice from the same breath. This is called a *two-stage cough*. The first cough raises secretions; the second facilitates expectoration.
• With a postoperative patient, you may want to use a splinting pillow or incisional support. Also, flexing the hips decreases abdominal pain from coughing.

• If the patient has neurologic impairment resulting in weak abdominal muscles, provide abdominal support while coughing.
• If the patient expectorates, examine the secretions, noting the color, odor, viscosity, and amount.
• Document patient teaching, treatment, and any noticeable change in auscultation.

Clinical considerations
Besides patients with respiratory or neurologic problems (such as cerebrovascular accident or multiple sclerosis), all surgical patients and those on bed rest longer than a day or two should be taught how to perform deep-breathing exercises. Time spent teaching the patient properly—especially when he's pain-free and not in pulmonary distress—can help prevent or improve pulmonary problems.

If your patient has trouble understanding what deep diaphragmatic breathing means, you may want to have him sniff rapidly through his nose three times while he palpates diaphragmatic movement (below the xiphoid process). Then have him gradually lengthen the sniff until it's a full deep breath. A patient who has trouble producing a cough because of pain or other problems may be helped by alternative methods. Have him "huff" (exhale forcefully through an open mouth) or even say "huff" forcefully. You can also tell him to mimic the maneuver of forcing the breath as if trying to see his breath in cold air. Adequate hydration also helps loosen secretions for better expectoration.

Occasionally a patient has trouble stopping a coughing spell. A hacking cough irritates the throat and can stimulate more coughing. To help break this cycle, have the patient breathe through his nose instead of gasping through his mouth. Covering the mouth *after* the cough may help the patient inhale through his nose. The

Positioning Patients for Bronchial Drainage

To drain *the posterior basal segments of the lower lobes,* elevate the foot of the table 18″ (45 cm), or 30 degrees, or change the elevation of the foot of the bed to simulate the table. Instruct the patient to lie on his abdomen with his head lowered. Then, position pillows as shown here. Percuss his lower ribs on both sides of his spine.

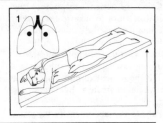

To drain *the lateral basal segments of the lower lobes,* elevate the foot of the table 18″ (45 cm), or 30 degrees. Instruct the patient to lie on his abdomen with his head lowered and his upper leg flexed over a pillow for support. Then have him rotate a quarter turn upward Percuss his lower ribs on the uppermost portion of his lateral chest wall.

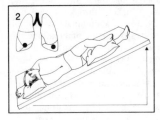

To drain *the anterior basal segments of the lower lobes,* elevate the foot of the table 18″ (45 cm), or 30 degrees. Instruct the patient to lie on his side with his head lowered. Then, place pillows as shown here. Percuss with a slightly cupped hand over his lower ribs just beneath the axillia. *Note:* If an acutely ill patient experiences breathing difficulty in this position, adjust the angle of the bed or table to one he can tolerate. Then, begin percussion.

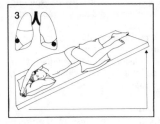

To drain *the superior segments of the lower lobes,* make sure the table is flat. Then, instruct the patient to lie on his abdomen, and place two pillows under his hips. Percuss on both sides of his spine at the lower tip of his scapulae.

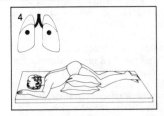

Positioning Patients for Bronchial Drainage *(continued)*

To drain *the medial and lateral segments of the right middle lobe,* elevate the foot of the table 14″ (35 cm), or 15 degrees. Tell patient to lie on his left side with head lowered and knees flexed. Then, have him rotate a quarter turn backward. Place a pillow beneath him. Percuss with your hand moderately cupped over the right nipple. In women, cup your hand so its heel is under the armpit and your fingers extend forward beneath the breast.

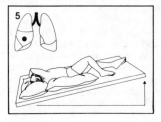

To drain *the superior and inferior segments of the lingular portion of the left upper lobe,* elevate the foot of the table 14″ (35 cm), or 15 degrees. Have the patient lie on his right side with his head lowered and his knees flexed. Then have him rotate a quarter turn backward. Place a pillow behind him from his shoulders to his hips. Percuss as above, but on the left side.

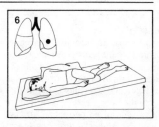

To drain *the anterior segments of the upper lobes,* make sure the table is flat. Instruct the patient to lie on his back with a pillow folded under his knees. Then, have him rotate slightly away from the side being drained. Percuss between his clavicle and nipple.

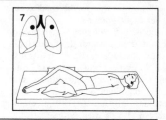

To drain *the apical segment of the right upper lobe and the apical subsegment of the apical-posterior segment of the left upper lobe,* keep the table flat. Have the patient lean back on a pillow at a 30-degree angle against you. Percuss between clavicle and top of each scapula.

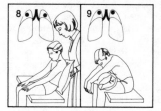

To drain the *posterior segment of the right upper lobe and the posterior subsegment of the apical-posterior segment of the left upper lobe,* have the patient lean over a folded pillow at a 30-degree angle. Stand behind him; percuss and clap his upper back on each side.

slower inspiratory rate via the nose decreases laryngeal irritation and is less likely to stimulate a cough reflex.

Complications
Deep breathing or coughing rarely causes complications. If the patient takes too many deep breaths, however, he may deplete his carbon dioxide supply and become light-headed; deep breathing can also exacerbate untreated pneumothorax. Also, too much coughing can irritate the throat.

Postural drainage

Description
Also known as bronchial drainage, postural drainage uses gravity to enhance secretion clearance from the lungs. Optimal drainage occurs when the segmental bronchus is perpendicular to the floor. Secretions then move from the involved peripheral airways toward the segmental bronchus and up the bronchial tree to the trachea for easier expectoration.

Any patient with lung secretions can benefit from postural drainage. Indications include chronic conditions, such as cystic fibrosis, chronic bronchitis, emphysema, and asthma, and acute conditions, such as pneumonia and lung infiltration. Postural drainage can also be used postoperatively. Studies show that greater success occurs when the secretions are less viscous and when percussion and vibration are performed along with postural drainage.

In most cases, contraindications for postural drainage apply only when the method is performed in Trendelenburg's position. This position causes increased intracranial and intrathoracic pressure and decreased venous return, cardiac output, and arterial oxygen tension. Therefore, postural drainage while in Trendelenburg's position is contraindicated for patients with severe shortness of breath or dyspnea, continuous tube feedings, significant cardiac dysrhythmias, and postoperative craniotomy. Other patients who shouldn't be placed in Trendelenburg's position include neurologically impaired patients with decreased respiratory muscle strength (for example, quadriplegics and patients with Guillain-Barré syndrome) and those with large abdominal obesity, because this position compromises oxygenation.

Purpose
• Assists with mucociliary transport and secretion clearance
• Allows for maximal ventilation to the most superior lung segments

Procedure
• Check the patient's chart to determine involved lung segments.
• Explain to the patient what you will be doing and why.
• Auscultate the lungs to accurately identify the involved areas.
• Have tissues available.
• Unless contraindicated, position the patient in a postural drainage position. (See *Positioning Patients for Bronchial Drainage,* pages 230 and 231.)
• If the patient can't tolerate full Trendelenburg's position or prone positioning, then modify the position. Decrease the foot elevation, lower just the head of the bed, or have the patient lie on his side. However, a modified position may limit the effectiveness of treatment.
• Use pillows as support under the knees, arms, abdomen, or chest so that the patient's comfortable and relaxed during the procedure.
• When positioning, take care not to disrupt equipment, such as I.V. lines and tubes.
• Drain only the involved segments. Optimally, the patient should maintain a drainage position no longer than 20 minutes; some patients may tolerate

only 10 to 15 minutes. If indicated, perform percussion and vibration while the patient's in this position, to expedite secretion clearance.

• Encourage the patient to use diaphragmatic breathing while in the postural drainage position.

• Be prepared with tissues in case the patient expectorates. Suction as needed.

• Auscultate the lungs after treatment.

• Document segments drained, length of session, character and amount of sputum, and any noticeable change in auscultation.

Clinical considerations

Wait 30 minutes to 1 hour after the patient has eaten before starting postural drainage. Also keep in mind that postural drainage is rarely used as the sole treatment. Usually, the patient's receiving instruction in deep diaphragmatic and segmental breathing. After or even during drainage, you may perform percussion and vibration, if indicated. (Preferably, allow 10 minutes of postural drainage before beginning percussion and vibration.) If your patient can receive percussion and vibration but can't tolerate a full 20-minute postural drainage session, begin percussion and vibration as soon as the patient's in the drainage position.

Complications

This procedure rarely causes complications. The most common are shortness of breath, headache, and nausea. Assess the patient's condition before treatment to avoid these complications.

Percussion and vibration

Description

Percussion and vibration are the most dramatic and well-known CPT procedures, mainly because of the noise created by the "clapping" of percussion. These procedures are preferably performed sequentially while the patient is in the postural drainage position for the involved segment. Occasionally, they may be performed independently.

Most effective in treating atelectasis and retained secretions, percussion involves cupping the hand to create the maximum air pocket, then clapping over the involved segment to cause rhythmic waves that help loosen secretions. Both hands are used to create the wave. Studies indicate that the speed or force of the percussion is not as important as the rhythm. Some researchers believe alveolar oxygenation increases during and after percussion.

Vibration usually follows percussion, helping to mobilize secretions from the bronchial tree to the trachea. Here the clinician creates a vibration through the chest wall by vibrating his arms with his hands against the patient.

Percussion and vibration appear simple but require much practice for efficient use. In fact, poor technique can even harm the patient.

Percussion has many contraindications. Typically, they include conditions that could be worsened by forceful contact. These conditions include flail chest or recent rib fracture; unstable angina; potentially lethal dysrhythmias; frank hemoptysis; cancer metastases to the ribs or vertebrae; open wounds; or recent skin grafts. Percussion shouldn't be performed on any lung segment if deep-breathing exercises can achieve the same therapeutic results.

Causing fewer adverse reactions than percussion, vibration is still contraindicated in rib fracture and flail chest, bony metastasis to the ribs or vertebrae, hemoptysis, and bronchospasm. However, if not contraindicated, vibration may be performed with deep-breathing exercises in place of percussion.

Both percussion and vibration should be used cautiously in hemodynamic lability, low platelet count (which may be evidenced by petechiae), osteoporosis, prolonged steroid therapy, severe dyspnea, bronchospasm, pulmonary embolism (until the patient has been on anticoagulation therapy for 4 days), pneumothorax, and untreated tuberculosis. Be sure to consult with the doctor if you have any doubts about performing these procedures.

Purpose
Percussion
• Loosens secretions
• Prevents atelectasis
• Helps reexpand alveoli
• Increases alveolar oxygenation.

Vibration
• Helps move secretions up the tracheobronchial tree
• Assists with expectoration of upper airway secretions.

Procedure
Percussion
• Explain the importance and desired effect of the treatment to the patient.
• Review patient's chart to determine involved lung segments.
• Auscultate the lungs.
• Position the patient in either the postural drainage position or a modified position for the involved segment. Make sure that you and the patient are facing each other.
• Place a layer of towel or gown over the area to be percussed.
• Make sure your position allows for good body mechanics.
• Cup your hands with fingers closed, thumbs against the hands, and all finger joints slightly bent.
• Relax wrist and elbow.
• Bend at the elbow and clap lightly on the patient's chest wall.
• Begin slowly and lightly, and increase speed and pressure gradually (to patient's tolerance).

• Continue percussing over the involved segment.
• Don't percuss over bone or the kidneys. Position your hand for optimal contact with the chest wall.
• Listen to the sound of the percussed region—the more hollow and resonant, the better.
• Check the patient's tolerance to the treatment. Ask him how he feels throughout the session.
• Percuss each segment for about 3 to 4 minutes.
• Preferably, begin percussing after 10 to 20 minutes of postural drainage.
• When you stop to rest, have the patient take a few deep breaths. Some practitioners suggest deep breathing *during* percussion. Although this can be helpful, clapping on the chest and the postural drainage position may make it hard for the patient to perform.
• Examine skin color. A pink blush is normal; redness suggests the percussion was too hard.
• Auscultate the lungs after the treatment.
• If indicated, reposition the patient for proper drainage of other involved segments and begin percussion.
• Document the treatment, noting the segments involved and any changes.

Vibration
• Explain the importance and desired effect of the treatment to the patient.
• Review the patient's chart to determine the involved lung segments.
• Auscultate the lungs.
• Position the patient in either the postural drainage position or a modified position, with the involved segment at the highest point the patient can tolerate. (This may be semi-Fowler's position if the patient has significant shortness of breath.)
• Position the bed so that you're above the patient. Your outstretched arms should be at an angle no greater than

45 degrees from your body. This allows you to create sufficient force during the procedure and prevents arm strain.

• Place your hands flat, in full contact with the patient's chest one on top of the other, over the involved segment.

• Bend your elbows to about a 90-degree angle.

• Vibrate your arms and hands by contracting the biceps and triceps as you slowly extend your elbows.

• Take a breath and blow out as you vibrate. This difficult maneuver may cause you to hold your breath.

• Have the patient take a deep breath. Vibrate as the patient exhales.

• Vibrate three times in a row.

• Have the patient do a two-stage cough on the fourth deep breath. Be prepared with a tissue.

• Repeat the sequence three times.

• Check the patient's tolerance to the procedure.

• If the patient has more than one lung segment to vibrate, reposition him as you would for percussion before proceeding.

• Auscultate the lungs after vibration and assess for any changes.

• Document patient teaching and treatment, noting the involved segments and any changes.

Clinical considerations

Because both percussion and vibration require motor skill for successful use, practice them before using them on a patient. You can practice percussion best on your own lateral thigh. Position your leg for optimal contact. Note your hand position and the sound created. Try for the most hollow resonant sound. But remember—don't clap the patient as hard as you clap your thigh.

Use a pillow or mattress to practice vibration. Try to produce shaking without denting the pillow or mattress more than an inch or two.

Some clinicians advocate the use of mechanical percussors in young, oth-

erwise healthy patients with viral or fungal pneumonia. These patients can tolerate the equipment's force and occasional irritatingly rhythmic claps. For cystic fibrosis patients, mechanical percussion is also pratical. These patients may require chest physical therapy daily or even a few times a day to clear tenacious secretions. A mechanical percussor allows them to treat themselves, to a degree.

Otherwise, manual percussion is preferable because you can better control the amount of pressure exerted. Also, the hand conforms to the odd shapes of the areas being percussed. Perhaps most important, manual percussion allows you to interact with the patient.

Occasionally, vibration can be used to promote upper secretion removal. For example, if a patient has an inefficient, congested cough, you can place a hand over each anterior side of the upper chest while he's in semi-Fowler's or a sitting position. Have him take a large breath through his nose and vibrate as he exhales out his mouth through slightly pursed lips. On the third or fourth breath, have him perform a two-stage cough.

Complications

Fractured ribs are the major complication of percussion. Percussion done too low posteriorly can cause kidney pain or damage. Percussion and vibration can increase bronchospasm, especially if combined with postural drainage. One of the most common problems is patient discomfort from too much force or other problems stemming from poor technique. If you suspect that the patient may have complications from these procedures, avoid them and concentrate instead on appropriate breathing exercises, coughing, and postural drainage, if indicated. Be sure to report this to the doctor.

Incentive spirometry

Description

Incentive spirometry involves use of a device that promotes maximal inspiration. The device provides a relative measure of inspiratory volume or inspiratory flow, thereby encouraging the patient to inhale to a maximal volume. Unless contraindicated, he should hold the deep breath for 3 seconds. This creates alveolar hyperinflation for an extended time, which helps prevent or reverse alveolar collapse that could produce atelectasis and pneumonitis.

Incentive spirometry benefits patients on prolonged bed rest. It's especially useful for postoperative patients who may have trouble recovering normal respiratory function because of pain; narcotic or anesthetic effects; location of incisions; and swelling—all of which limit inspiratory effort. Bedridden patients may be susceptible to pulmonary complications because of advanced age, inactivity, smoking, or decreased ability to cough effectively and expel secretions. (See *Incentive Spirometer.*)

Purpose

- Increases alveolar ventilation, thereby preventing atelectasis and pneumonia
- Improves respiratory muscle strength
- Increases lung volume
- Increases surfactant production
- Involves the patient in his recovery

Procedure

- Assemble the necessary equipment at the patient's bedside.
- Read the manufacturer's instructions for spirometer set-up and operation.
- Remove the sterile flow tube and mouthpiece from the package and attach them to the device.
- Set the flow rate or volume goal, as determined by the doctor or respiratory therapist, based on the patient's preoperative performance. (If no predetermined setting exists, wait until the patient goes through the steps, and then set the goal at a challenging but attainable volume or rate.)
- Assess the patient's condition before he proceeds.
- Explain the procedure to the patient, making sure he understands the importance of performing this exercise regularly to maintain alveolar inflation and to help prevent lung collapse and pneumonia.
- Assist the patient to a comfortable sitting or semi-Fowler's position to promote optimal lung expansion. If you're using a flow-incentive spirometer and the patient can't assume or maintain this position, have him perform the procedure in any position, as long as the device remains upright. Tilting a flow-incentive spirometer decreases patient effort and thus reduces the procedure's effectiveness.
- Auscultate the patient's lungs to obtain a baseline for later comparison.
- Teach the patient how to do deep diaphragmatic breathing (see "Deep breathing and coughing," page 226). The success of the procedure will improve if the patient can take large, deep breaths.
- Have the patient insert the mouthpiece and close his lips tightly around it (a weak seal may alter flow or volume readings). Some patients may need noseclips to prevent air leakage.
- Instruct the patient to exhale normally and then inhale to the predetermined level. If you're using a flow-incentive spirometer, inhalation either causes one, two, or three balls to rise to the top of the meter or makes ⌐ bellows rise, depending on the equipment. If you're using a volume spirometer, inhalation causes a light to go on (with most models).

• When the patient inhales to the predetermined level, instruct him to hold his breath for 3 seconds or, with a volume spirometer, until the light goes off, to achieve maximal alveolar inflation. If the patient has a history of cardiac problems or cardiac precautions, don't let him hold his breath, because this may cause decreased venous return and increased intrathoracic and pulmonary pressures.

• Next, have the patient remove the mouthpiece and exhale normally. Allow him to relax and take several normal breaths before he attempts another breath with the spirometer.

• Encourage him to cough after every third or fourth effort, because deep lung inflation may loosen secretions and facilitate their removal. Observe any expectorated secretions.

• Have the patient take the prescribed number of deep breaths. Note tidal volumes. Instruct him to take 10 deep breaths with the spirometer every waking hour.

• Auscultate the patient's lungs and compare your findings to baseline findings.

• At the end of the session, have the patient remove the mouthpiece. Wash the device in warm water, and shake it dry. Avoid immersing the spirometer, because this enhances bacterial growth and impairs the internal filter's effectiveness in preventing inhalation of extraneous material.

• Place the mouthpiece in a plastic storage bag between exercises. If appropriate, label the mouthpiece and spirometer with the patient's name to avoid inadvertent use by another patient.

• Document the procedure thoroughly.

Clinical considerations

If the patient's scheduled for surgery, make a preoperative assessment of his respiratory pattern and function to develop appropriate postoperative goals. Then, teach him to use the spirometer before surgery so that he can concentrate on your instructions and practice

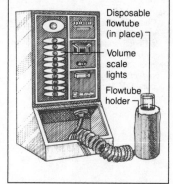

Incentive Spirometer

As it measures inspiratory flow volume, this incentive spirometer shows the patient how deeply he's breathing.

Disposable flowtube (in place)

Volume scale lights

Flowtube holder

the exercise. Avoid exercising at mealtime to prevent nausea. If the patient has difficulty breathing through his mouth, provide a noseclip to fully measure each breath. Provide paper and pencil so the patient can note exercise times. Exercise frequency varies with the patient's condition and ability.

After surgery, monitor the exercise frequently to ensure patient compliance with the instructions and to assess his achievement level. However, don't expect him to do as well postoperatively as he did before surgery, especially after thoracic or upper abdominal surgery.

Complications

Hyperventilation can occur if the patient takes more than three to four deep breaths in a row. In an effort to complete the exercises, the patient may not stop and breathe normally between spirometer trials. This may cause decreased venous return and increased intrathoracic and pulmonary pressures.

Selected References

Batemen, J.R., et al. "Is Cough as Effective as Chest Physiotherapy in the Removal of Excessive Tracheobronchial Secretions?" *Thorax* 36:683-87, September 1981.

Hammon, W.E., and Martin, R.J. "Chest Physical Therapy for Acute Atelectasis: A Report on Its Effectiveness," *Physical Therapy* 61:217-20, February 1981.

Irwin, S., and Tecklin, J.S. *Cardiopulmonary Physical Therapy.* St. Louis: C.V. Mosby Co., 1984.

Kigin, C.M. "Chest Physical Therapy for the Postoperative or Traumatic Injury Patient," *Physical Therapy* 61(12):1724-36, December 1981.

MacKenzie, C.F., et al., eds. *Chest Physiotherapy in the Critical Care Unit.* Baltimore: Williams & Wilkins Co., 1981.

Procedures. Nurse's Reference Library. Springhouse, Pa.: Springhouse Corp., 1983.

OXYGEN AND AEROSOL THERAPIES

Introduction

First identified by Joseph Priestley in 1774, oxygen was used therapeutically for the first time in 1800. More than 100 years later, in 1907, the oxygen catheter was introduced. Oxygen therapy provides tissues with sufficient oxygen to carry on metabolic processes.

Oxygen has become so commonplace that many people forget that it's a drug and requires a doctor's order. Although it's essential to life, it does pose potential dangers. While nonflammable, it will support combustion—a flame will burn hotter and faster in an oxygen-enriched environment. Several physiologic complications are also connected with its use. One seen in newborns is retrolental fibroplasia (RLF). The severity of RLF uniquely relates to PaO_2, not FIO_2. As PaO_2 increases, the retinal blood vessels constrict. Massive constriction in these tiny vessels can lead to thrombus formation and eventually fibrosis. Therefore, PaO_2 levels must be monitored carefully in infants receiving supplemental oxygen therapy.

Two other complications of oxygen therapy affect the lungs and relate directly to FIO_2. Absorption atelectasis occurs with high FIO_2. The increasing oxygen percentage displaces nitrogen in inspired air. Normally, some alveoli are intermittently underventilated. When this happens, nitrogen in the inspired air stays in the alveolus rather than diffusing into the capillary and keeps the alveolus from collapsing until it's ventilated again. When an alveolus receives high oxygen percentages, oxygen readily diffuses into the blood, leaving nothing in the alveolus to keep it expanded.

The other major hazard is pulmonary oxygen toxicity. The risk of oxygen toxicity relates to FIO_2 and length of exposure. Oxygen molecules act on lung tissues and can cause damage in as little as 48 hours at an FIO_2 of 1.0. An FIO_2 of 0.4 or below is usually considered nontoxic to lung tissue.

Patients who need supplemental oxygen fall into four categories:
• those with decreased PaO_2 levels
• those with decreased cardiac output
• those with decreased blood oxygen-carrying capacity
• those with an increased oxygen demand.

The causes of *decreased PaO_2 levels* vary widely. In some patients, such as those with massive intrapulmonary shunt, increasing the FIO_2 will not increase the PaO_2 level. Patients with *decreased cardiac output* may have acceptable PaO_2 levels; however, less blood reaches the tissues per minute. Supplemental oxygen can increase the amount of oxygen available to those tissues despite decreased blood flow volume. Patients with *decreased blood-oxygen-carrying capacity* include those with anemia, carbon monoxide poisoning, methemoglobinemia, and sickle cell disease. Increasing the amount of oxygen dissolved in the blood slightly increases the oxygen amount available to

Hyperbaric Oxygen Therapy

Hyperbaric oxygen therapy has been used to treat compression sickness ("the bends"). Recently, however, it has received increasing attention in treating such conditions as osteomyelitis, skin ulcers, and sickle cell disease.

Hyperbaric oxygen therapy provides additional oxygen to the tissues because the high pressure gradient of O_2 makes tissues absorb more oxygen. Thus, an even greater oxygen concentration reaches diseased or damaged tissue. Oxygen dissolves in blood in direct proportion to the partial pressure of the atmosphere. At three atmospheres, for example, blood has approximately 6.5 ml of dissolved oxygen per 100 ml, compared to 2 ml per 100 ml at one atmosphere.

Hyperbaric chambers can accommodate several patients. The chamber must be sealed so that the inside can be pressurized. This presents a problem because pressure changes occur in all air spaces, including bubbles in I.V. lines, endotracheal tube cuffs, and Foley catheter balloons. Pulmonary oxygen toxicity poses a great risk. To help prevent this complication, keep the FIO_2 as low as possible to protect the lung tissue.

Be sure specific guidelines have been established for hyperbaric chamber treatment and that all personnel are thoroughly familiar with them before any patient undergoes pressurization or depressurization.

Patients with compression sickness may receive *hyperbaric oxygen therapy*. Recently, this therapy has been used successfully to treat several other conditions. (See *Hyperbaric Oxygen Therapy*.)

Oxygen therapy can be delivered through various devices, classified into two categories: high-flow and low-flow systems. *High-flow systems,* which require use of Venturi adapters, entrain relatively large amounts of room air for each liter of flow from the flowmeter. For example, a system that administers an FIO_2 of 0.4 through a Venturi device with the flowmeter set at 10 liters/minute entrains room air at a ratio of 3 to 1—3 liters of room air entrained for each liter of oxygen. The total flow of the device would thus be 40 liters/minute, an amount adequate to meet virtually any patient's inspiratory efforts.

In *low-flow systems,* oxygen flows from the flowmeter directly to the patient. If the flowmeter's set at 2 liters/minute for a nasal cannula, for example, that's what the patient will receive. This can lead to a serious problem if you need to know precise FIO_2. No set answer exists because low-flow systems (catheter, cannula, and various non-Venturi masks) can deliver FIO_2 from 0.22 to 1.0, depending on the patient's respiratory rate and depth. A patient with Kussmaul's respirations—rapid, deep breaths—takes in a lot of room air, diluting the eventual FIO_2 delivered by a low-flow system. On the other hand, a patient who's had a drug overdose and takes slow, shallow respirations dilutes the delivered liter flow with less room air and has a correspondingly higher FIO_2. When reviewing the FIO_2s listed for these devices, remember that they apply to the average adult taking approximately 12 to 16 breaths/minute with a tidal volume of approximately 500 ml. Devices most vulnerable to variations in the percentage of oxygen delivered to the patient are the cannula and simple mask; least vulnerable de-

the tissues. Although only 3% of oxygen in the blood is dissolved, even a minimal increase can make a difference in a borderline patient.

Patients with an *increased need for oxygen* or increased oxygen consumption include those with increased metabolism from hyperthyroidism, fever, or massive tissue repair, as is seen in multiple trauma and burns.

vices are the partial and nonrebreathing masks.

Oxygen therapy can be used at home because oxygen's readily available for home use in most areas. (See *Home Oxygen Therapy.*)

Humidification and nebulization involve addition of moisture to inspired air. Humidification refers to the addition of molecular water; nebulization, to the addition of particulate water, which appears as a mist.

Supplemental moisture is essential to any patient with an artificial airway, because these devices bypass the nose and sinuses, which normally humidify inspired air. Additional supplemental moisture can be administered to help loosen secretions, but parenteral hydration is critical in keeping secretions from becoming inspissated. Supplemental moisture, especially in the form of a cool mist, can be soothing to raw, irritated mucous membranes after throat surgery or extubation or when the patient must breathe through his mouth after nasal trauma or surgery.

Contamination is the greatest hazard of supplemental moisture administration. Contamination may occur from water reservoirs, especially if the water's heated and the container's dark.

In some hypersensitive patients, particulate water, such as in an ultrasonic nebulizer, can cause bronchospasm. With large volumes of nebulized water, patients with borderline fluid status may experience fluid overload from a combination of increased fluid intake through the respiratory system and the elimination of insensible fluid loss.

With the advent of new technology and the economic motivation to keep patients out of the hospital, more and more patients are using home oxygen and aerosol therapy. Good communication between hospital and community

Home Oxygen Therapy

Oxygen therapy is perhaps the prime example of a hospital procedure introduced for home use. Home oxygen therapy is available in three basic forms. The oxygen tank, the traditional form, is typically used for a patient who needs oxygen on a standby basis or who needs a ventilator at home. Tanks have several disadvantages:
• They need to be refilled frequently.
• They're cumbersome and therefore not easily movable.
• Oxygen's stored under high pressure.

The second form, the oxygen concentrator, is a device that works off electrical current and extracts oxygen molecules from room air. It can be used for low-oxygen flow (less than 4 liters/minute) and doesn't need to be refilled with oxygen. However, it won't work during a power failure.

Liquid oxygen, the third home oxygen form, has become popular with patients who are oxygen-dependent but still mobile. This system includes a large liquid reservoir. If the patient wants to leave the house, he can fill a portable unit that he wears over his shoulder; this supplies oxygen for a few hours, depending on liter flow.

You may want to find out in advance which services the home oxygen suppliers in your area offer, types of home oxygen available, and their service schedules. If your patient will be discharged with oxygen for the first time, be sure someone checks his insurance coverage to make sure it covers home oxygen; if not, find out what criteria he has to meet to obtain coverage. Without third-party payment, home oxygen therapy may be prohibitively expensive.

care providers can help develop a comprehensive plan of care for these patients, decreases disease exacerbations, and keeps them out of the hospital.

Oxygen administration by nasal cannula

Description

The nasal cannula delivers low-flow oxygen by means of two plastic prongs that fit into the nostrils and attach to flexible tubing.

Inexpensive and comfortable, the nasal cannula doesn't interfere with eating, coughing, or talking. This system delivers oxygen at the equivalent of up to 0.4 FIO_2 in a normally breathing adult in situations in which accuracy isn't crucial. (No direct correlation exists between liters/minute and FIO_2.) A nasal cannula can't be used when the patient has complete nasal obstruction. The patient must cooperate to help keep the cannula in place.

Purpose

• To prevent or reverse mild hypoxia
• To improve tissue oxygenation

Procedure

• Explain the procedure to the patient.
• Make sure the patient's room is safe for oxygen administration and explain necessary oxygen precautions. (See *Preparing and Maintaining Oxygen Equipment.*)
• Wash your hands.
• Using a flashlight, check the patency of each nostril. As you gently move the tip of the patient's nose, observe for a deviated septum, polyps, edema, or other nasal obstruction. If both nostrils are blocked, you'll have to use a mask to administer oxygen.
• After the humidifier, tubing, and cannula have been connected, set the flow rate, as ordered, reading the flowmeter at the center of the ball, but avoid exceeding the safe limit of 6 liters/minute. If a humidifier isn't used,

simply connect the tubing and cannula. (Humidifiers aren't always used if oxygen flow is low and ambient humidity is considered adequate.) If you're using a cylinder, you must also turn on the oxygen.

• Examine the cannula prongs for straight or curved surfaces. Place straight prongs into the patient's nostrils with either surface up, unless one side is flatter and smoother than the other. In this case, place the smoother, flatter side against the skin, because it produces less friction and pressure in this position. Direct curved prongs in toward the floor of the nostrils, thus following the nostrils' natural curve. (If the curve faces out, the mucous membrane can occlude the prong openings, thereby reducing oxygen flow.)

• Hook the cannula tubing behind the patient's ears and under his chin; then slide the adjuster upward under the chin to secure the tubing. When using an elastic strap to secure the cannula, position it over his ears and around the back of his head. Avoid too tight an application, which can result in pressure areas in the nostrils, on the nose, upper lip, and cheeks, behind the ears, and, with cannula tubing, under the chin. Excessively tight application can also occlude the cannula prongs.

• Document the procedure thoroughly. Be sure to describe the patient's condition before and after treatment.

Clinical considerations

Place an OXYGEN PRECAUTION sign on the outside of the patient's door and another sign over his bed. Remove and clean the cannula with a wet cloth whenever it's soiled, but at least every 8 hours. Give good mouth and nose care. Moisten the patient's lips and nose with water-soluble jelly, but take care not to occlude the cannula. Check the position of the cannula prongs frequently. Also check for pressure areas under the patient's nose and over his ears. Apply gauze padding, if necessary.

Preparing and Maintaining Oxygen Equipment

Assemble the necessary equipment. Check the expiration date on each sterile package and inspect for tears. If you're using a wall unit, plug or screw the flowmeter into the wall outlet, turn the control knob to ensure that the meter's working, and shut it off again.

If you're using an oxygen cylinder, check the cylinder gauge to ensure an adequate oxygen supply. When full, the gauge should read 2,200 psi on a large or small tank. Remove the valve cover. With the oxygen spout pointing away from you, "crack" the cylinder by opening the valve slightly to blow any dust from the spout lip; then immediately shut the valve. Connect the pressure-reduction gauge to equalize pressure between the tank and the flowmeter. Attach a flowmeter if the pressure gauge lacks one. Turn the gauge's flow-control knob counterclockwise to open it, and slowly open the valve on top of the cylinder until the pressure gauge needle stops moving. Then turn the flow-control knob clockwise until the flowmeter dial shows the prescribed flow rate in liters/minute. Next, turn the flow-control knob counterclockwise until the flowmeter needle falls to zero. Transport the cylinder to the patient's bedside in a cylinder cart. Keep the cylinder secured and away from heat to prevent breakage and possible explosion.

If a humidifier will be used, fill the humidity bottle two-thirds full with sterile distilled water. (See Cold bubble-diffusion humidifier, page 252, for more information on humidifiers.) Screw the filled humidity bottle to its adapter and connect it to the flowmeter.

Turn on the oxygen to 2 or 3 liters/minute and watch for bubbles in the distilled water to ensure humidifier patency. Then place your hand at the bottle opening to check for the airflow. If you can't feel the flow of air, increase the flow-control knob setting to 10 or 15 liters/minute; check again for airflow to verify patency of the equipment. Then return the control knob to the prescribed flow setting.

If necessary, attach the cannula or mask to the connecting tubing; then attach the tubing to the humidifier port. Test the patency of the cannula or mask by holding it next to your hand or cheek to feel for airflow. Turn up the flow to 10 or 15 liters/minute for a moment to flush the equipment. Then turn it off until the patient's ready.

If you're using an oxygen cylinder, calculate the length of time that the cylinder will supply oxygen. (See Appendix 2, Equations, page 397.) If the duration of flow is low, have a second cylinder available for quick switching when the first is spent. Change the humidity bottle setup and sterile distilled water according to hospital policy. Replace the water in a reusable bottle to prevent bacterial growth in the water. Discard and replace a commercially prepared bottle. Make sure the patient is comfortable, because some humidification systems produce a strong chill.

Warn the patient, his roommate(s), and all visitors not to smoke or use an improperly grounded radio, TV, or electric razor while the oxygen's in the room.

Check hospital policy on taking oral temperatures when the patient's using a cannula. Recent studies show that oxygen administration lowers body temperature a maximum of 0.4° F. (0.2° C.). Many hospitals regard this drop as minimal and not worth the discomfort that rectal temperature measurement causes in some patients; nor is it worth interruption of oxygen administration during temperature recording.

When oxygen therapy's being discontinued, watch for signs of hypoxia, such as tachycardia, restlessness, and confusion. Immediately notify the doctor if these occur. After therapy, discard disposable equipment properly or send reusable equipment to the proper department for sterilization.

The patient with chronic obstructive pulmonary disease (COPD) should receive a low flow of oxygen/minute until arterial blood gas measurements are obtained. Delivering much oxygen to COPD patients, who chronically retain carbon dioxide, may inhibit their hypoxic stimulus to breathe. (See *The Hypoxic Drive.*)

Complications
Complications include headache or dry mucous membranes if the flow rate exceeds 6 liters/minute. Skin irritation and necrosis can result from pressure and irritation. Sinus irritation can also result from pressure.

Oxygen administration by mask

Description
An oxygen mask is a cone-shaped device that fits over the patient's nose, mouth, and chin. Secured by an adjustable head strap, it connects to flexible oxygen tubing. Depending on the type, an oxygen mask can deliver an FIO_2 of up to 1.0. It can be used in patients who require high humidity or higher amounts of oxygen and in those with total nasal obstruction. Because the mask is confining, prevents eating, and hampers speech, it may reduce patient compliance. The patient may remove his mask when he's not in crisis or when he's confused and restless secondary to hypoxemia. (See *Oxygen Masks*, pages 246 and 247.) A mask

The Hypoxic Drive

Increased $PaCO_2$ provides the primary breathing stimulus. When the $PaCO_2$ level increases, central chemoreceptors signal the brain's respiratory centers to increase the respiratory rate or depth.

A secondary system exists when PaO_2 levels decrease: peripheral chemoreceptors stimulate the respiratory centers to increase respiratory rate or depth. These two systems work together to maintain normal arterial blood gas (ABG) levels.

In patients with chronic lung disease, such as chronic obstructive pulmonary disease (COPD), the $PaCO_2$ level increases over a period of years. Because this occurs gradually, the kidneys can respond by retaining bicarbonate to maintain arterial pH within acceptable limits. However, hypercapnia constantly stimulates the central chemoreceptors. Eventually, these chemoreceptors become insensitive to such constant stimulation and no

longer control respiration. Hypoxia then becomes the stimulus for respiration. When the PaO_2 level drops to about about 60 mm Hg, peripheral chemoreceptors signal the brain's respiratory centers to trigger breathing (the hypoxic drive for respiration).

The hypoxic drive requires cautious oxygen administration in patients with COPD. Severe arterial hypoxemia warrants treatment, but if the PaO_2 level gets much higher than about 60 mm Hg, the patient will have no stimulus to breathe and can become apneic. Low-flow oxygen by nasal cannula or precise oxygen administration via a Venturi mask should be used. ABG monitoring and close respiratory assessment to detect respiratory rate or tidal volume decrease associated with oxygen administration are essential. Too much oxygen can kill the patient whose breathing depends on a hypoxic drive.

may also be used to deliver continuous positive airway pressure (CPAP). (See *CPAP Mask.*)

Purpose

- To prevent or reverse hypoxia
- To improve tissue oxygenation

Procedure

- Explain the procedure to the patient.
- Make sure the patient's room is safe for oxygen administration; explain necessary oxygen precautions.
- Wash your hands.
- Obtain the mask ordered and select the size that offers the best fit.
- After connecting the humidifier, tubing, and mask, set the flow rate. The doctor usually sets the flow rate for simple masks, but for other masks you can use these guidelines to set the proper rate. Follow the instructions that accompany the Venturi mask. Set the flow rate on a rebreathing or nonrebreathing mask so that the bag doesn't totally deflate at peak inspiration; no specific flow rate applies. Flow rates below 5 liters/minute for all but the Venturi mask can't flush exhaled CO_2 from the mask.
- Place the mask over the patient's nose, mouth, and chin, and press its flexible metal nosepiece so that it fits the bridge of the nose. Adjust the elastic band around the head to hold the mask firmly but comfortably over the cheeks, chin, and bridge of the nose. For elderly, cachectic, or toothless patients with sunken cheeks, tape gauze pads to the mask over the cheek area to create the most airtight seal possible. Without this seal, room air dilutes the oxygen, preventing delivery of the maximum possible FIO_2.
- If you're using the nonrebreathing mask, make sure the one-way valves or flaps are secure and functioning to ensure correct oxygen delivery and CO_2 exhalation.
- If you're using a nonrebreathing or partial rebreathing mask, observe the reservoir bag as the patient breathes. If it collapses more than slightly dur-

ing inspiration, raise the flow rate until you see only a slight deflation. Marked or complete deflation means that the flow rate's too low.

- Keep the reservoir bag from twisting or kinking, and make sure it lies outside the gown, sheet, and blankets so it's completely free to expand.

Clinical considerations

Place an OXYGEN PRECAUTION sign on the outside of the patient's door and another sign over his bed. Avoid using high humidity with a mask equipped with a reservoir bag unless the equipment has an in-line water trap, because water tends to collect in the bag. If water does accumulate in the bag, empty it. Check the mask's position frequently, and readjust as needed.

When using a partial or nonrebreathing mask, arterial blood gas

---

CPAP Mask

Continuous positive airway pressure (CPAP) supplies constant positive pressure to the airway when the patient is breathing spontaneously.

In a CPAP mask setup, flow comes from an air/oxygen source to the patient. He then exhales against resistance—that's what causes the positive pressure—creating back pressure in the lungs.

When setting up CPAP, make sure the system accommodates enough flow to flush out exhaled carbon dioxide. Two other hazards relate directly to the mask itself. To maintain pressure in the lungs, the mask must fit snugly around the mouth and nose. This can cause significant facial skin breakdown. Also, if the patient vomits, the mask's snug fit can cause aspiration of vomitus, especially if he's comatose or for some reason unable to remove the mask quickly. Positive pressure can also push vomitus back down the airway. Finally, the constant flow can cause gastric distention.

Oxygen Masks

Type	Description
Simple face mask (Low-flow system) 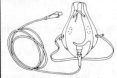	This mask is designed for short-term administration of moderate FIO_2.
Partial rebreathing mask (Low-flow system) 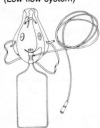	This mask is designed to conserve roughly the first third of a patient's exhaled air, which flows into the reservoir bag. Because this air comes from such passages as the trachea and bronchi, where no gas exchange occurs, the patient essentially rebreathes his exhaled air, which has a high oxygen concentration. This increases his FIO_2.
Nonrebreathing mask (Low-flow system) 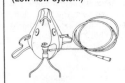	The mask has 3 one-way valves: one located between the reservoir bag and the mask, the others located on the mask itself. These valves prevent room-air entrainment and allow the patient to breathe only the source gas from the bag. It provides the highest possible, FIO_2 and can be used for administration of other gas mixtures (such as CO_2 and helium).
Venturi mask (High-flow system) 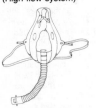	This mask delivers precise oxygen concentration to within 1%. Oxygen enters the tubing at a prescribed flow rate. When it reaches the Venturi device, it meets a restricted orifice. To maintain the same flow rate, the velocity increases, causing a decrease in pressure on the tubing walls and allowing room air to be drawn in through the ports of entrainment. The same amount of air is always entrained. Therefore, the oxygen concentration is very accurate. The amount of air entrained is determined by the size of the orifice: the smaller the orifice, the larger the increase in velocity, the larger the decrease in pressure, and the larger the amount of room air entrained. This results in greater oxygen dilution and lower FIO_2.

Advantages	Disadvantages
• Effectively delivers moderate oxygen concentrations to patients who cannot tolerate a cannula	• Hot and confining; may irritate skin • Tight seal, necessary for higher oxygen concentration, may cause discomfort • Interferes with eating and talking • Impractical for long-term therapy because it's imprecise
• Openings in mask allow room air to be inhaled if oxygen source fails • Effectively delivers higher oxygen concentrations (35% to 60%)	• Tight seal, necessary for accurate oxygen concentration, may cause discomfort • Interferes with eating and talking • Hot and confining; may irritate skin • Bag may twist or kink • Impractical for long-term therapy
• Delivers the highest possible oxygen concentration (60% to 90%) short of intubation and mechanical ventilation • Effective for short-term therapy • Doesn't dry mucous membranes • Can be converted to a partial rebreathing mask, if necessary, by removing one-way valve	• Requires a tight seal, which may be difficult to maintain; may cause discomfort • May irritate skin • Impractical for long-term therapy
• Delivers highly accurate oxygen concentrations despite patient's respiratory pattern because the same amount of air is always entrained • Diluter jets can be changed or dial turned to change oxygen concentration. • Doesn't dry mucous membranes • Humidity or aerosol can be added to the Venturi stream. • Never delivers more than the prescribed oxygen concentration even if knob on flowmeter is accidentally bumped and liter flow is increased	• Confining and may irritate skin • FIo_2 may be altered if mask doesn't fit snugly, if tubing's kinked, if oxygen intake ports are blocked, or if less than recommended liter flow is used • Interferes with eating and talking • Condensation may collect and drain on patient if humidification is being used.

Other Oxygen and Humidification Delivery Systems

Type	Advantages
Trach collar or mask (Humidification system) 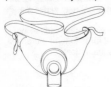	• Device can be used to administer high humidity. • Swivel adapter allows tubing to attach on either side. • Frontal port permits suctioning. • Elastic ties allow you to pull mask from tracheostomy without removing it.
Face tent (Humidification system) 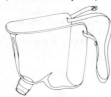	• Can be used to administer high humidity • Functions as a high-flow system when attached to a Venturi nebulizer • Substitutes for face mask if patient can't tolerate having his nose covered: for example, if his nose is broken or if he has facial burns • Doesn't dry mucous membranes
T-tube (Humidification system) 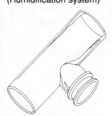	• Offers high humidity when connected to a nebulizer • Allows greater patient mobility • Can be used for tracheostomy or endotracheal tube • Functions as a high-flow system when attached to a Venturi system
Oxygen hood (Humidification system) 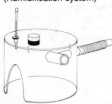	• Enclosed and compact • Provides more precise oxygen concentration than isolette can by itself. Lets you care for infant's lower torso while upper torso's inside hood. • Functions as a high-flow system when connected to a Venturi delivery system • Offers high humidity

Disadvantages	To avoid complications
• If condensation's allowed to collect, it can drain into tracheostomy. • If secretions collect in the collar, stoma can become infected. • Heated aerosol may cause bleeding if used on fresh tracheostomy.	• Empty condensation buildup at least once every 2 hours. • Remove and clean mask every 4 hours with *water*. • Don't cover exhalation port. • Make sure nebulizer delivers constant mist.
• May irritate skin • Interferes with eating and talking • Doesn't deliver precise oxygen concentrations without Venturi attachment; patient can rebreathe CO_2 unless Venturi system is used. • Impractical for long-term therapy	• Don't use on patient with chronic obstructive pulmonary disease. • Place pads between mask and bony facial parts. • Periodically massage face with fingertips. • Wash and dry face every 2 hours. • Don't adjust strap too tightly. • Remove and clean mask every 8 hours with a wet cloth.
• May stick to tracheostomy (from humidity or secretions) • Condensation can collect in tube and drain into tracheostomy. • Weight of T-tube can pull on the tracheostomy tube.	• If tube sticks to tracheostomy, gently twist off. Then, clean tube with hydrogen peroxide, rinse with water, and replace. • Empty condensation buildup at least once every 2 hours. • Keep chimney extension in place. If you don't, FIo_2 will drop drastically. • Make sure humidifier or nebulizer has enough water to create mist.
• Can irritate skin • Can be used with a nebulizer or a cascade humidifier • Can't feed infant while he's inside hood • Active infant can move hood.	• Pad hood with towel or foam rubber. • Keep bedding around head dry. • Empty condensation buildup from tubing every 2 hours. • When using heated nebulizer, check hood temperature every 4 hours so it stays between 94° and 96° F. (34.4° and 35.6° C.).

(continued)

Other Oxygen and Humidification Delivery Systems *(continued)*

Type	Advantages
Isolete (standard) (Low- or high-flow system) 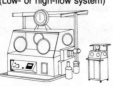	• Enclosed and compact. • Can provide enriched oxygen without restricting the infant
Croupette (Low-flow system) 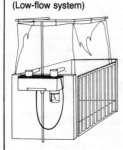	• Usually used for children • Delivers high humidity and aerosolized therapy • Allows child to move freely • Disposable canopy

(ABG) levels should be checked at least daily to assure the continued need for a high FIO_2. These masks can cause pulmonary oxygen toxicity because they deliver oxygen concentrations greater than 40%.

Keep the skin under the oxygen mask dry to prevent breakdown caused by humidity and perspiration. Every 2 hours—more often with high-humidity masks—wipe moisture from the patient's face and mask or encourage the patient to do so. Periodically wash and dry the face, but don't use powder, because the patient may inhale it. When necessary, but at least every 8 hours, wash the mask with soap and water and dry it thoroughly.

At least every 8 hours, check the skin under the elastic straps to detect necrosis from pressure, irritation, and moisture. Remember that discomfort can make the patient resist treatment. Apply gauze padding, if necessary.

Watch for signs of oxygen toxicity, such as dyspnea, decreased lung compliance, and paresthesias in extremities in the patient receiving concentrations above 40% for over 24 hours. To prevent atelectasis, which may occur during therapy with high oxygen concentrations, frequently remind the patient to cough and deep-breathe to keep his lungs inflated. Because prolonged treatment with high oxygen concentrations can also cause serious lung damage, make sure ABG levels are measured fre-

Disadvantages	To avoid complications
• When used without oxygen hood, isolette can deliver only 40% or 100% oxygen. Also, oxygen concentration can fluctuate depending on how often unit's opened.	• If 100% oxygen concentration is desired, keep port flaps tightly closed. • If oxygen hood isn't used, check oxygen concentration every 4 hours. • If you're using an oxygen hood with isolette, see instructions listed above. • Arterial blood gas monitoring is critical to prevent retrolental fibroplasia.
• If you must open tent, for any reason, remember it'll take 15 to 20 minutes to restore oxygen concentration. • Water or ice reservoir must be filled every 6 to 8 hours • High humidity promotes bacterial growth • System isolates patient • Significant FIO_2 increase is hard to achieve.	• Check temperature and oxygen concentraion every 4 hours. • Use rubber sheet on bed under linen to keep the mattress dry and prevent oxygen from escaping through mattress. • Use bath blanket over bottom sheet to absorb excess moisture. Change linen and gown as necessary to keep patient warm and dry. • Give patient care through tent opening whenever possible. When giving bath or changing linen, tuck tent under pillow to conserve oxygen. • Prevent patient from feeling isolated by talking to him. Use a normal tone; the tent doesn't impair hearing. • No electrical devices should be used in the tent because of the oxygen-enriched environment.

quently to determine continued need for high concentrations.

Because the patient must remove the mask for eating, suggest that the doctor order a cannula for use during meals.

Unless contraindicated, take the rectal temperature of a patient who is receiving oxygen by mask. Removing the mask to take an oral temperature can cause the blood oxygen level to drop precipitously.

When oxygen therapy's being discontinued, watch for signs of hypoxia, such as tachycardia, restlessness, and confusion. Immediately notify the doctor if these occur. After therapy, discard disposable equipment properly or send reusable equipment to the appropriate department for sterilization.

Always use a Venturi mask on a patient with chronic obstructive pulmonary disease. Other masks deliver an FIO_2 high enough to prevent the hypoxic drive to breathing and can thereby cause apnea.

Complications
• Skin irritation and necrosis can result from a tight-fitting mask (also see *Other Oxygen and Humidification Delivery Systems*, pages 248 to 251).
• Pulmonary oxygen toxicity can occur with an FIO_2 above 0.4 for several days. The higher the FIO_2, the faster oxygen toxicity can occur.
• Aspiration can occur if a patient vomits with the mask in place, especially if he is comatose.

Humidifiers

Description

Humidifiers add water vapor to inspired air. Some humidifiers also heat the water vapor, thereby enhancing its moisture-carrying capability and increasing its humidity. Supplemental humidity must accompany delivery of a therapeutic gas such as oxygen, because the gas is totally dry and extremely irritating to mucous membranes. Supplemental humidity's used with every oxygen-delivery device except the Venturi mask and, in some cases, the cannula. If the patient with a Venturi mask requires humidification, entrained room air—not the oxygen—is humidified. Supplemental humidity's also used for patients with particularly thick, tenacious secretions and for those who need relief from croup or tracheitis.

Humidity may be added to a room using a room humidifier or combined with inspired-gas lines and delivered directly to the patient. In-line devices include the cold bubble-diffusion humidifier for patients with an intact upper airway, and the cascade humidifier, which can deliver 100% of needed body humidity when heated and connected to a ventilator. Many humidifiers are available commercially. In addition, many are at least partially disposable. (See *Humidifiers.*)

Purpose

• To prevent drying and irritation of the respiratory mucosa
• To help loosen respiratory secretions for easier removal

Procedure

Explain the procedure to the patient.

Room humidifier

• Open the unit reservoir. Add sterile distilled water to the fill line and close the reservoir.

• Close windows and doors to maintain the humidity level in the room.
• Plug the unit in and direct the nozzle toward the patient to promote effective treatment. A mist should be visible at the nozzle.
• Frequently check the unit's water level and refill as necessary. When refilling, first unplug the unit to prevent electric shock. Discard any water in the reservoir, and refill it with sterile distilled water to prevent bacterial growth. Plug in the unit again.
• Continue the treatment for the prescribed time.
• Rinse the unit's reservoir after each use and return it to the central supply department for sterilization.
• Document the procedure.

Cold bubble-diffusion humidifier

• Unscrew the humidifier reservoir from the humidifier lid and add sterile distilled water to the fill line on the reservoir. Avoid overfilling, because this can cause condensation to collect in the small-bore oxygen tubing, increasing airflow resistance for the patient.
• Screw the reservoir back onto the humidifier. Then attach the flowmeter to the oxygen source, and connect the humidifier to the bottom of the flowmeter. If you're using a commercially prepackaged humidifier, simply break the seal and attach it to the flowmeter.
• To prevent delivery of dry gas to the patient, set the flowmeter to 2 liters/minute.
• Check humidifier function at this point. To determine if the gas is being delivered to the unit and properly humidified, be sure the flowmeter is set at 2 liters/minute. Bubbling should be visible in the reservoir. To determine if the pressure release system is operating, occlude the port where the oxygen delivery device will be connected to the humidifier and observe for audible pressure release from the pressure release valve on the humidi-

Humidifiers

Type	Advantages	Disadvantages
Cold bubble diffuser	• May be used with all oxygen masks (except the Venturi mask), nasal cannulas, and nasal catheters	• Provides only 20% to 40% humidity • Cannot be used for patient with bypassed upper airway
Cascade humidifier	• Provides 100% humidity at body temperature • Functions as mainstream humidifier with ventilator • Most effective of all evaporative humidifiers • May be used with oxygen hood or in isolette	• Temperature control may become defective from constant use. • If correct water level isn't maintained, patient's mucosa can become irritated from breathing hot, dry air.
Room humidifier (cool mist or steam vaporizer)	• May be used with all oxygen masks, nasal cannulas, and nasal catheters	• Produces humidity inefficiently • Cannot be used for patient with bypassed upper airway

fier. Decreased bubbling in the reservoir while the port's occluded indicates that the device is patent.
• Attach the oxygen-delivery device to the bubble-diffusion humidifier.
• Turn the oxygen flowmeter to the prescribed flow rate.
• Position the oxygen-delivery device on the patient.
• Frequently check the unit's reservoir. When water runs low or the bubbling stops, discard any remaining water and refill the chamber with fresh sterile distilled water. If you're using a commercially prepackaged humidifier, discard the entire unit and replace it with a fresh one when the water runs low. At low oxygen flow rates, when water isn't used rapidly, change the water according to hospital policy (usually at least once a day) to prevent bacterial growth.
• Regularly change the humidifier and its tubing, according to hospital policy, to prevent respiratory infection from bacterial growth in the equipment.

• When changing the apparatus or discontinuing treatment, return the used equipment to the proper department for resterilization.
• Document the procedure.

Cascade humidifier
• Unscrew the bottom of the cascade reservoir, add sterile distilled water to the reservoir's fill line, and reattach it. Remember—the cascade's heater control serves only as a guide; the in-line thermometer gives a more precise temperature of delivered vapor.
• Plug in the heater unit and set the temperature dial at mid-range (usually at 5). If the temperature's too low at a setting of 5, slowly adjust the dial upward one number at a time. Some temperature dials on cascade humidifiers allow selection of the desired temperature of delivered gas.
• Check the in-line thermometer to verify that the desired temperature has been reached. Instead of an in-line thermometer, some ventilators use a probe placed in the line with the thermometer located in the machine itself. Usually, strive for a reading slightly below body temperature, which results in a body humidity of 100%.
• If you're using the optional temperature alarm to detect gas temperature changes near the patient, turn it on and set it slightly above (usually +2° to 3° F.) normal body temperature.
• Frequently check the thermometer; the temperature should be slightly below or at body temperature. If at any time you suspect that the inspired-gas temperature may be too high for the patient's comfort or safety (when, for example, the tubing or the bottom of the cascade is hot to the touch), turn down the temperature control and arrange for a respiratory therapist to evaluate the equipment.
• If dangerously hot, empty the hot water in the cascade and replace it with room-temperature distilled water. Remember, the thermometer's only a

guide to inspired-gas temperature, because it averages both inspired and expired air temperatures.
• Arrange the tubing so that condensation can't flow toward the patient and be aspirated. Periodically drain condensation from the tubing to prevent backflow, maintain vapor temperature, and reduce the resistance to oxygen flow.
• Frequently check the cascade's water level and refill as necessary. When refilling, unscrew the bottom water reservoir. Discard any water left in the cascade reservoir and refill it with sterile distilled water to prevent bacterial growth in the residual water. Be sure to keep the cascade's water level well above the minimum line to prevent the administration of warm, dry air.
• Regularly change the cascade and its tubing, according to hospital policy, to prevent respiratory infection from bacterial growth in the equipment. To prevent burns, let the heater cool off before changing the apparatus.
• When changing the cascade or discontinuing treatment, return the used cascade to the appropriate department for resterilization.
• Document the procedure.

Clinical considerations
Check the humidifier cord for fraying or other electrical defects. Use only a three-pronged (grounded) plug to avoid electric shock.

Tell the patient who's using a room humidifier at home that he can fill it with plain tap water but that he should periodically run the unit with distilled water to dissolve the mineral deposits left by the tap water. Instruct him to run the unit occasionally with white vinegar or a solution of chlorine bleach and distilled water in the reservoir. This should be done in a well-ventilated room every 5 days to prevent the otherwise rapid accumulation of mold and bacteria.

Never allow a heated humidifier to run dry, because hot, dry gas can severely dry and burn the respiratory mucosa. Also, check thermometer readings regularly to ensure that inspired air remains at body temperature. Constant use or insufficient water in the humidifier can cause the heating device to overheat, raising the temperature of inspired gas. Although water in a heated humidifier container may reach temperatures up to 140° F. (60° C.), it cools and condenses as it passes through the tubing and should be close to body temperature as the patient breathes it. A range of 90° to 100° F. (32.2° to 37.8° C.) is acceptable.

If you're using a cascade humidifier to treat an oliguric patient, observe him for signs of pulmonary edema and congestive heart failure, because the system decreases insensible loss. Notify the doctor immediately if such signs occur.

Complications
• Fluid overload can occur. This is very important in the premature newborn because his fluid status is so critical.
• Burns can occur if the humidifier temperature isn't maintained at a safe level or if a heated humidifier is allowed to run dry and hot, dry gas reaches the respiratory mucosa. (See also *Other Oxygen and Humidification Delivery Systems*, pages 248 to 251.)

Nebulizers

Description
Nebulizers provide 100% humidity in a fine aerosol mist of fluid droplets that, ideally, slowly settle deep into the lungs.

The large-volume nebulizer, used for long-term therapy, delivers a heated or cool mist. Cool mist can be more comfortable for the recently extubated patient. It's also indicated for the patient with trauma or a recent tracheotomy, because a heated mist may in-

crease bleeding. Heated mist is indicated for neonates and patients with an artificial airway. (Cool mist blowing on a neonate can cause a significant decrease in body temperature.)

The ultrasonic nebulizer is used in short therapeutic sessions for patients with thick secretions to mobilize secretions and facilitate a productive cough.

Small-volume nebulizers deliver aerosolized medication. For a patient with chronic respiratory disease, a metered-dose inhaler (MDI) provides a more effective alternative to hand-held nebulizers. The self-contained MDI unit consists of an inhaler attached to a unit-dose pressurized canister or capsule containing medications, such as bronchodilators or steroids. The doctor may prescribe an MDI to treat chronic respiratory disease or acute conditions, such as asthma attacks. The side-stream nebulizer attaches to a ventilator or an intermittent positive-pressure breathing (IPPB) machine; the mini-nebulizer and the MDI are hand-held.

Continuous nebulization therapy with large-volume nebulizers is contraindicated in patients with delicate fluid balance. It should be used cautiously in asthmatic patients with active bronchospasm. (See *Nebulizers: Comparing Types*, pages 256 and 257.)

Purpose
To deliver moisture or medication into the lungs

Procedure
Explain the procedure to the patient.

Large-volume nebulizer
• Unscrew the water chamber and fill it to the indicated level with sterile distilled water. Avoid using sterile saline solution.
• Add a heating device, if ordered. Place an in-line thermometer between the outlet port and the patient, pref-

Nebulizers: Comparing Types

Type	Advantages	Disadvantages
Large-volume nebulizer (heated or cool) 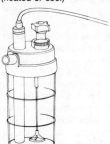	• Provides 100% humidity with cool or heated devices • Provides both oxygen and aerosol therapy • Is useful for long-term therapy	• Nondisposable units increase risk of bacterial growth. • Condensation can collect in large-bore tubing. • If correct water level in reservoir isn't maintained, mucosal irritation can result from breathing hot, dry air. • Infants easily become overhydrated from mist.
Mini-nebulizer or Maxi-mist 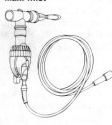	• Conforms to patient's physiology, allowing him to inhale and exhale on his own power • Can cause less air trapping than medication administered by intermittent positive-pressure breathing (IPPB) • May be used with compressed air, oxygen, or compressor pump • Compact and disposable	• Procedure takes a long time if patient needs nurse's assistance. • Medication's distributed unevenly if patient doesn't breathe properly.
Ultrasonic nebulizer 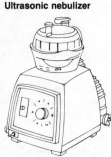	• Provides 100% humidity • 90% of particles reach lower airways • Loosens secretions	• May precipitate bronchospasms in the asthmatic patient • May cause overhydration

Nebulizers: Comparing Types *(continued)*

Type	Advantages	Disadvantages
Side-stream nebulizer Nebulizer portion	• Delivers medication to patient on ventilator or during IPPB therapy	• Those associated with ventilators or IPPB therapy • Adverse reaction to medication
Metered-dose inhaler 	• Delivers small, precise dose directly to the lungs • Minimizes the systemic effects of medication	• Requires good coordination • May lead to overdose if patient uses it too frequently when in respiratory distress

erably closer to the patient, to monitor the actual temperature of the inhaled gas and to detect and correct excess heat before the patient can be burned.

• After the equipment's prepared, attach the flowmeter to the gas source, and attach the nebulizer to the flowmeter. Turn the flowmeter to 10 to 14 liters/minute (these devices require at least 10 liters/minute to operate), and vent as excess any flow above 14 liters/minute.

• Make sure an ample quantity of mist emanates from the outflow port.

• Set the prescribed FIO_2, according to the doctor's order.

• Attach the large-bore tubing to the outlet port and the appropriate delivery device to the tubing's distal end.

• When giving oxygen, use the oxygen analyzer to evaluate gas flow at the patient's end of the tubing to ensure delivery of the prescribed FIO_2.

• If you're using a heater, instruct the patient to report warmth, discomfort, or hot tubing, because these may indicate a heater malfunction. Use the in-line thermometer to monitor the temperature of the gas the patient's inhaling. If you turn off the flow for more than 5 minutes, be sure to unplug the heater so the water doesn't overheat and burn the patient when the flow's turned back on.

• Attach the delivery device to the patient.

• Encourage and help the patient to cough and expectorate periodically, or suction him, if necessary.

• Check the water level frequently and refill or replace the container to prevent complications from inhaling dry, hot air, especially if the patient has an artificial airway. When refilling a 0reusable container, discard the old water and refill the container to the indicator line with fresh sterile distilled water to retard bacterial growth.

• Change the nebulizer unit and tubing daily to help prevent bacterial contamination.

• Document the procedure.

Ultrasonic nebulizer

• Fill the nebulizer cup with sterile distilled water or, if using a disposable sterile distilled water container, spike, hang, and attach the container of sterile distilled water to the nebulizer.

• If using a continuous-feed system, hang the large-volume continuous-feed bag or sterile distilled water on the hook provided on the nebulizer stand.

• Attach the tubing from the nebulizer bottle to the bag, open the clamp on the tubing, and allow the sterile distilled water to flow into the nebulizer bottle.

• After the equipment has been prepared, attach the appropriate large-bore tubing and gas-delivery device.

• Turn on the machine and check the outflow port for proper misting.

• Instruct the patient to breathe slowly and deeply to provide maximum aerosol distribution into the lower bronchial tree.

• Remain with the patient during the treatment (usually 15 to 20 minutes), and observe for side effects, such as bronchospasm and dyspnea. Take vital signs and auscultate for crackles or wheezes, if indicated, because increased water absorption may cause overhydration and lead to pulmonary edema or increased cardiac workload—conditions that may show up only after extended treatment.

• Encourage and help the patient to cough and expectorate, or suction him as necessary, because secretions may become thin and copious. Stop suctioning and allow the patient to rest as necessary.

• Document the procedure.

Small-volume nebulizers

Two types of commonly used small-volume nebulizers are the side-stream nebulizer and the mini-nebulizer. (See also *Nasal Inhaler.*)

For the side-stream nebulizer:

• Use unit-dose medication or draw up the medication and diluent, if required, into the syringe. Or draw the medication into the syringe and use a premeasured container of sterile saline solution or water.

• Take the patient's vital signs to establish a baseline.

• Remove the nebulizer cup, inject the medication, and replace the cup. If using an IPPB machine, attach the mouthpiece or mask to the machine.

• If possible, place the patient in a sitting or high Fowler's position to promote full lung expansion and aerosol dispersion. Encourage him to take slow, deep, even breaths. Turn on the machine and check for an ample quantity of mist, indicating proper operation.

• Remain with the patient during treatment (usually 15 to 20 minutes), and take vital signs to detect adverse reactions to the medication. If the patient must rest, turn off the nebulizer to avoid wasting medication.

• Encourage and assist the patient to cough and expectorate, or suction him as necessary.

For the mini-nebulizer:

• Draw up the medication into the syringe, and inject it into the medication cup.

• Take the patient's vital signs to establish a baseline.

• If possible, place the patient in a sitting or high Fowler's position to facilitate lung expansion and aerosol dispersion.

• Attach the free end of the oxygen tubing to the pressurized gas source. Turn on the gas source and check the outflow port for proper misting. If you're using a flowmeter, adjust it to provide proper misting. Usually a setting of 5 to 6 liters/minute is adequate.

• Instruct the patient to breathe slowly, deeply, and evenly through his mouth and to hold his breath for 2 to 3 seconds on full inspiration to receive the full benefit of the medication.

• If possible, remain with the patient during treatment (usually 15 to 20 minutes). Take vital signs to detect adverse reactions to the medication.

• Encourage and help the patient to cough and expectorate, or suction him as necessary. Briefly stop the treatment if he needs to rest.

Metered-dose inhaler

• Remove the mouthpiece and cap from the bottle. (See *Nasal Inhaler.*)

• Insert the metal stem on the bottle into the small hole on the flattened portion of the mouthpiece. Then turn the bottle upside down.

• Have the patient exhale fully and place the mouthpiece between his lips. Tell him to make sure neither his tongue nor his teeth block the opening. (*Note:* Some doctors recommend the open-mouth technique, in which the patient opens his mouth wide and positions the mouthpiece 2″ to 4″ from his lips.)

• Now, instruct the patient to press down on the canister after beginning a slow, deep inhalation. Inhaling slowly and deeply ensures maximum medication delivery. Your patient may need practice to master this step. (If your patient's using the open-mouth technique, have him release medication at the beginning of an inhalation that lasts about 5 seconds.)

• After the patient has inhaled fully, tell him to hold his breath for 10 seconds, then to slowly exhale through his nose or pursed lips.

Nasal Inhaler

The nasal inhaler is a metered-dose system designed to allow topical application of medication to the nasal mucosa. It's usually used for topical application of steroid preparations.

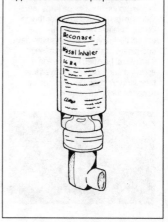

• If the doctor has ordered two doses, have the patient wait 2 minutes and repeat the procedure.

Completing nebulizer procedures

• After treatment with *any* nebulizer, make sure the patient's comfortable and breathing easily before you leave.

• Check vital signs for baseline comparison after medication administration.

• Clean all equipment, as appropriate, and return it to the proper area.

• Document the procedure.

Clinical considerations

When using a high-output nebulizer, such as an ultrasonic nebulizer in a pediatric patient or in a patient with a delicate fluid balance, stay alert for signs of overhydration, such as unexplained weight gain over several days after therapy begins, pulmonary edema, crackles, and electrolyte imbalance.

If a heated nebulizer overheats, unplug the heater and replace the hot water with fresh sterile distilled water.

Breathancer

One of the newest extenders on the market, the Breathancer consists of three interlocking plastic components that telescope together for convenient carrying between uses. Easily opened in one motion, the device traps medication in its middle portion for the patient to inhale. This device is especially helpful to patients who have coordination problems, because it eliminates the need to coordinate spraying and inhaling. Sprayed into the reservoir chamber, the medication's then inhaled.

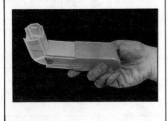

If you're using a T-piece for the patient with an artificial airway, watch for mist at the open end of the tube. If the mist disappears, the patient's inspiratory flow rate exceeds nebulizer output, causing inspiration of room air and, if he's receiving oxygen, reduction of FIO_2. To correct this, add a piece of large-bore oxygen tubing to the open end of the T-piece. Keep adding large-bore tubing until mist remains visible throughout inspiration.

Drug manufacturers can provide placebo inhalers that dispense only saline solution for patient practice and teaching.

Be sure to teach the patient to take only the prescribed dose and frequency. Tell him to call the doctor if shortness of breath persists. Self-administration of more than the prescribed medication dosage can cause serious cardiac dysrhythmias. To use an MDI effectively, the patient must synchronize medication delivery with inhalations. If he can't—for example, because he has arthritis—he may need an extender (or spacer) to delay medication delivery. (See *Breathancer*.)

Complications

• With the large-volume nebulizer, pulmonary burns can result from excessive heating caused by a short circuit or low water levels. Bacterial contamination also can occur. Increased upper airway edema can result from use of a heated aerosol in a patient with laryngeal edema.
• With an ultrasonic nebulizer, overhydration can occur, with resultant pulmonary edema or increased cardiac workload. Bronchospasm, a reduced PaO_2 level, or vital signs changes also are possible.
• With a side-stream nebulizer, metered-dose inhaler, or mini-nebulizer, adverse reactions to the drug can occur.

Selected References

Blodgett, L.C. *Manual of Respiratory Care Procedures,* 2nd ed. Philadelphia: J.B. Lippincott Co., 1987.
Caring for Surgical Patients. Nursing Photobook series. Springhouse, Pa.: Springhouse Corp., 1982.
Eggland, E.T. "Teaching the ABC's of COPD," Nursing87 17(1):60-64, January 1987.
Procedures. Nurse's Reference Library. Springhouse, Pa.: Springhouse Corp., 1983.

Providing Respiratory Care. Nursing Photobook series. Springhouse, Pa.: Springhouse Corp., 1982.
Ross, M.C. "Healing Under Pressure," *American Journal of Nursing* 86(10):1118-20, October 1986.
Shapiro, B.A., et al. *Clinical Applications of Respiratory Care,* 3rd ed. Chicago: Year Book Medical Pubs., Inc., 1985.

12 AIRWAY MANAGEMENT PROCEDURES

Introduction

If the lungs are the tree of life, the airways are the vital roots that carry life-giving substance. The airways must be kept patent, humidified, and free from bacterial contamination and injury. Like most aspects of respiratory care, methods for preserving a patent airway have changed markedly in the past 10 years.

The emergency action required to deal with a sudden complete airway obstruction from a foreign body in the pharynx, trachea, or bronchus is common knowledge among most health care professionals—and among much of the lay population. (See Appendix 1, *Basic Life Support*, pages 394 to 398.) Some specially trained health care professionals also know how to perform other emergency measures, such as cricothyrotomy and percutaneous transtracheal catheter ventilation, if a patent airway cannot be maintained. (See *Performing Cricothyrotomy and Percutaneous Transtracheal Catheter Ventilation*, pages 262 and 263.)

Changes also have occurred in the management of patients with artificial airways. Although no artificial airway can be considered totally harmless to the tissues, the degree of irreversible damage that an artificial airway inflicts on the trachea and upper airway has been reduced by emphasizing scrupulous tube care and by improving techniques and equipment for detecting complications and infection.

Advances in the selection and design of endotracheal and tracheostomy tubes, replacement of rigid tubes with more flexible plastic tubes, use of high-volume/low-pressure cuffs, and minimal-leak inflation technique have been especially significant. They've helped eliminate the severe tracheal stenosis and malacia that once commonly followed prolonged compromised arterial and venous circulation in the tracheal wall.

The use of disposable equipment for many respiratory procedures has practically eliminated the danger of treating patients with contaminated equipment, especially during an emergency. The skilled use of sterile, less traumatic suctioning techniques; maintenance of adequate humidification; and improvements in tracheostomy care have helped minimize the incidence of nosocomial infection in patients with an artificial airway.

Tracheostomy care has improved so dramatically that home management of tracheostomy, unheard of 10 years ago, is now commonplace. Similarly, the development of patient-teaching programs; community, professional, and lay support; and portable equipment, such as home oxygen units, have permitted home care of the patient with severe respiratory impairment.

In all of these patient-care efforts, clinical expertise plays a major role. With skilled assessment of airway patency and clearance, current respiratory patterns, and gas exchange effectiveness, the skilled practitioner can provide the most complex respi-

Performing Cricothyrotomy and Percutaneous Transtracheal Catheter Ventilation

If all your efforts to relieve your patient's airway obstruction fail and he still has inadequate air exchange, you may have to perform cricothyrotomy or percutaneous transtracheal catheter ventilation to gain rapid entry into his airway until the doctor can establish a definitive airway. (Of course, you'd do this only if you were specially trained and if no doctor was available.) Cricothyrotomy is the more effective method of providing short-term ventilation, but the procedure may interrupt cardiac compression. Transtracheal catheter ventilation takes only about 30 seconds to perform and can be done without hindering cardiopulmonary resuscitation. To begin either procedure, place the patient on his back and hyperextend his head and neck. Locate the cricothyroid membrane by palpating his neck, starting at the top. (The first prominence you'll feel is the thyroid cartilage; the second, the cricoid cartilage. The space between the two is the cricothyroid membrane.) Prepare the incision site with a broad-spectrum antimicrobial, such as povidone-iodine. Then proceed as follows, depending on the procedure you're performing.

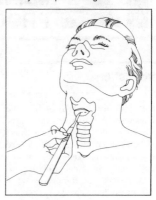

• For *cricothyrotomy* (shown above), make a horizontal incision, less than ½" (1.3 cm) long, with the scalpel, cutting through the patient's skin and the membrane. Then insert the scalpel handle and rotate it 90 degrees to spread the cartilage.
• Insert a small tube (#6 tracheostomy tube or similar-sized device) into the opening, and secure it.

ratory care and help maintain the physiologic integrity of this vital and delicate system.

Nasopharyngeal airway

Description
In nasopharyngeal airway insertion, a soft rubber or latex catheter follows the curvature of the nasopharynx, passing through the nose and extending from the nostril to the posterior pharynx. The bevel-shaped pharyngeal end of the airway facilitates insertion, and its funnel-shaped nasal end helps prevent slippage. (See *Nasopharyngeal Airway,* page 264.) Use of a nasopharyngeal airway is contraindicated in patients with a predisposition to nosebleeds and in those with a nasal obstruction, hemorrhagic disorder, or sepsis.

Purpose
• To prevent or relieve soft-tissue upper airway obstruction when an oropharyngeal airway is contraindicated
• To protect the nasal mucosa when frequent nasotracheal suctioning is necessary

• Attach the tube to a hand-held resuscitation bag or other ventilation device to provide positive-pressure ventilation with high oxygen concentration.

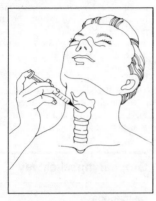

• For *percutaneous transtracheal catheter ventilation* (shown above), attach a 14G (or larger) plastic I.V. catheter with a needle to a 10-ml syringe.
• Carefully insert the needle and catheter through the patient's skin and membrane, aiming downward and caudally at a 45-degree angle to the trachea.
• Maintain negative pressure on the syringe as you advance the needle and catheter. You'll know the needle has entered the patient's trachea when air enters the syringe.
• When the needle is in his trachea, advance the catheter over the needle and carefully remove both needle and syringe.
• Here's how to provide jet insufflation (a temporary technique of providing intermittent ventilation to a patient with a percutaneous transtracheal catheter). Attach I.V. extension tubing to the catheter hub and attach a hand-operated release valve and then a pressure-regulating adjustment valve to the other end of the I.V. tubing. Connect the entire assembly to an oxygen source.
• Press the release valve to introduce an oxygen jet into the patient's trachea to inflate his lungs. When his lungs are visibly inflated, release the valve to allow passive exhalation. Adjust the pressure-regulating valve to the minimum pressure needed for adequate lung inflation.

Procedure
• Wash your hands thoroughly.
• In nonemergency situations, explain the procedure to the patient.
• Measure the diameter of the patient's nostril and the distance from the tip of his nose to his earlobe. Select an airway of slightly smaller diameter than the nostril and of slightly longer length (about 1″ [2.5 cm] longer) than measured.
• Lubricate the exterior of the entire airway with a water-soluble lubricant to prevent trauma during insertion. If possible, use lidocaine gel. Its anesthetic properties on the mucosa will make insertion much more comfortable.
• To insert the airway, hyperextend the patient's neck, if not contraindicated. Then push up the tip of his nose and pass the airway into his nostril. Avoid pushing against any resistance to prevent tissue trauma and airway kinking.
• To check for correct airway placement, first close the patient's mouth. Then place your finger over the tube's opening to detect air exchange. Also, depress the patient's tongue with a tongue depressor and look for the airway tip behind the uvula.

Nasopharyngeal Airway

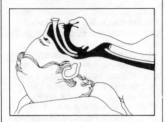

Advantages
• Tolerated better than oropharyngeal airway by conscious patients
• Allows for suctioning without displacing the patient's nasal turbinates

Disadvantages
• May cause severe nosebleed if inserted too forcefully
• May kink and clog, obstructing airway
• May cause pressure necrosis of nasal mucosa
• May cause air passage obstruction if artificial airway is too large

To remove a nasopharyngeal airway
Evaluate the patient's condition. If his natural airway is patent, remove the nasopharyngeal airway in one smooth motion. If it sticks, apply lubricant around the nasal end of the tube and around the nostril; then gently rotate the airway until it's free.

Clinical considerations
If the patient coughs or gags, the tube may be too long. If so, remove the airway and insert a shorter one.

To increase oxygen availability during respiration, place a nasal cannula just under the nose. Rarely, a nasal catheter may be inserted. To prevent mucus from creating an obstruction, humidify administered oxygen. Adequate parenteral hydration also helps prevent mucus obstruction. If suctioning's necessary, try

to elicit a strong cough, which may help remove mucus, by instilling saline solution through the suction catheter and toward the vocal cords.

Check the airway regularly to detect dislodgment or obstruction. Clean the airway by placing it in a basin and rinsing it with hydrogen peroxide and then with water. If secretions remain, use a pipe cleaner to remove them. Reinsert the clean airway into the other nostril, if it's patent, to avoid skin breakdown. Thoroughly document the procedure and associated care.

Complications
The use of a nasopharyngeal airway can cause nosebleed, pressure necrosis of the nasal mucosa, and sinus infection from obstruction of sinus drainage.

Oropharyngeal airway

Description
A curved rubber or plastic device, an oropharyngeal airway is inserted through the mouth into the posterior pharynx. Because the tongue usually obstructs the posterior pharynx of an unconscious patient, insertion of this airway, which conforms to the palate's curvature, corrects this obstruction and allows air to pass around and through the tube. (See *Oropharyngeal Airway.*) Trauma to the lower face, recent oral surgery, or loose or avulsed teeth contraindicate oropharyngeal airway use.

Purpose
• To provide short-term prevention or relief of soft-tissue upper airway obstruction in an unconscious patient
• To facilitate oropharyngeal suctioning

Procedure
• Select the appropriate-sized airway for your patient; an oversized airway can obstruct breathing by depressing

the epiglottis into the laryngeal opening. Usually, select a small size for an infant or child, a medium size for an average adult, and a large size for a large or obese adult. Confirm the correct size by placing the airway flange beside the patient's cheek, parallel to his front teeth. If it's the right size, the airway curve should reach to the angle of the jaw.

• Explain the procedure to the patient, even though he may not appear alert. Provide privacy, and wash your hands thoroughly. If the patient's wearing dentures, remove them so they don't cause further airway obstruction.

• If necessary, suction the patient.

• Place the patient in a supine position with his neck hyperextended, unless contraindicated.

• To insert the airway, use the cross-finger or tongue-depressor technique.

For the *cross-finger technique*, place your thumb on the patient's upper teeth and your index finger on his lower teeth. Gently open his mouth by pushing his teeth apart. Next, insert the airway, preferably by pointing the tip toward the cheek, gently advancing it, and then rotating it by sliding the tip back over the tongue's surface until it's pointing downward. Be careful that the tongue isn't pushed back with the airway, if you're using this method.

For the *tongue-depressor technique*, open the patient's mouth and depress his tongue with the blade. Guide the artificial airway over the back of the tongue as for the cross-finger technique, until it's in place.

• Position the patient on his side to decrease the risk of vomitus aspiration.

To remove an oropharyngeal airway

• Evaluate the patient's behavior for signs that he no longer needs the airway. As he becomes more alert, for example, he's likely to cough or gag.

• When the patient regains consciousness and can swallow, remove the airway by pulling it outward and down-

Oropharyngeal Airway

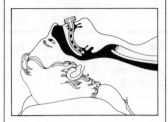

Advantages
• Easily inserted
• Holds tongue away from pharynx

Disadvantages
• Dislodges easily
• May cause obstruction if airway size is incorrect
• Poorly tolerated by most conscious patients
• May stimulate gag reflex

ward, following the mouth's natural curvature.

• Once the airway is removed, test the patient's cough and gag reflexes to ensure that removal wasn't premature.

Clinical considerations

Frequently check airway position for removal or dislodgment. Perform mouth care every 2 to 4 hours, as needed. Begin by holding the patient's jaws open with a padded tongue depressor and gently removing the airway. Place the airway in a basin and rinse it with hydrogen peroxide followed by water. If secretions remain in the airway, use a pipe cleaner to remove them. Complete standard mouth care and reinsert the airway.

While the airway's removed for mouth care, observe the mouth's mucous membranes to detect ulceration, because tissue damage can result from prolonged airway use. Thoroughly document the procedure and associated care.

Complications
Tooth damage or loss and tissue damage or bleeding may result from oropharyngeal airway insertion.

Esophageal airways
(esophageal gastric tube airway and esophageal obturator airway)

Description
The esophageal gastric tube airway (EGTA) and the esophageal obturator airway (EOA) are used to maintain ventilation for up to 2 hours during an emergency. They prevent tongue obstruction, air from entering the stomach, and stomach contents from entering the trachea. They can be inserted only after successful mouth-to-mouth resuscitation has established airway patency.

Use of esophageal airways is contraindicated in children (pediatric sizes aren't currently available); conscious or semiconscious patients, because they will reject them; patients who've undergone recent oral surgery; patients with trauma to the lower face, esophageal disease, or damage from ingestion of toxic chemicals; and patients with a suspected narcotic overdose that can be reversed by naloxone. (See *Esophageal Airways.*)

Purpose
To maintain ventilation during cardiac or respiratory arrest when endotracheal intubation isn't feasible

Procedure
• Assess the patient's condition to determine if he's a good candidate for an esophageal airway.
• Quickly gather and assemble the equipment, including the esophageal tube, face mask, #16 or #18 French nasogastric (NG) tube for EGTA, 35-ml syringe, stethoscope, intermittent gastric suction equipment, and oral suction equipment. Fill the mask with air and check for leaks. Inflate the esophageal tube cuff with 35 ml of air and check for leaks; then, deflate the cuff. Connect the esophageal tube to the face mask (the lower opening on an EGTA) and listen for the tube to click, indicating proper placement.
• Lubricate the first inch (2.5 cm) of the tube's distal tip with a water-soluble lubricant, I.V. fluid, the patient's saliva, or tap water. For an EGTA, also lubricate the first inch of the NG tube's distal tip.
• If the patient's condition permits, place him supine with his neck in a neutral or semiflexed position. Neck hyperextension may cause the tube to enter the trachea instead of the esophagus. Remove dentures, if applicable.
• Insert your thumb deeply into the patient's mouth behind the base of his tongue. Place your index and middle fingers of the same hand under the patient's chin and lift his jaw straight up.
• With your other hand, grasp the esophageal tube just below the mask in the same way you'd grasp a pencil. This promotes gentle maneuvering of the tube and reduces the risk of pharyngeal trauma.
• Still elevating the patient's jaw with one hand, insert the tip of the esophageal tube into his mouth. Gently guide the airway over the tongue into the pharynx and then into the esophagus, following the natural pharyngeal curve. No force is required for proper insertion; the tube should easily seat itself within 10 seconds. If you encounter resistance, withdraw the tube slightly and readvance it. When the tube's fully advanced, the mask should fit snugly over the patient's mouth and nose. If it isn't snug, the mask may need to be inflated more.
• Holding the mask firmly in place, immediately blow into the ventilatory port of the face mask (the upper opening on an EGTA). Watch for chest movement, or auscultate both lungs with a stethoscope.

Esophageal Airways

Advantages
• Quickly and easily inserted by personnel with minimal training
• Prevents aspiration of stomach contents while tube's in place
• Useful for patients with suspected spinal injuries because these devices don't require visualization of the trachea or neck hyperextension

Disadvantages
• May cause pharyngeal trauma during insertion
• May be accidentally inserted into trachea
• May cause gastric distension and may impair ventilation if cuff is improperly inflated
• May cause aspiration if tube is removed without endotracheal intubation

Esophageal gastric tube airway

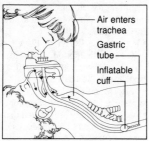

The *esophageal gastric tube airway* consists of an inflatable face mask and an esophageal tube. The transparent face mask has two ports: a lower port for insertion of an esophageal tube and an upper port for ventilation. The inside of the mask is soft and pliable; it molds to the patient's face and makes a tight seal, preventing air loss.

The proximal end of the esophageal tube has a one-way nonrefluxing valve that blocks the esophagus. This valve prevents air from entering the stomach, thus reducing the risk of abdominal distension and aspiration. The distal end has an inflatable cuff that rests in the esophagus just below the tracheal bifurcation, preventing pressure on the noncartilaginous back of the tracheal wall.

During ventilation, air is blown into the upper port in the mask and, with the esophagus blocked, enters the trachea and lungs. (See illustration at left.)

A gastric (Levin) tube can be used to suction stomach contents before extubation. It's inserted through the mask's lower port into the esophageal tube, then through a small hole in the end of the tube.

Esophageal obturator airway

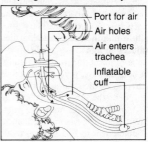

The *esophageal obturator airway* consists of an adjustable, inflatable, transparent face mask with a single port, attached by a snap lock to a blind esophageal tube.

When properly inflated, the mask prevents air from escaping through the nose and mouth. (See above illustration.)

The esophageal tube has 16 holes at its proximal end through which air or oxygen, blown into the port of the mask, is transferred to the trachea. The tube's distal end is closed and circled by an inflatable cuff. When the cuff's inflated, it occludes the esophagus, preventing air from entering the stomach and acting as a barrier against vomitus and involuntary aspiration.

• If chest movement or breath sounds are absent, immediately remove the tube, because it may be lodged in the trachea. Reestablish mouth-to-mouth resuscitation or use a hand-held resuscitation bag for 1 minute; then reinsert the esophageal tube.

Once the tube is properly in place in the esophagus, draw 35 ml of air into the syringe, connect the syringe to the tube's cuff-inflation valve, and inflate the cuff. Avoid overinflation, as this can cause esophageal trauma.

• If you've inserted an EGTA, insert the NG tube through the lower port on the face mask and into the esophageal tube, and advance it to the second marking so that it reaches 6″ (15 cm) beyond the tube's distal end. Suction stomach contents using intermittent gastric suction to decompress the stomach (particularly necessary after mouth-to-mouth resuscitation, which introduces air into the stomach). Leave the tube in place during resuscitation.

• For both airways, perform mouth-to-mouth resuscitation through the face mask port (the upper port on the EGTA), or connect the mask to a hand-held resuscitation bag or to a mechanical ventilator delivering FIO_2 of up to 1.0.

• Monitor the patient to ensure adequate ventilation. Watch for chest movement, and suction the patient if mucus blocks the EOA tube perforations or interrupts respiration in any way.

To remove an esophageal airway
• Assess the patient's condition to determine if you can remove the airway. The airway may be removed if the patient has spontaneous respirations and a respiratory rate of 16 to 20 respirations/minute. If 2 hours have elapsed since airway insertion and respirations aren't spontaneous or at the normal rate, the patient must be switched to an artificial airway that can be used for long-term ventilation, such as an endotracheal tube.

• Detach the mask from the esophageal tube.

• If the patient is conscious, place him on his left side, if possible, to avoid aspiration during removal of the esophageal tube. If he's unconscious and requires an endotracheal tube, insert the tube (or assist with its insertion) and inflate its cuff before removing the esophageal tube. With the esophageal tube still in place, you can easily place the endotracheal tube into the trachea; the patient's less likely to aspirate gastric contents when the tube is removed this way.

• Deflate the esophageal tube cuff by removing the tip of the cuff-inflation valve. Don't try to remove the tube with the cuff inflated, because this may cause esophageal perforation.

• Turn the patient's head to the side, if possible, to avoid aspiration.

• If necessary, insert an NG tube into the esophagus beside the EOA, if used. Decompress the stomach by gravity flow, or connect the NG tube to intermittent gastric suction, and suction stomach contents to prevent aspiration during extubation.

• Remove the EGTA or EOA in one swift, smooth motion, following the natural pharyngeal curve to avoid esophageal trauma.

• Perform oropharyngeal suctioning to remove any residual secretions.

• Assist the doctor as required in monitoring and maintaining adequate patient ventilation.

Clinical considerations
For easy insertion, you may prefer to direct the airway along the right side of the patient's mouth, because the esophagus is located to the right of and behind the trachea. Alternatively, you may advance the tube tip upward toward the hard palate, then invert the tip and glide it along the tongue surface and into the pharynx. This procedure keeps the tube centered, avoids snagging it on the sides of the throat, and eases insertion in the patient with clenched jaws.

Watch the unconscious patient as he regains consciousness. Restrain his hands if he tries to remove the airway. Explain the procedure to him, if possible, to reduce his apprehension. Observe also for retching and, if it occurs, immediately remove the airway; vomitus accumulation blocked by the airway cuff may cause esophageal perforation. Thoroughly document the procedure and associated care.

Complications
Insertion of an esophageal airway can result in airway obstruction if the tube enters the trachea; pharyngeal trauma; or esophageal perforation, which can lead to abscess formation, mediastinal and subcutaneous emphysema, mediastinitis, hemorrhage, fistula formation, pneumonia, or death.

Endotracheal intubation

Description
Endotracheal intubation involves oral or nasal insertion of a flexible, cuffed tube through the larynx into the trachea. The procedure may be performed by a doctor, physician's assistant, anesthetist, respiratory therapist, or specially trained nurse. Recently, endotracheal tubes have been used as a medication administration route in emergency situations. (See *Giving Medications through an Endotracheal Tube*, page 270.)

Oral endotracheal intubation is contraindicated in patients with trauma to the lower face or mouth and those who have recently undergone oral surgery. Nasal endotracheal intubation is contraindicated in patients with nasal obstruction, a fractured nose, sinusitis, or bleeding disorders. It should be used with caution in patients with basal skull fractures when communication exists between the nasopharyngeal mucosa and the brain. Oral and nasal intubation are contraindicated in patients with epiglottitis; acute, unstable cervical spine injury; or laryngeal obstruction caused by tumor, infection, or vocal cord paralysis. Tracheostomy is the alternative treatment for such patients. (See *Endotracheal Tubes*, page 272.)

Purpose
Oral endotracheal tube
• Provides an open airway during cardiopulmonary resuscitation and airway obstruction when all other efforts have failed
• Provides a controlled airway for mechanical ventilation when the patient has nasal obstruction or a predisposition to nosebleed

Nasal endotracheal tube
• Relieves airway obstruction when all other efforts to maintain an open airway have failed and when the patient has facial or oral trauma, cervical trauma, or a jaw movement problem
• Provides a controlled airway for mechanical ventilation
• Improves patient comfort when long-term intubation is necessary

Procedure
• In nonemergency situations, provide patient teaching.
• To prepare equipment, quickly gather the supplies you'll need. (Many institutions use intubation trays that contain most necessary supplies.)
• Check the battery-operated light in the laryngoscope handle by snapping the appropriate-sized blade into place for intubation. If the light fails to flash immediately, replace the laryngoscope bulb or the batteries, whichever is faster.
• Open sterile packages. Squeeze water-soluble lubricant onto a sterile field.
• Attach the endotracheal tube and its accompanying adapter so that the tube can be attached to a hand-held resuscitation bag or mechanical ventilator.
• Attach the syringe to the port of the tube's exterior pilot cuff and inflate the cuff slowly, observing for uniform infla-

Giving Medications through an Endotracheal Tube

If an I.V. line can't be established quickly, an endotracheal tube offers an alternate access route for such emergency drugs as epinephrine hydrochloride, atropine sulfate, and lidocaine hydrochloride. Once in the lungs, these drugs pass through the alveoli and into the circulation. (Other drugs you can give through an endotracheal tube include naloxone hydrochloride and metaraminol bitartrate.)

Endotracheal administration has distinct advantages over intracardiac injection, which interrupts resuscitation efforts and risks such complications as coronary artery laceration, cardiac tamponade, and pneumothorax. Current guidelines recommend intracardiac injection only as a last resort, when I.V. and endotracheal routes aren't available.

Onset of action varies according to the patient's hemodynamic status and other factors. Duration of action, however, typically lasts longer with endotracheal administration because of sustained absorption by the alveoli—a phenomenon called the *depot effect.* Consequently, you may need to adjust repeat doses and continuous infusions to prevent adverse drug effects.

Give the same initial drug dose through an endotracheal tube that you'd give through a peripheral I.V. line. Dilute the dose to 5 to 10 ml to enhance absorption—with greater volume, a larger proportion of drug leaves the endotracheal tube and contacts lung tissue. Use sterile water or normal saline solution as a diluent.

Caution: Don't give bretylium, calcium, diazepam, isoproterenol, norepinephrine, or sodium bicarbonate through an endotracheal tube.

tion. Check the cuff for leaks. Use the syringe to completely deflate the cuff.
• For nasal insertion, lubricate the tube cover with water-soluble lubricant to ease insertion. For oral intubation, a lubricant is rarely used.
• Lubricate the entire stylet if it will be used so that it may be easily removed from the tube after intubation. Insert it so that its distal tip lies about ½″ (1 cm) inside the endotracheal tube's distal end. To prevent vocal cord trauma, make sure it doesn't extend beyond the tube.
• Prepare the humidified oxygen system and the suctioning equipment for immediate use.

To insert an endotracheal tube
• Check the doctor's written order and assess the patient's condition.
• Administer medication, as ordered, to decrease respiratory secretions, induce amnesia or analgesia, and help calm and

relax the conscious patient. Remove any dentures.
• Administer oxygen until the tube is inserted, to prevent hypoxia.
• Suction the patient, if necessary, just before tube insertion to allow visualization of the pharyngeal and vocal cord structure. Use a tonsil suction tip to suction at the vocal cords if secretions and visualization pose a problem.
• Place the patient in a supine position with his neck hyperextended to straighten the pharynx and trachea.
• Spray local anesthetic into the posterior pharynx to help quell the gag reflex and to reduce patient discomfort during intubation.
• Grasp the laryngoscope handle in your dominant hand and gently slide the blade into the right side of the patient's mouth. Then center the blade, pushing the tongue to the left. Hold the patient's lower lip away from his

teeth to prevent it from being caught and traumatized.

• Advance the blade, bringing the handle toward you, to expose the epiglottis. Avoid using the patient's teeth as a pivotal point for the laryngoscope, because you may damage them.

• Continue to lift the laryngoscope handle toward you to reveal the vocal cords.

• Keeping the vocal cords in view, guide the endotracheal tube into the right side of the mouth and down along the laryngoscope blade into the vertical larynx opening between the vocal cords. Don't mistake the horizontal esophageal opening for the larynx. If the vocal cords are closed in spasm, wait a few seconds for them to relax, then guide the tube gently past them to avoid trauma.

• Advance the tube until the cuff disappears beyond the vocal cords. Further insertion may occlude a major bronchus and precipitate lung collapse.

• Holding the endotracheal tube in place, quickly remove the stylet, if present.

• Inflate the tube cuff until you feel resistance. Once the patient is on the ventilator, use the minimal-leak technique to establish correct cuff inflation.

• To ensure proper tube placement, feel the tube's tip for warm exhalations and listen for air movement. If the patient is breathing spontaneously, observe for chest expansion and auscultate the chest for bilateral breath sounds. If he's unconscious or uncooperative, use a hand-held resuscitation bag and observe for upper chest movement. If his stomach distends and belching occurs, the tube is in the esophagus. Immediately deflate the cuff, remove the tube, and repeat insertion, using another sterile tube to prevent tracheal contamination.

• Auscultate bilaterally to exclude the possibility of endobronchial intubation. If you fail to hear breath sounds on both sides of the chest, you may have inserted the tube into a mainstem

bronchus (usually the right one, because it's more vertical than the left and has a wider angle at the bifurcation). Such insertion occludes the other bronchus and lung and results in atelectasis on the obstructed side. If the tube is resting on the carina, the patient will cough and fight the ventilator, alerting you to the problem. To correct these problems, deflate the cuff, withdraw the tube ½" to 1" (1.3 to 2.5 cm), auscultate for bilateral breath sounds, and reinflate the cuff.

• Once you've confirmed correct tube placement, administer oxygen or initiate mechanical ventilation, and provide suction.

• To secure tube position, apply compound benzoin tincture to each cheek and let it dry for enhanced tape adhesion. Tape the tube firmly with adhesive or nonallergenic tape, but not paper tape. Initially, tape the tube in the middle of the mouth. This decreases mucosal pressure in the mouth corners, allows for mouth care on either side of the tube, and keeps the tube as straight as possible to the hypopharynx. Be careful not to get the patient's lips caught in the tape.

• Inflate the cuff using minimal-leak technique (also called minimal occlusive volume). Attach a 10-ml syringe to the port on the tube's exterior pilot cuff and place a stethoscope on the side of the patient's neck. Inject small amounts of air during the inspiratory phase of ventilation until you hear no leak. Then, aspirate 0.1 ml of air from the cuff to create a minimal air leak. Record the amount of air needed to inflate the cuff for subsequent monitoring for tracheal dilation or erosion.

• Note the tube's exit point by noting the marking (centimeter number) on the tube at the mouth corner. If the tube doesn't have centimeter marks on the proximal end, clearly mark the tube's exit point from the mouth with pen or tape. Periodic monitoring of the mark can reveal tube displacement.

Endotracheal Tubes

Oral endotracheal tube

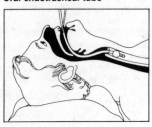

Nasal endotracheal tube

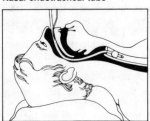

Advantages
- Quickly and easily inserted
- Causes less intubation trauma than nasal endotracheal airway or tracheostomy tube
- Permits positive-pressure ventilation and prevents aspiration of stomach contents, if cuff is inflated
- Permits removal of tracheobronchial secretions in patients who can't cough effectively

Disadvantages
- May damage teeth or lacerate lips, mouth, pharyngeal mucosa, or larynx during insertion
- Activates gag reflex in conscious patients
- May be bitten or chewed
- May cause pressure necrosis

Advantages
- More comfortable than oral endotracheal tube
- Permits good oral hygiene
- Can't be bitten or chewed
- Provides a channel for suctioning
- May be adapted easily if patient requires continuous ventilation
- Can be anchored in place easily
- Permits positive-pressure ventilation and prevents aspiration of stomach contents, if cuff is inflated

Disadvantages
- May lacerate pharyngeal mucosa or larynx during insertion
- Kinks and clogs more easily than an oral endotracheal tube
- Increases airway resistance because of small lumen size needed to fit nasal passages
- May cause pressure necrosis
- More difficult and time-consuming to insert
- Poses increased risk of infection because it introduces nasal bacteria into the trachea

- Make sure a chest X-ray is taken to verify tube position.
- If available, place a swivel adapter between the tube and the humidified oxygen source to allow for intermittent suctioning and to reduce tube tension.
- Place the patient with his head in a comfortable position to avoid tube kinking and airway obstruction.

Clinical considerations

Because of airway differences, you intubate a child differently from an adult. (See *Intubating a Child: Points to Remember.*)

Auscultate both sides of the chest and check chest movement hourly to ensure correct tube placement and full lung ventilation. Give frequent oral care and position the endotracheal tube

Intubating a Child: Points to Remember

A child's airway becomes narrowest at the cricoid cartilage (rather than at the glottic opening, where an adult's airway narrows). Consequently, the doctor may have difficulty advancing an endotracheal tube at the cricoid level. Other differences from adult anatomy include a more flexible and proportionately smaller airway, a proportionately larger tongue, and a glottic opening located higher in the neck. Using appropriate equipment and techniques minimizes insertion problems.

Indications for endotracheal intubation include inability to ventilate an unconscious patient, cardiac or respiratory arrest, and a need for prolonged artificial ventilation. Follow these guidelines:

• Choose a tube appropriate for the child's size. Usually an uncuffed tube is used for a child under age 8, a cuffed tube for older children. However, the tube size and type depend on the child's size and ventilatory needs. Use of high positive end-expiratory pressure may warrant a cuffed tube.

• Obtain a stylet or a straight or curved laryngoscope blade to help provide rigidity and guide the tube through the child's vocal cords. (The doctor will probably prefer a straight blade for an infant.)

• Give artificial ventilation with supplemental oxygen, before insertion.

• During insertion, constantly monitor heart rate. If it falls below 60 beats/minute (below 80 beats/minute for an infant), stop the procedure and provide artificial ventilation. *Important:* Don't allow more than 30 seconds to pass without ventilating the patient.

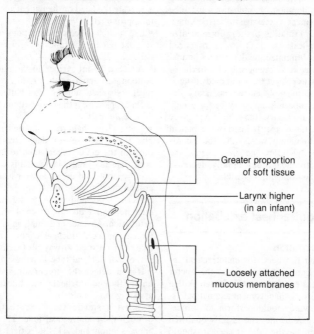

— Greater proportion of soft tissue

— Larynx higher (in an infant)

— Loosely attached mucous membranes

to avoid pressure sores from excess pressure on the sides of the mouth.

Suction secretions through the endotracheal tube when necessary to clear secretions and prevent mucus plugs from obstructing the tube. Retape the tube only when necessary (for example, when the tape becomes loose).

Keep intubation equipment easily accessible to reintubate the patient if accidental extubation occurs. Thoroughly document the procedure and associated care.

Complications

Potential complications include apnea caused by reflex breath-holding; bronchospasm; aspiration of blood, secretions, or gastric contents; tooth damage or loss; trauma to the lips, mouth, pharynx, or larynx (vocal cord damage); laryngeal edema and erosion; and tracheal stenosis, erosion, and necrosis.

Complications relate directly to tube size, duration of intubation, and tube movement (excessive tube movement can traumatize tissue). To minimize complications, don't use an oversized tube. Minimize the duration of intubation by encouraging use of a tracheostomy to protect the vocal cords if long-term intubation becomes necessary. Reduce tube movement by retaping only when necessary (the tube moves every time it's retaped). Instruct the patient not to mouth words (the vocal cords move by reflex and press against the endotracheal tube). Finally, decrease head movement, if possible.

Endotracheal extubation

Description

When the need for endotracheal intubation no longer exists, the doctor orders extubation. A clinician skilled in airway management and patient assessment should perform the procedure. Someone who is fully qualified to replace the tube, if needed, should be readily available. Similarly, the necessary supplies for tube replacement also should be readily available.

Purpose

To remove an endotracheal tube safely when the patient no longer needs mechanical ventilation, has a patent natural airway, and can protect his own airway via gag and cough reflexes

Procedure

• If you're authorized to remove the tube, have another nurse assist you to help prevent unnecessary tube manipulation during untaping, which can be traumatic.

• Gather necessary equipment, including suction equipment, hand-held resuscitation bag with mask, supplemental oxygen source with mask, and equipment for reintubation.

• Wash your hands and explain the procedure to the patient.

• Elevate the head of the patient's bed to approximately 90 degrees.

• Use suction to remove secretions inside and outside the tube (as described earlier).

• Attach a 10-ml syringe to the pilot balloon port and aspirate air until you meet resistance and the pilot balloon deflates. Never cut the pilot balloon to deflate the cuff.

• Using a hand-held resuscitation bag, give the patient several deep breaths through the endotracheal tube to hyperinflate his lungs, increase his oxygen reserve, and detect any air leaks around the deflated cuff. If you fail to detect a leak, notify the doctor immediately, and do not proceed with extubation. Absence of an air leak may indicate marked tracheal edema and can result in total airway obstruction if the endotracheal tube is removed.

• If you detect the proper air leak, untape the endotracheal tube while the assisting nurse holds it.

• Insert a sterile suction catheter through the endotracheal tube. Then, apply suction and ask the patient to open his mouth fully and pretend to cry out. This causes vocal cord abduction and reduces the risk of laryngeal trauma during tube withdrawal.

• Simultaneously remove the endotracheal tube and the suction catheter in one smooth outward and downward motion, following the natural curve of the patient's mouth. Suctioning during extubation removes secretions retained at the end of the tube and prevents aspiration.

Clinical considerations

Give the patient supplemental oxygen. For highest humidity, use a cool-mist, large-volume nebulizer to help decrease airway irritation, patient discomfort, and laryngeal edema. Encourage the patient to cough as needed and remind him that his sore throat and hoarseness are expected adverse reactions that will gradually subside.

Frequently auscultate the patient's lungs and check for signs of respiratory distress. Be especially alert for stridor or other evidence of upper airway obstruction. If ordered, draw an arterial blood specimen for blood gas analysis. Keep supplies needed for reintubation readily available for at least 12 hours or until you're sure that the patient can tolerate extubation. Thoroughly document the procedure and associated care.

Complications

Complications that can occur during endotracheal tube extubation include laryngospasm (especially in infants and children), marked tracheal edema, or ventilatory failure.

Tracheostomy care

Description

A tracheostomy is an external opening to the trachea that has been created surgically to maintain a patent airway in patients with complete upper airway obstruction when endotracheal intubation is impossible. An indwelling tracheostomy tube is inserted into the opening to prevent its closure. A tracheostomy minimizes the risk of vocal cord damage from an endotracheal tube during long-term airway support. Usually preferred for long-term intubation, it also can be used to provide airway access in the patient with unmanageable secretions.

Metal and plastic tracheostomy tubes come in various sizes to accommodate patients of all ages. The metal tube, used mainly for the long-term tracheostomy patient who isn't receiving mechanical ventilation, has three parts: an outer cannula, an inner cannula, and an obturator that serves as a guide for outer cannula insertion. Some plastic tubes have the same three parts; most, however, consist of the obturator and one single-walled tube that doesn't require removal for cleaning, because incrustations are less likely to form on nonmetal materials. (See *Tracheostomy*, page 276.)

Tracheostomy care must be performed using sterile technique to prevent infection, especially until the stoma has healed (usually 4 days). Care may be given as frequently as every 30 minutes immediately after tracheotomy; it should never be suspended for more than 8 hours.

Purpose

• To ensure airway patency by keeping the tracheostomy tube free of blood clots after insertion and free of mucus buildup

• To maintain mucous membrane and skin integrity while helping to prevent infection

Procedure

• Explain the procedure to the patient, even if he's unresponsive.

• Assess the patient's condition and provide privacy.

• Wash your hands and assemble all equipment and supplies, including suc-

Tracheostomy

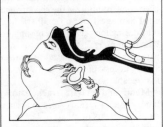

Advantages
- Suctioned more easily than endotracheal tube
- Reduces dead air space in respiratory tract
- Causes less trauma to upper airway
- Permits patient to swallow and eat more easily
- More comfortable than other tubes
- Permits positive pressure ventilation and prevents aspiration of stomach contents, if cuff is inflated

Disadvantages
- Requires surgery to insert
- May cause laceration or pressure necrosis of trachea
- May cause tracheoesophageal fistula
- Increases risk of tracheal and stomal inflammation, infection, and mucus plugs

tion equipment, in the patient's room. (Prepackaged commercial tracheostomy care sets are readily available.)
- Place a cuffed trash bag adjacent to your working area.
- Establish a sterile field near the patient's bed and place sterile equipment and supplies on it.
- For cleansing, pour sterile solutions into sterile containers.
- For double-cannula care, you may use an additional basin to hold your gauze sponges and swabs saturated with cleansing solution.

- Prepare new tracheostomy ties from twill tape, if indicated.
- If you're using a spare sterile inner cannula, unscrew the cap from the top of the sterile container, but don't remove it.
- Assess the patient's condition.
- Unless contraindicated, place the patient in semi-Fowler's position.
- Remove any humidification or ventilation device.
- Using sterile technique, suction the entire length of the tracheostomy tube to clear the airway of any secretions that may impair oxygenation. Follow appropriate suctioning guidelines.
- Reconnect the patient to the humidifier or ventilator, if necessary.
- Remove and discard the patient's tracheostomy dressing.
- Put a sterile glove on your dominant hand.

To cleanse a single-cannula tube
- With your gloved hand, wet a sterile 4″ x 4″ gauze sponge with the cleansing solution. Squeeze out excess liquid to prevent accidental aspiration. Then, wipe the patient's neck under the tracheostomy tube flanges and twill tapes.
- Saturate a second sponge and wipe until the skin surrounding the tracheostomy is cleansed. Use additional sponges or cotton-tipped applicators to cleanse the stoma site and the tube flanges. Wipe from the stoma outward only once with each sponge and then discard the sponge.
- If incrustations resist removal, cleanse with a sterile cotton-tipped applicator saturated in hydrogen peroxide and press to remove excess liquid. Use each applicator only once and wipe gently, especially if the surrounding skin's excoriated.
- Rinse debris and any hydrogen peroxide with one or more sterile 4″ x 4″ gauze sponges dampened in sterile normal saline solution. Dry the area thoroughly with additional sterile gauze sponges. Remove and discard your glove.

To cleanse a double-cannula tube

• With your ungloved hand, disconnect the ventilator or humidification device. Then, with the same hand, unlock the tracheostomy tube's inner cannula. Next, remove the inner cannula with your ungloved hand.

• Place the inner cannula in the hydrogen peroxide container, and allow it to soak to remove incrustations.

• For the mechanically ventilated patient, use your ungloved hand to remove the lid from the container with the spare inner cannula. Pick up the cannula with your gloved hand and insert it into the outer cannula of the patient's tracheostomy tube. Use your ungloved hand to reconnect the patient to the ventilator.

• Put a sterile glove on your nondominant hand and cleanse the skin, stoma, and tracheostomy tube flanges with the presoaked gauze sponges and cotton-tipped applicators, as previously described.

• Pick up the inner cannula from the soaking container. Using the sterile nylon brush, scrub the cannula. If the brush doesn't slide easily into the cannula, use a sterile pipe cleaner.

• Immerse the cannula in the container of sterile normal saline solution and agitate it for about 10 seconds to rinse it thoroughly and provide a thin film of solution to lubricate it for replacement.

• Hold the cannula up to the light and inspect it for cleanliness. If incrustations are still present, repeat the cleaning process. If not, grasp the clean cannula and tap it gently against the inside edge of the sterile container to remove excess liquid, preventing possible aspiration by the patient. Use three sterile pipe cleaners twisted together to dry the inside of the cannula. Refrain from drying its outer surface because a thin film of moisture acts as a lubricant during insertion.

• If the patient isn't on a ventilator, gently reinsert the inner cannula into his tracheostomy tube. Lock it in place and pull on it gently to ensure secure positioning. For a patient on a ventilator, place the cleaned inner cannula in the sterile storage container.

• Apply a new sterile tracheostomy dressing. If you're not using a commercially prepared dressing, avoid using cotton-filled gauze or a trimmed gauze sponge, because aspiration of lint and fibers can cause a tracheal abscess. Instead, open a sterile 4" x 4" gauze pad to its full length and fold it in half lengthwise to form a long, thin rectangle. With the folded edge facing downward, find the center of the edge; then fold each side straight up from this point to create a U-shaped pad. Slip the pad under the flanges of the tracheostomy tube so that the pad's flaps encircle and cushion the tube.

• Remove and discard your gloves. Replace and tighten the lid on the container with the clean inner cannula, if applicable.

To conclude tracheostomy care

• Replace the tracheostomy ties if they're soiled, loose, or too tight (see below).

• Replace any humidification device.

• Give oral care, as needed, because the oral cavity can become dry and malodorous and can develop sores from incrusted secretions.

• Make sure that the patient is comfortable and that he can easily reach the call signal and communication aids.

• Observe soiled dressings and any suctioned secretions for amount, color, consistency, and odor.

To change tracheostomy ties

• Obtain assistance from another nurse or a respiratory therapist, because of the risk of accidental tube expulsion during this procedure. Patient movement or coughing can dislodge the tube.

• Wash your hands thoroughly.

• If you're not using commercially packaged tracheostomy ties, prepare new ties from a 30" (75-cm) length of twill tape by folding one end back 1" (2.5 cm) on itself. Then, with the ban-

Occluded Tracheostomy Tube

The situation
While working the night shift on a medical-surgical unit, you see a patient who had a total laryngectomy a week ago come out of his room. He's stooped over and in obvious distress. When you reach him, he points to his tracheostomy tube and hands you his notepad with the message, "Something's wrong!"

You immediately see that he's pale and diaphoretic, and you hear a whistling sound with each breath he takes. His labored respirations are rapid and shallow. You feel minimal airflow at the stoma.

The problem
A postlaryngectomy patient is in respiratory distress. His signs indicate that a mucus plug is lodged in his tracheostomy tube.

The worst case
Mucus continues to accumulate until it completely occludes the tube. Lack of air exchange leads to respiratory arrest.

The best case
Either the patient coughs out the mucus plug or you're able to remove it, thereby restoring air exchange.

The assessment
The patient has a mucus plug partially occluding his tracheostomy tube—his only airway. Because you

hear a whistling sound and feel a minimal airflow, you know he's still receiving some air. You must act quickly to remove the mucus plug before he develops further respiratory distress.

Call for help as you get the patient back to bed. Have him sit upright. Remove the tube's inner cannula and have him try to cough out the plug. (This may be difficult; because his glottis has been removed, he can't perform Valsalva's maneuver or cough with an effective force.)

If this doesn't work, quickly attach a humidified oxygen source to his tracheostomy tube and assemble a tracheal suction setup. Prepare a syringe of 2 ml sterile isotonic saline solution (without preservatives). Remove the oxygen source, quickly instill the saline solution, then vigorously suction. Apply suction for no longer than 10 seconds at a time, and replace the oxygen source between each suctioning attempt.

If the mucus plug still hasn't come out, call for the anesthesiologist, then cut the ties and gently remove the entire tube. Don't worry about the stoma closing; it's been permanently sutured open.

If the plug doesn't come out with the tube, use a flashlight to examine inside the tracheal stoma. If you see that the mucus plug is near the stoma, *carefully* try to remove it us-

dage scissors, cut a ½″ (1.3-cm) slit down the center of the tape from the folded edge. Alternatively, you may fold the end of the tape and cut a small hole at each end of the tie.
• Prepare the other end of the tape in the same way.
• Hold both ends together and, using scissors, cut the resulting circle of tape so that one piece is approximately 10″ (25 cm) long, and the other is about 20″ (50 cm) long.

• Assist the patient into semi-Fowler's position, if possible.
• After your assistant puts on sterile gloves, instruct her to hold the tracheostomy tube in place to prevent its ejection during replacement of the ties. If you must perform the procedure without assistance, fasten the clean ties in place before removing the old ties to prevent tube expulsion.
• With the assistant's gloved hand holding the tracheostomy tube in place,

ing a pair of sterile hemostats. *Don't* blindly grasp at it; you could push it down the trachea or damage the tracheal mucosa.

Repeat the procedure of instilling saline solution and applying suction. If these actions fail to remove the plug, replace the oxygen source and wait for the anesthesiologist.

Remember to stay calm, continually reassuring the patient throughout this ordeal. *Don't* leave him alone until the plug's been removed.

After the doctor has removed the plug, reassess the patient. Is he breathing without difficulty? Are his breath sounds clear? Are his vital signs stable? Does he require medication for anxiety? Is arterial blood gas analysis indicated?

Later actions
Closely assess the patient for formation of new mucus plugs. Stay alert for tenacious, blood-tinged tracheal mucus and the telltale whistling sound and decreased airflow at the stoma during respirations.

Consider how this incident could have been prevented. Did the patient receive frequent tracheostomy care? Was his inspired air well humidified to keep his secretions liquefied? Remember that the postlaryngectomy patient can no longer use his nose as a source of humidification and thus requires other sources, such as humidified oxygen or ultrasonic nebulization. You also can instill sterile normal saline solution regularly into his trachea. This helps liquefy tracheal secretions, making their removal easier.

Were other preventive actions taken? For example, did the patient routinely perform coughing and deep-breathing exercises? Was he well hydrated? Especially important: Did he know to alert you at the first sign of trouble?

Consider also whether the patient's potential complications were identified and appropriate nursing interventions documented on his care plan. Standardized postlaryngectomy care plans that incorporate humidification procedures may be helpful to minimize development of mucus plugs in these patients.

Ask yourself if you handled the emergency smoothly. Did you have tracheal suction, normal saline solution, flashlight, scissors, and hemostats readily available? Determine whether the patient's call bell was at his bedside. Why did he have to leave his room to seek help?

Your final follow-up action should be thorough discharge teaching. Show the patient how to prepare and instill saline solution, and emphasize the importance of humidifying his air. Be sure he uses a humidification source at home, particularly during winter months, when indoor air is hot and dry.

---

cut the soiled tracheostomy ties with the bandage scissors or untie them and discard the ties. Before cutting, be certain that the pilot balloon for the tube cuff is away from the scissors.

• Thread the slit end of one new tie a short distance through the eye of one tracheostomy tube flange from the underside; use the hemostat, if necessary, to pull the tie through. Then, thread the other end of the tie completely through the slit end and pull it taut so that it loops firmly through the tube's flange. This avoids knots that can cause discomfort and lead to throat tissue irritation, pressure, and necrosis.

• Fasten the second tie to the opposite flange in the same manner.

• Instruct the patient to flex his neck while you bring the ties around his neck to the side and tie them together. Flexion produces the same neck circumference as coughing and helps prevent an overly

Dislodged Tracheostomy Tube

The situation

When the call light for room 366 goes on, you go to the room immediately because you know the patient can't speak. Eight hours ago he underwent an emergency tracheotomy for an obstructive pharyngeal tumor. As you enter the room, you see him struggling to sit up while he's making a high-pitched crowing sound and clutching his neck, which is bleeding at the stoma. His face looks dusky and his tracheostomy tube's on the floor.

The problem

The tracheostomy tube is dislodged and, because the incision is new, the stoma has closed. Because the patient's pharynx is obstructed by the tumor and edema from the tracheotomy, he doesn't have a patent airway.

The worst case

You can't open the stoma, and the patient stops breathing.

The best case

You open the stoma and insert a new tracheostomy tube. Or you open the stoma and calm the patient so that he can take in air through the stoma while you wait for the doctor to insert a new tube under controlled conditions.

The assessment

You observe a restless, cyanotic patient in respiratory distress, with stridor and suprasternal retractions. He's bleeding slightly from the stoma, which has closed. You know from report that a tumor is obstructing his pharynx. You conclude that he doesn't have a patent airway and is already suffering from lack of oxygen. Call for help as you place him in the supine position and hyperextend his neck. Reassure him that you're going to help him.

If his chest isn't moving, listen for breath sounds or feel for air movement at the stoma. If you detect no signs of air movement or if he's just gurgling around the stoma, you'll have to reestablish his airway. Adjust the bedside light so that it shines directly on the stoma. Look for stay sutures. (Some surgeons place these sutures at the top and bottom of the incision so that you can pull them up and out to open the stoma in an emergency.) If the patient doesn't have stay sutures, use a sterile Kelly clamp. Place the closed clamp into the center of the incision, then open it, spreading the incision. Hold the clamp in place.

If the clamp doesn't provide an adequate airway, you'll have to replace the tracheostomy tube. By now, at least one other nurse should have arrived to help. Tell her to unwrap the spare tracheostomy tube (also kept at the patient's bedside), place the obturator in the outer cannula, and hand you the assembled tube.

tight tie. Have your assistant place one finger under the tapes as you tie them to ensure that they're tight enough to avoid slippage, but loose enough to prevent choking or jugular vein constriction. Place the closure on the side to allow easy access and to prevent pressure necrosis at the back of the neck when the patient is recumbent.

• After securing the ties, cut off the excess tape with the scissors and instruct your assistant to release the tracheostomy tube.

• Make sure the patient's comfortable and can easily reach the call signal and communication aids.

Clinical considerations

Perform tracheostomy care at least once every 8 hours, or more often as needed. Change the dressing as often as necessary, whether or not you also perform

Ask this nurse to monitor the patient's vital signs and to get the suction equipment ready. Then, trying not to touch the end of the new tube, insert it into the incision. Remove the clamp. Hold onto the tube as you remove the obturator. You should hear a rush of air and see the patient's breathing become less labored. Anchor the tube with trach ties.

If the patient's breathing doesn't improve, the tube may be in the interstitial space. Remove it (keeping the incision open with the Kelly clamp) and reinsert it. If you can't get the tube inserted or you no longer detect a pulse, call a code.

When the patient is breathing more easily, attach the humidity source to the new tracheostomy tube and determine whether he needs supplemental oxygen. Continue to monitor vital signs, skin color, and level of consciousness. Elevate the head of the bed, unless contraindicated by vital signs. Assure the patient that he's out of danger, and give him paper and a pen so that he can communicate his feelings. Notify the surgeon.

Later actions

After the new tube is in place, make sure an X-ray is taken to confirm that the tube is positioned correctly. Then document what happened and what actions you took.

Make sure someone stays with the patient until his condition stabilizes. Monitor his vital signs and provide reassurance. Be alert for increased bloody secretions and slight bleeding from the stoma, which is likely to occur because reinsertion is traumatic. Profuse bleeding, especially blood that's bright red, indicates vascular damage; call the surgeon immediately.

Determine whether the patient should be transferred to the intensive care unit. Because the tube wasn't inserted under controlled conditions, the patient is at high risk for infection. Observe the stoma for at least a week for induration, redness, and purulent drainage.

Replace the Kelly clamp and spare tracheostomy tube (one size smaller than the original one) at the patient's bedside. Check the suctioning apparatus. If any emergency equipment was not at the bedside, restock it and find out why it wasn't there. Then find out what caused the tube to dislodge. Did the patient's coughing eject it because it was secured inadequately? Did the patient loosen his tracheostomy ties because they were too tight?

Check the patient's chart and Kardex to make sure they clearly state why the patient needed the tracheotomy and whether he has stay sutures. Update your care plan.

Finally, assess how you and other staff members reacted to the emergency. Ask yourself how your response could have been improved, and implement any necessary changes.

---

the entire cleansing procedure. A dressing wet with exudate or secretions predisposes the patient to skin excoriation, breakdown, and infection. Thoroughly document tracheostomy care.

Diligently check for complications that can follow tracheostomy tube insertion. Within the first 48 hours, the following complications are most likely: hemorrhage at the operative site, causing drowning; bleeding or edema within tracheal tissues, causing airway obstruction; aspiration of secretions, resulting in pneumonia; introduction of air into the pleural cavity, causing pneumothorax; hypoxia, acidosis, or sudden electrolyte shifts, triggering cardiac arrest; and introduction of air into surrounding tissues, causing subcutaneous emphysema.

After the first 48 hours, infection at any site distal to and including the stoma can lead to pneumonia from aspirated secretions. Secretions may collect under dressings and twill tape, producing skin excoriation and infection. Hardened mucus or a slipped cuff on a metal tube can occlude the cannula opening and obstruct the airway. Tube displacement can cause blood vessel erosion and hemorrhage. Tracheal erosion and necrosis can result from the tube's presence or cuff pressure.

Always have the following emergency equipment ready and in full view in the patient's room: all equipment and supplies for suctioning, as the patient may need his airway cleared at any time; the sterile obturator originally used to insert the patient's tracheostomy tube, for quick reinsertion if the tube is expelled; an additional sterile tracheostomy tube (with obturator) of the size currently being used, to replace a contaminated or expelled tube; and a spare sterile inner cannula, to replace a contaminated or expelled inner cannula. Optional emergency equipment includes a sterile tracheostomy tube (with obturator) one size smaller than the one in current use, to replace an expelled tube when the trachea immediately begins to close (this makes insertion of a tube of the original size difficult); and a sterile tracheal dilator or sterile hemostat, to maintain an open airway before insertion of a new tracheostomy tube.

To make sure you're prepared for an emergency, consult the doctor about first-aid measures you can use for your tracheostomy patient. Follow hospital policy regarding tracheostomy emergency procedures. (See *Occluded Tracheostomy Tube*, pages 278 and 279, and *Dislodged Tracheostomy Tube*, pages 280 and 281.)

If the patient is being discharged with a tracheostomy, start self-care teaching as soon as he's receptive. Teach him at-home tracheostomy care using clean technique. If he's being discharged with suction equipment, also make sure he and his family are knowledgeable and feel comfortable about using the equipment.

Refrain from changing tracheostomy ties unnecessarily during the immediate postoperative period before the stoma track is well formed (usually 4 days) to avoid accidental dislodgment and tube expulsion. Unless secretions or drainage pose a problem, ties can be changed once daily.

Refrain from changing a single-cannula tracheostomy tube or the outer cannula of a double-cannula tube. Because of the risk of tracheal complications, the doctor usually changes the cannula, with the frequency of change depending on the patient's condition (usually once weekly or every other week). For the patient going home with a metal tracheostomy tube, teach him to change the tube and clean it daily, as indicated.

Measure tracheal cuff pressure, as ordered. (See "Tracheal cuff pressure measurement.") If the patient's neck or stoma is excoriated or infected, apply a water-soluble topical lubricant or antibiotic cream, as ordered. Remember not to use a powder or an oil-based substance on or around a stoma, because aspiration can cause infection and abscess.

Regularly replace all equipment, including solutions, according to hospital policy, to reduce the risk of nosocomial infections.

Tracheal cuff pressure measurement

Description
The endotracheal (or tracheostomy) cuff provides a closed system for mechanical ventilation, so that the desired tidal volume can be delivered to the patient's lungs. It also protects the lower respiratory tract from secretions or gastric contents that may accumulate in the pharynx.

To perform these functions, the cuff must exert enough pressure on the tracheal wall to seal the airway. Too much pressure, however, can compromise arterial, capillary, or venous blood flow to the tracheal mucosa. The ideal cuff pressure is the lowest amount needed to seal the airway—an amount known as minimal occlusive volume (MOV). Many authorities recommend maintaining cuff pressure lower than capillary perfusion pressure—usually about 15 to 20 mm Hg. Although that's a good general principle to follow, optimal cuff pressure varies with each patient.

Purpose
To measure pressure within the tracheal cuff to minimize risk of injury to the tracheal mucosa

Procedure
• Gather the necessary equipment, including a stethoscope, three-way stopcock, 10-ml syringe partially filled with air, mercury manometer, and suction equipment. Wash your hands and explain the procedure to the patient.
• Suction the endotracheal tube. Then suction the patient's oropharynx to remove secretions that have accumulated above the cuff.
• Connect the ports of the three-way stopcock to the manometer tubing, syringe, and the cuff's pilot balloon. Close the port to the pilot balloon so that air can't escape from the cuff.
• Instill air from the syringe into the manometer tubing until the pressure reading reaches 10 mm Hg. (Later, when you open the stopcock to the cuff and the manometer, this air will prevent sudden cuff deflation.)
• With the stethoscope, auscultate the patient's trachea. A smooth, hollow sound indicates a sealed airway; a loud, gurgling sound indicates an air leak. (If you detect an air leak, proceed to the step describing cuff reinflation.)
• Turn off the stopcock to the manometer.
• If you don't hear an air leak, continue to auscultate the trachea while you slowly deflate the cuff. Stop deflating when you hear the loud, gur-

Measuring Tracheal Cuff Pressure

Minimize the risk of tracheal mucosa damage by measuring pressure within the tracheal cuff to ensure that it's within safe limits.

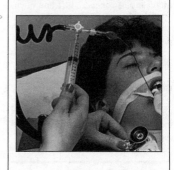

gling sound of a leak. (If deflating the cuff makes the patient cough, wait until he stops coughing before going on.)
• Reinflate the cuff until you no longer hear an air leak on inspiration. (Airways are larger on inspiration than on expiration. Therefore, if you stop reinflating the cuff when you no longer hear a leak on expiration, a leak still may occur on inspiration, especially with positive-pressure ventilation.)

Certain patients—those with high inspiratory pressure or positive endexpiratory pressure, for instance—may need extremely high cuff pressure to seal the airway.

If the tube is too small, you may be unable to seal the airway without overinflating the cuff. Report this to the doctor; the tube may need to be replaced with a larger one.
• Turn off the stopcock to the syringe.
• Record the manometer reading on expiration; this is the cuff pressure at MOV. (The mercury level will fluctuate as the patient inhales and exhales. The reading on inspiration reflects the effect of positive-pressure ventilation on the airways; the reading

on expiration reflects the effect of cuff pressure on the tracheal wall.)
• Turn off the stopcock to the pilot balloon, then disconnect the stopcock.

Clinical considerations
To ensure that your patient's cuff pressure is within safe limits, measure MOV at least once a shift and document results.

If the patient has a Lanz cuff, cuff pressure measurement isn't necessary, because a valve automatically keeps the pressure between 20 to 25 mm Hg.

Complications
Aspiration of upper airway secretions, underventilation, or coughing spasms may occur if cuff pressure measurement creates a leak.

Nasopharyngeal and oropharyngeal suctioning

Description
Nasopharyngeal and oropharyngeal suctioning maintain a patent airway by removing secretions from the pharynx with a suction catheter inserted through the mouth or nostril. This procedure promotes pulmonary gas exchange and prevents pneumonia caused by accumulated secretions.

Nasopharyngeal and oropharyngeal suctioning are usually clean procedures, because the catheter doesn't progress beyond the pharynx. However, sterile technique is indicated whenever the patient's oral, nasal, or pharyngeal mucosa has been impaired—for example, by burns, lesions, or local radiation treatment. Nasopharyngeal suctioning is contraindicated in patients with nasopharyngeal bleeding, a deviated nasal septum, a broken nose, nasal polyps, and spinal fluid leakage into the nasopharyngeal area. Both suctioning forms are contraindicated in patients who have blood dyscrasias or who are receiving anticoagulants.

Purpose
To clear the airway in patients who cannot clear it effectively via coughing and expectoration—for example, in unconscious or severely debilitated patients

Procedure
• Explain the procedure to the patient, provide privacy, and wash your hands.
• Assemble the equipment, if necessary. Place the suctioning equipment on the patient's overbed table or bedside stand. Position the table or stand on your preferred side of the bed to facilitate suctioning.
• Attach the collection bottle to the suctioning unit, then attach the connecting tubing to it.
• Pour 50 to 100 ml of tap water into the cup or disposable container. If the suction catheter doesn't have a control valve, connect the tail of the Y-connector to the connecting tubing. Let the patient know that suctioning may stimulate the cough or gag reflex.
• Place the patient in semi-Fowler's position to promote lung expansion and effective coughing.
• Instruct the patient to cough and breathe slowly and deeply several times before beginning to suction. Coughing helps loosen secretions and may decrease the amount of suctioning; deep breathing helps minimize or prevent hypoxia.
• To facilitate catheter insertion for oral suctioning, have the patient turn his head toward you; for nasal suctioning, hyperextend the patient's neck.
• Turn on the suction. If required, set the pressure according to hospital policy. Usually, pressure may be set at 100 to 120 mm Hg for adults, or 50 to 75 mm Hg for infants and children. To check suction pressure, occlude the catheter lumen by pinching it between your fingers. Place your thumb over the suction port to apply suction, then look at the gauge on the suction apparatus. Adjust suction pressure accordingly, but be sure to release and reapply suction between test adjustments.

• Put on the glove. Use your gloved hand to pick up the catheter and your ungloved hand to hold the connecting tubing. Attach the catheter to the connecting tubing or to the arm of the Y-connector.

• If nasal insertion is indicated, without allowing the catheter to touch the patient, measure the length of the catheter from the tip of the patient's nose to his earlobe to determine the correct insertion length and ensure that the catheter won't pass into the trachea. Mark the position on the tube with the thumb of your ungloved hand and make a mental note of the length required for proper insertion.

• With your gloved hand, dip the catheter tip into the tap water. With your ungloved hand, place a finger over the catheter's control valve or over the Y-connector's open end and suction a little water through the catheter to lubricate the inside (to facilitate passage of secretions through the catheter) and to test the suction apparatus.

• Lubricate the outside of the catheter to facilitate insertion and prevent nasal trauma. Dip the suction catheter tip into the tap water, or apply a water-soluble lubricant along the length of the catheter. Follow hospital policy.

• Tell the patient you're going to insert the catheter.

• To place the catheter for *oropharyngeal* suctioning, insert it into the patient's mouth and along one side until it reaches the back of the throat. To place it for *nasopharyngeal* suctioning, gently insert it through one nostril to the appropriate premeasured distance, directing the tip along the floor of the nasal cavity to avoid the nasal turbinates.

• Then, apply suction as you withdraw the catheter. Simultaneously roll the catheter between your thumb and index finger as you remove it. This rotating motion prevents tissue trauma. Apply suction for only 10 to 12 seconds at a time to minimize or prevent tissue trauma.

• If secretions are thick, clear the catheter lumen by dipping it in water and applying suction.

• Repeat the procedure until respirations become quiet and gurgling or bubbling sounds stop.

• After suctioning completely, instruct the patient to take several slow, deep breaths to relieve any hypoxia and to promote relaxation.

• Apply suction to clear the connecting tubing; then discard the catheter, disposable container of water, and used glove.

• Wash your hands and replace the above items so that they're ready for the next suctioning.

• Record the date and time of the procedure; the reason for suctioning; and secretion amount, color, consistency, and odor (if any).

Clinical considerations

Depending on the patient's condition, suctioning may be required as seldom as once every 8 hours or as often as every 15 minutes.

Remove, empty, rinse, and reattach the collection bottle every 8 hours (or more often, as necessary). Replace the suction bottle and tubing according to hospital policy. To avoid damaging the machine, do not allow the suction-collection bottle to fill past the three-quarter mark.

Let the patient rest after each 10- to 12-second suctioning period to reduce the risk of hypoxia.

To facilitate catheter insertion through a nostril, insert the catheter on a slight downward slant and ask the patient to take slow, deep breaths through his mouth. Avoid inserting the catheter further than the premeasured distance, because it could enter the trachea or esophagus. Also, avoid applying suction during catheter insertion, to prevent tissue trauma.

If the patient has no history of nasal problems, alternate suctioning between the left and right nostrils to reduce trauma to one nostril.

To facilitate catheter insertion for oropharyngeal suctioning, depress the tongue with a tongue depressor or ask another nurse to do so. This makes it easier to see the back of the throat and prevents the patient from biting the catheter.

Complications

Hypoxia can result because suctioning removes oxygen from the airway. Prolonged or traumatic suctioning can cause bloody aspirate.

Nasotracheal suctioning

Description

Nasotracheal suctioning removes secretions from the trachea via a suction catheter inserted through a nasopharyngeal airway. This airway is used to protect nasal mucosa from trauma during suctioning and to help direct the catheter anteriorly toward the trachea. Because nasotracheal suctioning may cause hypoxia, life-threatening dysrhythmias, or laryngospasm, it should be reserved for secretion removal when all other attempts short of intubation have failed. It should not be done routinely to stimulate a cough. Nasotracheal suctioning is contraindicated in patients with nasal polyps, deviated nasal septum, blood dyscrasias, or chronic liver disease; in patients receiving anticoagulants; and in those who have previously experienced laryngospasm during suctioning or endotracheal intubation.

Purpose

To clear the airway in patients who can't clear it effectively via coughing and expectoration—for example, in unconscious or severely debilitated patients

Procedure

• Auscultate the patient's breath sounds to determine whether he needs suctioning and to serve as a baseline

for assessing the procedure's effectiveness. If you hear loud rhonchi in the upper airway, the patient needs suctioning. Be aware that diminished breath sounds also may indicate a need for suctioning, because secretions may be blocking the airway. Also listen to heart sounds and take a baseline pulse.

• Explain the procedure to the patient, provide privacy, and wash your hands.

• Assemble the equipment, if necessary. Place the suctioning equipment on the patient's overbed table or bedside stand. Position the table or stand on your preferred side of the bed to facilitate suctioning.

• Attach the collection bottle to the suctioning unit and attach the connecting tubing to it.

• Pour 50 to 100 ml of tap water into the cup or disposable container. If the suction catheter doesn't have a control valve, connect the tail of the Y-connector to the connecting tubing. Let the patient know that suctioning may stimulate the cough or gag reflex.

• Place the patient in the semi-Fowler position to promote lung expansion and effective coughing.

• Instruct the patient to cough and breathe slowly and deeply several times before you begin to suction. Coughing helps loosen secretions and may decrease the amount of suctioning; deep breathing helps minimize or prevent hypoxia.

• Provide supplemental oxygen by placing an oxygen mask over the patient's mouth, leaving his nose outside the mask.

• Insert the nasopharyngeal airway. (See "Nasopharyngeal airway," pages 262 to 264, for information on how to insert this airway.)

• To facilitate suction catheter insertion, hyperextend the patient's neck.

• Turn on the suction. If required, set the pressure according to hospital policy. In most cases, pressure may be set at 100 to 120 mm Hg for adults, or 50 to 75 mm Hg for infants and children. To check suction pressure, occlude the catheter lumen by pinching it between your fingers. Place your thumb over the suction port to apply suction, then look at the gauge on the suction apparatus. Adjust suction pressure accordingly, but be sure to release and reapply suction between test adjustments.

• Put on the glove. Use your gloved hand to pick up the catheter and your ungloved hand to hold the connecting tubing. Attach the catheter to the connecting tubing or to the arm of the Y-connector.

• With your gloved hand, dip the catheter tip into the tap water. With your ungloved hand, place a finger over the catheter's control valve or over the Y-connector's open end and suction a little water through the catheter to lubricate the inside (to facilitate passage of secretions through the catheter) and to test the suction apparatus and catheter patency.

• Disconnect the catheter from the connecting tubing, and lubricate the outside of the catheter with a water-soluble lubricant to facilitate insertion into the airway.

• Tell the patient you're going to insert the catheter into the airway.

• Have the patient stick out his tongue as far as he can while you insert the catheter. This will help prevent him from swallowing the catheter. Throughout insertion, remind him to keep his tongue out. Watch his breathing, and advance the catheter during inspiration.

• When you've advanced the catheter past the tip of the airway, bring your ear down to the catheter opening as you continue inserting it. You should be able to hear the air moving in and out with each respiration, indicating that the catheter is still in the airway. If the sound of air movement stops, you've accidentally passed the catheter into the esophagus. (See *Assessing Catheter Placement in Nasotracheal Suctioning.*)

• As the catheter enters the trachea, past the epiglottis, the patient probably will cough violently. Continue to advance the catheter slowly, as toler-

Assessing Catheter Placement in Nasotracheal Suctioning

Sounds of air moving in and out with respirations indicate that the nasotracheal catheter is still in the airway, not in the esophagus.

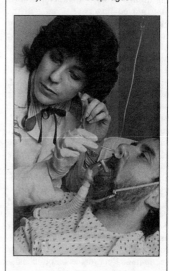

ated by the patient, until you meet resistance. Then pull it back ⅜″ (1 cm).

• Let the patient rest during the procedure whenever he indicates the need or when you note cyanosis, marked tachycardia, or tachypnea. Check his pulse again.

• Once the catheter is in place, tell the patient to relax and to take slow, deep breaths. Assess his condition. If he has a highly reactive respiratory tract, he may continue to cough. Tell him to swallow and to try to suppress his coughing. While he's resting, attach the connecting tubing to the catheter.

• To apply suction, slide your thumb over the suction port and ask him to cough as hard as he can. Rotate and slightly withdraw the catheter as you apply suction. Try not to withdraw it all the way out of the trachea. Don't suction for more than 15 seconds.

• When you've finished suctioning, remove the catheter. If the patient will need to be suctioned again soon, leave the airway in place, but not for more than 8 hours.

• Apply suction to clear the connecting tubing. Wrap the catheter around your gloved fingers. As you pull the glove off your hand, turn it inside out so that the catheter is inside it. Dispose of the catheter and glove according to hospital policy.

• Encourage the patient to relax and breathe deeply. Place the oxygen mask over his nose and mouth and ask whether he is having any trouble breathing. Auscultate his breath sounds again to determine whether suctioning was effective. Also, listen to his heart sounds and check his pulse for any changes. Make him comfortable, then turn the oxygen-delivery device back to the prescribed setting.

• Wash your hands and replace used items.

• Chart the procedure, including your assessment of the patient's breath sounds and vital signs before and after suctioning. Record the color, consistency, and amount of secretions. Be sure to record the amount in milliliters—*small* to you may be *moderate* to someone else. Note any complications and nursing actions taken.

Clinical considerations

Depending on the patient's condition, suctioning may be required as seldom as every 8 hours or as often as every 15 minutes. Ideally, you'll want to introduce the catheter into the trachea only once. But if you don't see secretions moving in the connecting tubing, thick mucus may have plugged the catheter's tip. Then, if you can't suction, you'll have to withdraw the catheter completely, rinse it with saline solution, and begin again.

Maintaining sterile technique and suctioning only when necessary (to reduce mucosal damage) decrease the risk of nosocomial infection.

Take care when using oxygen if the patient has chronic lung disease and depends on a hypoxic drive to breathe. Don't avoid using oxygen, however, or he'll become hypoxic during the procedure. Just monitor him closely for any indication of respiratory depression, lethargy, and other signs of carbon dioxide narcosis.

Let the patient rest after each 10- to 12-second suctioning period, to reduce the risk of hypoxia.

To prevent life-threatening cardiac dysrhythmias, give the patient supplemental oxygen before, during, and after suctioning. If he develops a dysrhythmia despite this precaution, stop suctioning immediately, remove the catheter, and begin appropriate measures, as indicated by the patient's condition.

Stay alert for signs of laryngospasm: stridor after passing the catheter through the patient's vocal cords, increased respiratory distress, or your inability to move the catheter.

If laryngospasm occurs, leave the catheter in place to maintain an airway. Increase supplemental oxygen. (Don't attach the oxygen source directly to the catheter—the patient won't be able to exhale.) Immediately call an anesthesiologist or anesthetist to evaluate the patient's condition and to intubate, if necessary.

If the laryngospasm resolves spontaneously, don't attempt nasotracheal suctioning again. Once laryngospasm occurs, it's more likely to recur from the repeated irritation of suctioning.

Remove, empty, rinse, and reattach the collection bottle every 8 hours (or more often, as necessary). Replace the suction bottle and tubing according to hospital policy. To avoid damaging the machine, don't allow the suction-collection bottle to fill past the three-quarter mark.

Complications

Hypoxia can result because suctioning removes oxygen from the airway and because catheter insertion stimulates the sympathetic nervous system, which increases the heart's oxygen demand. Hypoxia may lead to atelectasis and pneumonia.

Manipulating the catheter may stimulate the vagus nerve (located superficially in the hypopharynx), which can cause bradycardia, heart block, ventricular irritability, and even ventricular tachycardia and asystole.

The catheter also may irritate mucous membranes, causing bleeding and possibly infection. By irritating the larynx, suctioning may produce laryngospasm.

Endotracheal and tracheostomy suctioning

Description

Endotracheal or tracheostomy suctioning removes secretions from the trachea or bronchi via a suction catheter inserted through a tracheostomy or endotracheal tube. This procedure helps maintain a patent airway to promote optimal gas exchange and to prevent pneumonia resulting from secretion collection. Serious complications, such as hypoxia, infection, and life-threatening dysrhythmias, can result from suctioning. Action should be taken to minimize these risks. (See *Cardinal Rules of Suctioning*.)

Suctioning should be performed cautiously in patients with a recent tracheotomy or other tracheal or upper respiratory surgery, in those with blood dyscrasias, or in those who are receiving anticoagulant therapy (bleeding is more likely to occur).

Purpose

To maintain airway patency in patients who can't clear the lower airway effectively

Cardinal Rules of Suctioning

To reduce the risk of complications from suctioning, follow these rules:
● Determine the need for suctioning.
● Hyperinflate and oxygenate the patient's lungs before and after suctioning.
● Maintain sterile technique throughout the procedure.
● Complete the procedure quickly, applying suction for no more than 10 seconds, while closely monitoring the patient's vital signs.

Procedure

● Check the doctor's order for any instructions on suctioning.
● Collect all necessary equipment, wash your hands, and provide privacy.
● Attach the collection container to the suction unit and the connecting tube to the collection container. If the catheter doesn't have a control valve, connect the tail of the Y-connector to the connecting tubing.
● Explain the procedure to the patient, even if he's unresponsive. Tell him that suctioning usually causes transient coughing or gagging, but that coughing helps to remove secretions. If the patient has been suctioned previously, summarize the reasons for suctioning. Continue to reassure the patient throughout the procedure to minimize anxiety and promote relaxation.
● Unless contraindicated, place the conscious patient in semi-Fowler's position to promote lung expansion and productive coughing. Place the unconscious patient in the supine position with his head turned toward you; the supine position helps negate gravitational influence and allows easier aspiration of secretions; turning the head facilitates catheter insertion.
● Auscultate the patient's lungs bilaterally and take vital signs, if the patient's condition warrants, to serve as baseline data.

Checking Suction Catheter Patency

Before suctioning the patient, be sure to check the catheter's patency.

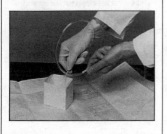

• Prepare equipment. Be sure the connecting tubing is within easy reach.
• Hook up the oxygen-delivery device, as needed.
• Remove the top of the normal saline solution bottle.
• Open the package containing the sterile solution container and, using sterile technique, pour the normal saline solution into the container.
• Place a sterile towel over the patient's chest, if desired, to provide an additional sterile area.
• Loosen the adapter on the endotracheal tube before gloving, to make it easier to remove with one hand later (when you're gloved).
• Open the catheter package (if the catheter is wrapped separately).
• Place the sterile glove on your dominant hand, and remove the sterile catheter from its wrapper. Keep it coiled so that it can't touch a nonsterile object. Attach the sterile catheter to the Y-connector or the connecting tubing. Hold the catheter in your gloved hand and the Y-connector and connecting tubing in your ungloved hand.
• Turn on the suction with your ungloved hand. If required, set the suction pressure according to hospital policy. In most cases, the pressure may be set at

100 to 120 mm Hg for adults, or 50 to 75 mm Hg for infants and children. To check suction pressure, occlude the catheter lumen by pinching it between your fingers. Place the thumb of your ungloved hand over the control valve to apply suction, then look at the gauge on the suction apparatus. Adjust the suction pressure accordingly, but be sure to release and reapply suction between test adjustments.
• Dip the catheter tip in the sterile saline solution to lubricate the outside of the catheter and to reduce tissue trauma during insertion.
• With the catheter tip in the sterile saline solution, occlude the control valve with the thumb of your ungloved hand. Suction a little solution through the catheter to test the suction equipment and catheter patency, and to lubricate the inside of the catheter to facilitate passage of secretions through it. (See *Checking Suction Catheter Patency*.)
• Before suctioning and unless contraindicated, hyperoxygenate the patient's lungs with 100% oxygen, using the sigh mode on the ventilator or a hand-held resuscitation bag for 1 to 2 minutes to help prevent hypoxia. (See *Hyperoxygenating before Suctioning*.) If available, have an assistant manage the patient's oxygen needs while you perform the suctioning. Also, if the patient is breathing spontaneously, have him cough and breathe slowly and deeply several times before you begin to suction. Coughing helps loosen secretions and may reduce the amount of suctioning required; deep breathing helps to minimize or prevent hypoxia.
• Disconnect the oxygen from the patient, if applicable.
• Tell the patient he may feel short of breath during the procedure and that he will probably cough.
• If the patient has an endotracheal tube in place, open the adapter's suction port.
• With the catheter's control valve uncovered, gently inset the catheter deep into the trachea (and into a bronchus, if

indicated) through the patient's tracheostomy or endotracheal tube.

• Stop advancing the catheter when it touches the carina—you'll feel resistance and the patient usually will cough. Do not apply suction during insertion, to avoid oxygen loss and tissue trauma.

• Withdraw the catheter about ⅜" (1 cm) from the carina, then apply suction for 5 to 10 seconds by placing the thumb of your ungloved hand over the control valve. Simultaneously, use your gloved hand to withdraw the catheter as you roll it between your thumb and forefinger. This rotating motion prevents the catheter from adhering to tissue as it exits and therefore prevents tissue trauma. If the catheter does adhere, stop the suction immediately to protect tracheal tissue. Even if the patient shows no sign of distress, never suction for more than 10 seconds at a time to prevent hypoxia.

• Withdraw the catheter completely and uncover the control valve to stop the suction.

• If applicable, resume oxygen delivery after suctioning by reconnecting the source of oxygen or ventilation, and hyperoxygenate the patient's lungs before continuing (unless contraindicated) to prevent or relieve hypoxia.

• Observe the patient and allow him to rest for a few minutes before the next suctioning. The timing of each suctioning and the length of each rest period depend on his tolerance for the procedure and on any complications.

• Repeat the above procedure until breathing becomes quiet and relatively effortless.

• If secretions are thick, clear the catheter periodically by dipping the tip in the sterile saline solution and applying suction.

• If the patient's heart rate and rhythm are being monitored, observe for dysrhythmias. Should they occur, stop suctioning and ventilate the patient.

• After the procedure is over, hyperoxygenate the patient's lungs for 1 to 2

Hyperoxygenating before Suctioning

Hyperoxygenating the patient's lungs before suctioning helps prevent hypoxia.

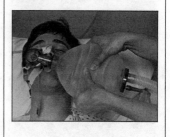

minutes (unless contraindicated) to relieve hypoxia and promote relaxation.

• Decrease the oxygen flow rate to the ordered setting after hyperoxygenation.

• If the patient has an endotracheal tube in place, close the adapter's suction port.

• Clear the connecting tubing by aspirating the remaining sterile saline solution. Then, turn off the suction and disconnect the catheter from the connecting tubing.

• Wrap the catheter around your gloved fingers. Pull off the glove so the catheter is inside it. (See *Removing Glove after Suctioning,* page 292.) Discard the glove and the catheter in the waterproof trash bag.

• Auscultate the patient's lungs bilaterally and take vital signs, if his condition warrants, to assess the procedure's effectiveness.

• Perform tracheostomy care or mouth care, as indicated.

• Observe the amount, color, and consistency of suctioned secretions.

• Wash your hands and replace all used items at the patient's bedside for possible emergency use.

• Document the procedure in your nurse's notes. Record the following: date and time of the procedure and the

Removing Glove after Suctioning

After suctioning, correctly dispose of the contaminated catheter.

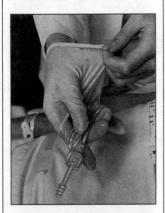

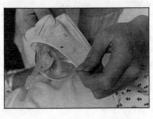

reason for suctioning; secretion amount, color, consistency, and odor (if any); vital signs and auscultation findings before and after suctioning; use of saline instillation, if ordered; hyperoxygenation before, during, and after suctioning; any complications and the nursing action taken; any inability to suction effectively and notification of this to the doctor; and pertinent data regarding the patient's subjective response to the procedure.

Clinical considerations

To facilitate catheter insertion to suction the right or left bronchus, ask the patient to turn his head in the direction opposite

the bronchus to be suctioned. A straight (not coiled) catheter can be used more successfully to enter the left bronchus, which diverges from the trachea at a sharper angle (45 degrees) than the right bronchus (25 degrees).

To help produce a cough, you may instill 3 to 5 ml of sterile normal saline solution into the trachea. (See *Instilling Saline Solution into the Trachea.*) Check to see if a doctor's order is required to instill saline solution.

Maintaining sterile technique and suctioning only when necessary (to reduce mucosal damage) decrease the risk of nosocomial infection. Increasing parenteral hydration helps to liquefy secretions but may be contraindicated in some patients.

If you can't suction effectively, notify the doctor.

Empty and rinse the collection container, as indicated by hospital policy. Replace the sterile solution, collection container, and connecting tubing according to hospital policy to minimize the risk of infection from bacterial growth.

Complications

Endotracheal and tracheostomy suctioning may cause hypoxia because it removes oxygen from the airway. Hypoxia, in turn, may lead to atelectasis and pneumonia.

Manipulating the catheter may stimulate the vagus nerve, which may cause hypotension, bradycardia, heart block, ventricular irritability, ventricular tachycardia, or asystole. The catheter also may irritate mucous membranes, causing bleeding and possible infection.

Introducing the suction catheter into the respiratory tract through the endotracheal tube bypasses the patient's normal upper airway defense mechanisms. Other factors—the patient's debilitated physical condition, use of antibiotics (which allow organism overgrowth), and unavoidable damage to mucous membranes occurring during suctioning—contribute to the infection risk.

Instilling Saline Solution into the Trachea

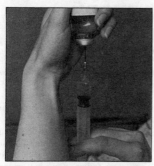

First, wipe the top of the vial with alcohol, then withdraw 10 ml of sterile normal saline solution into a sterile syringe.

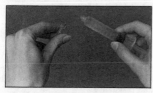

Remove the needle from the syringe. Never instill saline solution while the needle is still attached.

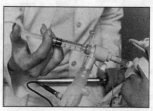

Hyperinflate and oxygenate the patient's lungs. Then instill the saline solution through the suction port, about 3 to 5 ml at a time. Immediately ventilate the patient with the hand-held resuscitation bag to disperse the saline solution. Suction his airway, then ventilate again.

If the patient has a highly reactive respiratory tract and coughs continuously, or if he has elevated intracranial pressure and you must minimize coughing spasms, you may (with a doctor's order) instill 1% or 2% lidocaine (lignocaine, Xylocaine) to anesthetize his respiratory tract. Do not remove this by suctioning.

Then, if you've used the ventilator sigh mechanism, return the ventilator controls to their original settings.

Selected References

Emergency Care Handbook. Springhouse, Pa.: Springhouse Corp., 1986.

Fuchs, P.L. "Streamlining Your Suctioning Techniques, Part 1, Nasotracheal Suctioning," *Nursing84* 14(5):55-61, May 1984.

Fuchs, P.L. "Streamlining Your Suctioning Techniques, Part 2, Endotracheal Suctioning," *Nursing84* 14(6):46-51, June 1984.

Fuchs, P.L. "Streamlining Your Suctioning Techniques, Part 3, Tracheostomy Suctioning," *Nursing84* 14(7):39-43, July 1984.

Hoffmann, L.A., and Maszkiewicz, R.C. "Airway Management for the Critically Ill Patient," *American Journal of Nursing* 87(1):39-53, January 1987.

Luce, J.M., et al. *Intensive Respiratory Care.* Philadelphia: W.B. Saunders Co., 1984.

Montanari, J., and Spearing, C. "The Fine Art of Measuring Tracheal Cuff Pressure," *Nursing86* 16(7):46-49, July 1986.

Procedures. Nurse's Reference Library. Springhouse, Pa.: Springhouse Corp., 1983.

Respiratory Emergencies. NursingNow series. Springhouse, Pa.: Springhouse Corp., 1984.

Shapiro, B.A., et al. *Clinical Applications of Respiratory Care,* 3rd ed. Chicago: Year Book Medical Pubs., Inc., 1985.

13 VENTILATORY SUPPORT PROCEDURES

Introduction

When a patient can no longer maintain ventilation or gas exchange, both functions can be assisted by a hand-held resuscitation bag or mechanical ventilator. (See *Why It's Called a Ventilator—Not a Respirator*.)

Manual ventilation with a hand-held resuscitation bag is used most commonly during emergencies or while a patient is being disconnected temporarily from a mechanical ventilator. A patient also may need mechanical ventilation when respiratory failure occurs from inadequate gas exchange.

Respiratory failure may occur in such conditions as adult respiratory distress syndrome, pneumonia, and chronic obstructive pulmonary disease. Ventilatory failure, which occurs when the body can't provide the mechanical means for respiration, also may warrant mechanical ventilation. Ventilatory failure may occur in some patients with neuromuscular disorders, head injuries, and conditions that decrease respiratory drive. (See Chapter 9 for a discussion of respiratory failure.)

Compliance and resistance

Of the many factors affecting airflow in the lungs, two are most important in mechanical ventilation: compliance and resistance.

Compliance reflects the stiffness or flexibility of lung tissue, indicating how easily air flows into the lungs. It's measured in units of volume per unit of pressure—ml/cmH_2O. As compliance increases, the lungs are easier to ventilate; thus, a ventilator can push a larger volume of air into the lungs with each cmH_2O of pressure. Compliance can be estimated roughly by using the ventilator tidal volume and peak inspiratory pressure. (See *Equations*, pages 399 to 401, in the Appendix.)

Resistance reflects how easily air flows through the airways leading to the alveoli. Any condition that narrows airways can increase resistance, the most common condition being bronchospasm. Small-lumen tubing and artificial airways also increase resistance.

Why It's Called a Ventilator— Not a Respirator

The terms *ventilator* and *respirator* often are used interchangeably, but ventilator is actually the correct term. Just think back to basic physiology—ventilation is the movement of air in and out of the lungs; respiration is the exchange of gases. The machines discussed in this chapter are ventilators; they move air in and out of the lungs. A true respirator would be a heart-lung machine in which gas exchange takes place.

Manual ventilation with a hand-held resuscitation bag

Description

Manual ventilation involves use of a hand-held resuscitation bag, such as an Ambu bag—an inflatable device that can be attached to a face mask or directly to an endotracheal or tracheostomy tube. Typically used in an emergency, manual ventilation with a resuscitation bag can be performed during temporary disconnection from a mechanical ventilator, such as during a tubing change, during transport, or before suctioning. Oxygen administration and hyperexpansion with a resuscitation bag can help improve the patient's compromised cardiorespiratory status.

Purpose

• To deliver oxygen or room air to the lungs of a patient who can't ventilate independently
• To hyperexpand the lungs, thereby improving alveolar ventilation
• To prevent hypoxia, which can lead to brain damage or death

Procedure

• Explain the procedure to the patient, if possible.
• Select a mask that fits snugly over the patient's mouth and nose, and attach the mask to the resuscitation bag.
• If oxygen is readily available, connect the hand-held resuscitation bag to the oxygen. Attach one end of the tubing to the bottom of the bag and the other end to the nipple adapter on the flowmeter of the oxygen wall unit or tank. Set up suction equipment if time allows.
• Before using the hand-held resuscitation bag, check the patient's upper airway for foreign objects. If present, remove them—in some instances, their removal alone may restore spontaneous respirations. Also, foreign matter or secretions can obstruct the airway and impede resuscitation efforts. If necessary, insert an oropharyngeal or nasopharyngeal airway to maintain airway patency.
• If appropriate, remove the bed's headboard and stand at the head of the bed to help hyperextend the patient's neck and to free space at the side of the bed for other emergency activities.
• Hyperextend the patient's neck, unless contraindicated, and pull his jaw forward to move the tongue away from the base of the pharynx and prevent airway obstruction.
• Place the mask over the patient's face so that the apex of the triangle covers the bridge of his nose and the base lies between his lower lip and chin. Or, if the patient has a tracheostomy or endotracheal tube in place, remove the mask from the bag and attach the hand-held resuscitation bag directly to the tube.
• Keeping your nondominant hand on the patient's mask, exert downward pressure to seal the mask against his face. For the adult patient, use your dominant hand to compress the bag every 5 seconds to deliver approximately 1 liter of air. For a child, compress the bag 15 times per minute, or once every 4 seconds; for an infant, 20 times per minute, or once every 3 seconds.
• Observe the patient's chest to ensure that it rises and falls with each compression. If ventilation fails to occur, check the fit of the mask and the patient's airway patency; if necessary, reposition the patient's head.

Clinical considerations

To facilitate neck hyperextension, you may place a rolled towel under the patient's neck. However, avoid neck hyperextension if the patient has a possible cervical injury; instead, use the jaw-thrust technique to open the airway. If you need both hands to keep the patient's mask in place and maintain hyperextension, use the lower part of your arm to compress the bag against your side. Observe for vomitus through the clear part of the mask. If vomiting occurs, stop the procedure immediately, lift the mask, remove the vomitus, and resume resuscitation.

Complications
Aspiration of vomitus can result in pneumonia. Gastric distension may occur after air is forced into the patient's stomach.

Mechanical ventilation: initiation and care

Description
Mechanical ventilation refers to use of a machine that takes over the patient's work of breathing. Patients may need total or partial ventilatory support. In the latter, the patient breathes on his own between breaths produced by the machine; the machine may provide only 20% to 40% of total ventilation.

Mechanical ventilators can be classified according to whether they deliver air with positive or negative pressure. (See *Mechanical Ventilators*, pages 298 and 299.)

Negative-pressure ventilators
Negative-pressure ventilators were the first widely used ventilators. The iron lung, invented in 1928, was used extensively during the polio epidemics of the 1950s. It works by encasing the patient's entire body in a sealed cylinder. The patient's head sticks out at the end, and a collar fits around the neck. A diaphragm at the foot of the cylinder is pulled out during inspiration, creating negative pressure within the cylinder; this pulls the chest wall up. Chest wall expansion increases thoracic volume, which creates negative pressure in the lungs. This, in turn, causes atmospheric air to be drawn into the lungs. Thus, the iron lung mimics the normal physiologic

process. When the cylinder's diaphragm resumes its normal position, pressure in the cylinder returns to baseline levels; the chest wall falls; and exhalation (a passive process) occurs.

Three basic problems diminish the usefulness of the iron lung:
• Access to patient is severely limited.
• Abdominal pooling of blood occurs because the abdomen is also subjected to negative pressure during inspiration.
• Diseased airways conduct airflow poorly.

The first two problems were resolved with the chest shell piece. Worn like a turtle's shell, the chest shell works by the same principles as the iron lung. The advent of positive-pressure ventilators helped resolve the challenge of ventilating patients with lung disease.

Positive-pressure ventilators
Positive-pressure ventilators provide much more control over ventilatory parameters and have proven superior in ventilating patients with lung disease. They work by pushing air into the chest—the opposite of normal physiologic function and negative-pressure ventilators. Exhalation occurs passively at the end of inhalation. (High-frequency ventilation, a new ventilation method, is being used on an experimental basis for patients who don't respond to conventional positive-pressure ventilation. See *High-Frequency Ventilation*, for more information.)

Positive-pressure ventilators can be grouped according to how they end the inspiratory phase—by limiting inspiratory volume, pressure, or time.

Volume-cycled ventilators end inspiration when a preset volume has been delivered to the patient. Inspiratory time and pressure may vary. The prime advantage of this ventilator is that the operator can control minute volume, which determines the $PaCO_2$ level. The ability to vary inspiratory pressure also allows for easier ventilation of the patient with decreasing

High-Frequency Ventilation

High-frequency ventilation (HFV) uses high ventilation rates (60 to 3,000 breaths/minute, depending on the type of HFV), low tidal volumes, brief inspiratory time, and low peak airway pressures.

HFV has three different delivery forms—high-frequency jet ventilation (HFJV), high-frequency positive-pressure ventilation, and high-frequency oscillation. You'll probably hear about HFJV most often. Here's how it works.

HFJV mechanics

• High-pressure gas jet-pulses through the narrow-lumen gas jet valve on inspiration and accelerates as it flows through the port's narrow lumen and into the patient's endotracheal tube.

• The pressure and velocity of the jet stream cause a drag effect that entrains low-pressure gases into the patient's airway.

• These gas flows combine to deliver 100 to 200 breaths/minute to the patient.

• The gas stream moves down the airway in a progressively broader wave front of decreasing velocity.

• Tidal volume is delivered to airways under constant pressure.

• The gas stream creates turbulence, which causes the gas to vibrate in the airways. Alveolar ventilation increases without raising mean airway pressure or peak inflation pressure.

Uses

• Treatment of bronchopleural fistulae
• Rigid bronchoscopy
• Laryngeal surgery
• Thoracic surgical procedures
• Treatment of infant and adult respiratory distress syndrome (limited clinical experience)

Benefits

• Improved venous return
• Decreased airway pressures and (possibly) improved pulmonary artery pressure
• Improved arterial gas exchange
• Decreased right ventricular afterload
• Reduced chance of pulmonary barotrauma and decreased cardiac output

Nursing interventions

• Regularly check the mechanical setup, parameter alarms, and tubing connections.
• Assess breath sounds regularly.
• Suction the patient as indicated by physical assessment. During suctioning, disconnect the patient from the ventilator. Turn off the humidification system to prevent fluid from accumulating in the tubing and then being inspired when you restart ventilation. Assess airway secretions. If they're extremely viscous, you may need to increase humidification to prevent mucus plug formation.

---

pulmonary compliance (as in adult respiratory distress syndrome [ARDS]). The main disadvantage is patient exposure to high intrathoracic pressures when the lungs are especially stiff. Volume-cycled ventilators are the most common in adult critical care. Examples include the Puritan Bennett MA1, MA2, and MA2 + 2; the 7200; and the Bear Models 2 and 5.

Pressure-cycled ventilators are technically simpler and were used initially for ventilation before volume-cycled ventilators were widely available. Pressure-cycled ventilators end inspiration when a preset pressure has been reached, regardless of the time needed or volume delivered. Examples include the Bird Mark series and the Puritan Bennett PR series. The most serious of this ventilator's *many* disadvantages is

Mechanical Ventilators

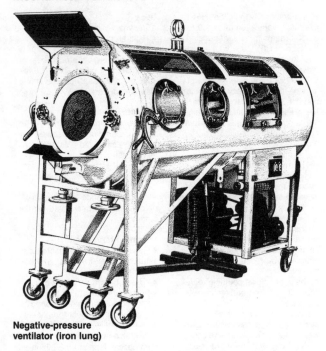

Negative-pressure ventilator (iron lung)

variation of delivered volume with changes in lung compliance, posing the risk of hypoventilation and respiratory acidosis, or hyperventilation and respiratory alkalosis. Also, with a leak in the system, the inspiratory phase may never end if the predetermined pressure isn't met; with an obstruction, the inspiratory phase may end abruptly after only a moment with minimal volume delivery.

Time-cycled ventilators end inspiration after a preset time interval has elapsed. Time-cycled ventilators are most commonly used with newborns and children. Their disadvantages include variable inspiratory volume—making control of $PaCO_2$ more difficult.

Based on the patient's condition, the doctor will choose one of the following ventilation modes:

• *Control mode* allows the ventilator to deliver breaths according to the machine settings and locks the patient out of any interaction with the machine. This mode is rarely used.

• *Assist/control (A/C) mode* allows the patient to initiate breaths; however, if the patient doesn't breathe on his own, the machine delivers breaths based on machine settings to guarantee minimum ventilation. Breaths the patient initiates, called assisted breaths, deliver the set tidal volume.

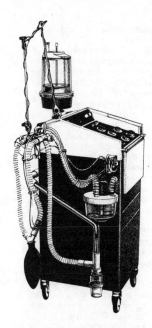

Volume-limited (volume-cycled) ventilator

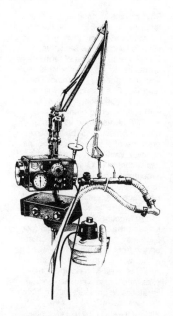

Pressure-limited (pressure-cycled) ventilator

• *Intermittent mandatory ventilation (IMV)* allows the patient to breathe totally on his own between machine breaths. Originally designed as a weaning mode, IMV is being used more frequently during initial ventilation.

• *Synchronized intermittent mandatory ventilation (SIMV),* now available on many ventilators, allows for intermittent machine breaths synchronized with the patient's own inspiratory efforts.

• *Continuous positive airway pressure (CPAP),* another option on many ventilators, provides no mechanical ventilation—just a flow of oxygen-enriched air at positive pressure. Many health care professionals now use this mode instead of the T-tube for final weaning stages before extubation be-

cause this mode has alarms to assist in patient monitoring. (See *Understanding PEEP and CPAP,* pages 300 and 301.)

Purpose

• To reestablish normal arterial blood gas levels

• To provide ventilation when the patient can't breathe because of a neurologic or neuromuscular condition or pharmacologically induced paralysis

• To provide hyperventilation in patients with head injuries

• To allow application of positive pressure to improve gas exchange and reverse hypoxemia

Understanding PEEP and CPAP

Physiologically, positive end-expiratory pressure (PEEP) and continuous positive-airway pressure (CPAP) function the same way. They differ in the use of terminology pertaining to mechanical ventilation and spontaneous breathing. The term PEEP is associated with mechanical ventilation; the term CPAP, with spontaneous breathing.

• *PEEP* refers to the addition of positive pressure to the baseline pressure of a patient receiving mechanical ventilation (in either the assist/control [A/C] mode or the synchronized intermittent mandatory ventilation mode). After the patient receives a machine-delivered breath, PEEP keeps a predetermined amount of pressure in his lungs at the end of exhalation (consequently, the pressure manometer on the front of the machine won't go all the way down to zero). Because PEEP is used with positive-pressure mechanical ventilation, mean intrathoracic pressure will be higher than with CPAP.

• *CPAP* refers to the use of positive pressure when the patient is breathing spontaneously without mechanical support. Positive pressure during inspiration may help the patient overcome the resistance of the artificial airway, and, even more importantly, it ensures that a predetermined amount

of pressure remains in his lungs at the end of exhalation.

PEEP and CPAP are used to increase the resting volume of air in the lungs. Air normally present in the lungs after exhalation—called functional residual capacity (FRC)—keeps the alveoli open, maximizing the area available for gas exchange. If FRC drops, so does the area available for gas exchange.

• Many ventilated patients have compromised FRC resulting from such problems as atelectasis (especially postoperative patients), secretions that occlude the airway, and fluid that may fill alveoli and cause pulmonary edema. If FRC drops, so does the area available for gas exchange, leading to decreased arterial oxygen partial pressure (PaO_2).

• PEEP and CPAP also can be used in patients who lack pulmonary surfactant, such as from adult respiratory distress syndrome (ARDS), smoke inhalation, toxic lung damage, and neonatal respiratory distress syndrome. Surfactant deficiency would allow alveoli to collapse; however, PEEP and CPAP can keep alveoli expanded while surfactant is being produced.

• In patients with pulmonary edema, PEEP and CPAP can help decrease the alveolar fluid/volume ratio. Expanding alveolar size while the amount of fluid remains the same increases the area available for gas ex-

Procedure

The following procedure applies to most positive-pressure, volume-cycled ventilators used for adults. When caring for a patient on a ventilator, be sure to check both the operator's manual for the machine you're using and hospital policy and procedure for instructions specific to the machine.

Preliminary ventilator check

Before bringing the machine to the bedside:

• Wash your hands.

• Attach the tubing to the ventilator, making sure the inner tubing and patient connector remain sterile.

• Attach the humidification device to the ventilator and tubing, making sure the inside of the water reservoir remains sterile.

• Fill the humidifier with sterile distilled water.

• Set the humidifier temperature control at the mid-range.

• Plug the machine into a grounded electrical outlet.

change. Some health care professionals also believe that positive pressure in alveoli helps to push fluid back into alveolar capillaries.

• PEEP and CPAP levels above 40 cmH₂O have been used to treat patients with severe ARDS; however, such levels should be used only by specially trained clinicians. Even patients receiving PEEP and CPAP levels of 10 cmH₂O should be weaned from positive pressure slowly to avoid rapid deterioration.

Possible problems
Although widely used, PEEP and CPAP pose certain risks. The risks are associated with increased intrathoracic pressure—primarily, circulatory compromise and barotrauma. PEEP's risks can be minimized by using the intermittent mandatory ventilator (IMV) instead of the A/C mode, because IMV allows the patient to breathe spontaneously between machine-generated breaths, which helps decrease overall intrathoracic pressure. CPAP's risks are not as great because spontaneous breathing allows lower intrathoracic pressures.

• *Circulatory compromise.* During normal spontaneous breathing, inspiration creates negative intrathoracic pressure. This helps draw venous return into the heart. Positive-pressure

ventilation disrupts this normal process, and PEEP compounds the problem. (CPAP is less risky because the patient is breathing spontaneously, which decreases overall intrathoracic pressure.) Although decreased venous return may be helpful in patients with increased preload, such as from congestive heart failure (CHF), it can be dangerous in patients with a delicate fluid balance who are borderline hypotensive, because it causes decreased cardiac output. Hemodynamic measurements must be monitored closely whenever PEEP or CPAP is increased or decreased and for 15 to 50 minutes afterward. For example, CHF may recur after a decrease in PEEP or CPAP because of increased venous return.

• *Barotrauma.* Barotrauma can occur whenever positive pressure is exerted within the chest. The risk increases as the magnitude of pressure and its duration increase. Barotrauma can cause pneumothorax and subcutaneous emphysema.

• *Alveolar rupture.* Use extreme caution while administering PEEP or CPAP to patients with chronic obstructive pulmonary disease. These patients already have an increased FRC from air trapping; PEEP and CPAP can cause alveolar overdistension, making alveoli more prone to rupture.

• Adjust the oxygen control to 100%, and listen for an alarm before the ventilator is attached to the gas source.
• Connect the ventilator to the air or oxygen source.
• Turn on the ventilator.
• Set the ventilator controls as shown below.
Tidal volume: 800 ml
Rate: 10
High-pressure alarm: As high as possible
Low-pressure alarm: Approximately 0 cmH₂O

Sensitivity: Off
Mode: A/C
Peak flow: 40 liters/minute
• Place a sterile 4″ x 4″ gauze square over the patient connector, occluding the tubing, and push the manual breath button or allow the machine to cycle and deliver a breath.
• Observe the pressure manometer—it should go all the way to the maximum if no leaks exist; the high-pressure alarm should sound and the indicator should light up.

Ventilator Settings

The controls most commonly set on a positive-pressure, volume-cycled ventilator are shown here and described below. Check your hospital's policy to determine which settings require a doctor's order. Remember that not all controls apply to every ventilator; the control panel of a Puritan-Bennett MA-2+2 ventilator is shown. On the new microprocessor ventilators, a keypad replaces traditional knobs, and settings are displayed digitally. Changes in settings can only be made by staff with the correct access code.

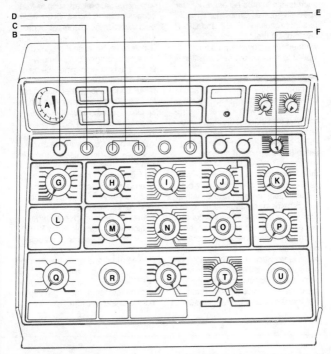

A. Pressure manometer
The needle registers inspiratory pressure as it rises during machine breaths, and shows PEEP/CPAP pressures as a baseline while the patient is exhaling. In the absence of PEEP/CPAP, the needle should return to zero during exhalation.

B. Power
In the "on" position provides power to the ventilator.

C. Lamp test
Test function of lights on the ventilator.

D. Mode selector
Choose A/C, SIMV, or CPAP
(spontaneous breathing).

E. Alarm reset
Used only after cause of alarm is
determined and corrected.

F. Temperature alarm
Usually set slightly above and
below the temperature setting.

G. Low-pressure alarm
Sounds when the set minimal
pressure is not reached on the
manometer.

H. Sigh pressure limit

I. Sigh volume
Sighs are extra-deep breaths
usually set at 1½ to 2 times the set
tidal volume.

J. Sigh rate
Preset the number of sighs the
patient has been ordered to receive
per hour. Some clinicians believe
these minimize the monotony of
ventilation and decrease atelectasis. *Note:* On most machines,
sighs only work during A/C ventilation, not during SIMV, because the
mandatory machine breaths act as
a sigh compared to the smaller
spontaneous breaths.

K. Temperature
Usually set at normal body temperature.

L. Manual breath button
Pushing this button delivers one
breath according to set parameters.

M. High-pressure alarm
Sounds and stops inspiration when
the set limit is reached on the
manometer.

N. Tidal volume
Amount of air delivered with each
machine breath. Set according to
doctor's order.

O. A/C respiratory rate
The number of breaths the machine
will deliver per minute. Set according to doctor's order.

P. FIo$_2$
Amount of oxygen delivered to the
patient with each breath, or the
amount available to the patient
breathing spontaneously during
IMV. Amount ordered by doctor.

Q. Plateau
Measured in tenths of a second, set
to simulate breath-holding at peak
inspiration. Plateau of 0.5 delays
exhalation for 0.5 sec., holding the
patient at peak inspiration for that
length of time.

R. PEEP/CPAP
The level of positive pressure
present as a baseline reading during ventilation or spontaneous
breathing; read on the ventilator
manometer.

S. Peak flow
Determines how fast air is delivered
to the patient. Needs to be increased as rate is increased.

T. SIMV respiratory rate
The number of SIMV breaths the
machine will deliver per minute. Set
according to doctor's order.

U. Sensitivity
Determines how easy it is for the
patient to trigger the machine.

• If pressure doesn't go to the maximum, check for leaks—especially in all tubing connections, the exhalation valve, and the humidifier.

• Open the tubing to air and turn the sensitivity on, increasing it until the machine self-cycles (chatters); then adjust the sensitivity (to make the machine less sensitive) until the chattering stops.

• When the tubing is open to air and the machine cycles, check for the low-pressure alarm to sound and the indicator to light up.

• Unplug the ventilator and disconnect it from the gas source before taking the machine to the patient's bedside.

Initiating mechanical ventilation

• Check the doctor's order for mechanical ventilation; particular settings that must be ordered vary from hospital to hospital, so check your policy and procedure manual.

• Check indications for mechanical ventilation, such as arterial blood gas (ABG) measurements, chest X-ray results, and spirometry results. (See Chapter 9 for specific parameters for respiratory and ventilatory failure.)

• Wash your hands.

• If possible, explain the procedure to the patient.

• Make sure that the patient has a patent artificial airway with an intact, inflated cuff. (See Chapter 12 for information on intubation technique.)

• Bring the ventilator to the bedside, and connect it to the appropriate gas source and electrical outlet.

• Turn on the ventilator.

• Adjust settings as ordered. (See *Ventilator Settings*, pages 302 and 303.)

• Connect the tubing to the patient's artificial airway.

• Monitor the pressure manometer on the front of the ventilator; if the needle doesn't rise smoothly, increase the flow rate until it does.

• Make sure all alarms are set before you leave the bedside. (Use the following parameters for guidelines, but be sure to check each ventilator for the location of available alarms and how to set them [usually by turning a dial or entering numbers on a keypad].)

• Note maximal inspiratory pressure, and set the high-pressure alarm approximately 10 to 15 cmH_2O above that pressure.

• Set the low-pressure alarm 10 to 15 cmH_2O below the maximal inspiratory pressure.

• Monitor the exhaled volume for machine-generated breaths; it should be within 100 to 200 ml of the set tidal volume.

• Set the exhaled volume alarm within 200 ml of the actual exhaled volume.

• Analyze the oxygen concentration, and compare it to the setting.

• Set the positive end-expiratory pressure (PEEP), if ordered. (See *Understanding PEEP and CPAP*, pages 300 and 301, and *Visualizing the Effects of PEEP and CPAP*.)

• If the patient can communicate, reassure him and explain why the ventilator is necessary.

• Explain how the ventilator works.

• Put the call bell within the patient's reach.

• Warn the patient that he won't be able to talk with the artificial airway, but assure him that you'll provide a means of communication (a letter board, flash cards, or a pad and pen).

• Describe the use of mechanical ventilation to the patient's family.

• If possible, stay with the patient for a few minutes after ventilation begins to provide reassurance, especially if he's awake and anxious.

• Complete the ventilator checklist according to hospital policy.

Clinical considerations

Monitoring the patient and ventilator

The underlying disease and the patient's clinical condition determine the monitoring frequency. Make sure you know why mechanical ventilation was initiated and whether the patient can maintain any spontaneous ventilation. Then, in case of machine failure, you'll know whether immediate manual ven-

Visualizing the Effects of PEEP and CPAP

Pressure Exerted with Various Types of Ventilation

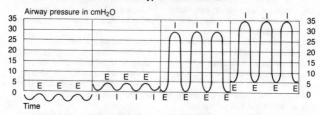

Airway pressure in cmH$_2$O

35
30
25
20
15
10
5
0

Time

Key: I = inspiration   E = expiration

| Intrathoracic pressure of patient with normal breathing | Intrathoracic pressure of patient breathing spontaneously, receiving CPAP of 5 | Normal airway pressure baseline of patient on A/C without PEEP | Normal airway pressure baseline of patient on A/C with PEEP of 5 |

PEEP/CPAP in the alveolus

Normal alveolus:
FRC provides volume that keeps the alveolus open for gas exchange.

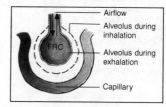

— Airflow
— Alveolus during inhalation
— Alveolus during exhalation
— Capillary

Alveolus with a decreased FRC:
Note that less area is available for gas exchange, and the color of blood in the capillary is darker, indicating a lower PaO$_2$.

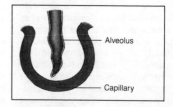

— Alveolus
— Capillary

The problem of diminished FRC has been resolved, using PEEP/CPAP.

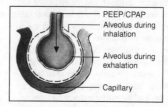

— PEEP/CPAP
— Alveolus during inhalation
— Alveolus during exhalation
— Capillary

Ventilator Alarm Checklist

The major alarms on a ventilator indicate high pressure, low pressure, and low exhaled volume. When a ventilator alarm goes off, remember that the problem might be with the machine, not the patient. The important questions to ask: How does the patient look? Is he gasping for breath? Is he diaphoretic or cyanotic? Always assess the patient first.

Or, if all the numbers are within normal limits but something just doesn't look right, keep a close eye on the patient, even if you can't determine exactly what's wrong.

If the cause of an alarm cannot be determined immediately, call for help and prepare to ventilate the patient manually.

High-pressure alarm
• Patient needs to be suctioned
• Kink in inspiratory tubing
• Obstruction in tubing (possibly from patient lying on it)
• Pneumothorax
• Patient coughing as ventilator delivers breath
• Patient holding his breath as ventilator delivers breath

• Displacement of artificial airway
• Water in tubing
• Increased airway resistance
• Decreased pulmonary compliance

Low-pressure alarm
• Patient "overbreathing" (drawing more air than ventilator delivers)
• Leak in the system (hole in tubing, disconnected tubing, leak around airway cuff, leak at humidifier)

Low exhaled volume alarm
This is indicated by high- or low-pressure readout or spirometer alarm:
• Leak in system preventing breath from being delivered
• Patient stops spontaneous respirations while on IMV
• Spirometer disconnected
• Increased airway resistance on pressure-cycled ventilator
• Decreased pulmonary compliance on pressure-cycled ventilator
• Any situation that triggers high- or low-pressure alarm on volume-cycled ventilator and prevents the full volume of air from being delivered

tilation is necessary. Keep a hand-held resuscitation bag, a flowmeter, and an oxygen source readily available at all times. Monitor ABG measurements regularly; obtain a blood specimen approximately 30 minutes after initiating mechanical ventilation, after a change in setting, or immediately if the patient's condition deteriorates. (Because insurance reimbursement requires orders for blood work, many hospitals have a standing order that blood specimens may be drawn for ABG analysis after a ventilator setting change or when the patient's condition changes.)

Pulmonary function test results, including tidal volume (TV), vital capacity, and negative inspiratory force, should be monitored routinely to determine the patient's respiratory re-

serve and to evaluate him for potential weaning.

Regularly monitor the patient's vital signs. To determine the respiratory rate, count the total number of breaths/minute and note whether they're machine-controlled breaths or a combination of machine-controlled and spontaneous breaths. (Simply noting a respiratory rate of 16 doesn't provide enough information.)

You also should perform periodic physical examinations. When taking vital signs or whenever the patient's condition changes, perform a respiratory assessment. Listen for breath sounds when the patient is receiving ventilator breaths and if he's breathing spontaneously (on the ventilator dial labeled IMV/SIMV). Especially listen for ventilation in the lung bases and dependent areas. Coordinate auscultation of posterior lung fields with turning to minimize patient discomfort. Inspect and palpate both sides of the chest during the machine's breath delivery to ensure symmetrical ventilation and to determine whether the patient's own respiratory efforts are synchronized with the machine. Use percussion as needed to evaluate consolidated, overinflated, or underventilated areas.

Also keep track of other parameters, such as peak inspiratory pressure. On a volume-cycled ventilator, peak inspiratory pressure reflects the machine's ability to deliver air into the patient's lungs. This pressure appears on the manometer on the front of the machine. Peak pressure is read as the highest pressure indicated by the manometer needle during inspiration. An increasing pressure reflects decreased pulmonary compliance from fluid accumulation caused by such conditions as pulmonary edema, secretion accumulation, or interstitial edema (as in ARDS). Increased pressure also may indicate increased airway resistance, such as that in bronchospasm. As with central venous pressure, one peak inspiratory pressure reading doesn't provide as much information as a series of readings over time. Consider *trends* in these readings especially important.

Make sure the ventilator operates according to the settings. Measure TV with a spirometer (either the machine's spirometer or a hand-held device), and analyze oxygen content with an oxygen analyzer. Frequently check to see that all ventilator alarms are properly set. These alarms alert you to changes in the patient's condition and in ventilator function. Always respond promptly to a ventilator alarm. (See *Ventilator Alarm Checklist*.)

Regularly check the humidification device. Be sure that it's filled and that it provides adequate moisture. When it's set correctly, condensation (commonly called "rainout") usually ap-

Pediatric Considerations

When caring for a newborn or young child who's on a mechanical ventilator, keep these special considerations in mind:

• Technological limitations make the small tidal volumes (TV) used to ventilate a 10-lb child (such as a 30-ml TV) difficult to measure. Instead of relying on numerical analysis, you'll need to carefully assess the patient's aeration and chest movement.

• Pressure applied to tubing causes expansion, which consequently results in some loss of air volume to the patient. In adults, TVs are high enough to make this loss insignificant. But in the child with a small TV, 50% of the set TV can be lost in tubing expansion before it ever reaches the child. This tubing compliance factor must be calculated and compensated for to avoid hypoventilation when small TVs and pediatric ventilators are used.

• Because artificial airways for children are so small, a tremendous amount of negative pressure must be exerted to breathe through them effectively. Therefore, small amounts of positive pressure (5 cmH$_2$O) should be applied to the airway at all times to make spontaneous breathing easier and to allow the child to overcome the resistance of the small tube's lumen.

pears in the tubing leading to the patient. This occurs when warm air from the humidifier comes in contact with the tubing, which is exposed to the cooler atmospheric air. Empty the water from the tubing regularly to prevent resistance to airflow from the ventilator and to decrease the risk of water aspiration when the patient turns in bed. Momentarily disconnect the tubing so that you can empty it. (An unstable patient or one on massive ventilatory support may need to be ventilated manually while the tubing

Patient and Family Teaching before Discharge

Teach patient and designated family member the following procedures.

Airway assessment
Show family member how to assess patient's respiratory rate and to recognize variations in breathing patterns, including shortness of breath and apnea. Then teach how to describe quality and amount of secretions.

Bagging technique
• Identify appropriate equipment.
• Connect hand-held resuscitation bag to oxygen.
• Connect hand-held resuscitation bag to tracheostomy tube.
• Use hand-held resuscitation bag to give oxygen at comfortable rate.

Sterile suctioning
• Explain need for sterile technique.
• Wash hands.
• Select appropriate equipment (catheter, gloves, hand-held resuscitation bag, sterile packet of normal saline solution).
• Use sterile suctioning technique.

Cleaning inner cannula of tracheostomy tube
• Review aseptic technique. Wash hands.
• Gather necessary supplies: gloves, mixture of ½ hydrogen peroxide and ½ normal saline solution or other appropriate solution, brush, pipe cleaners, sponges, tracheostomy tapes, and 4″ x 4″ dressing. Extra tracheostomy set will already be at bedside.
• Unwrap equipment and disconnect ventilator from patient. Then put on gloves.
• Remove inner cannula.
• Submerge inner cannula in mixture of ½ hydrogen peroxide and ½ normal saline solution. *Caution:* Assess patient's respiratory status continuously while cleaning inner cannula.
• Clean inner cannula with brush.
• Feed pipe cleaner through inner cannula.
• Shake excess fluid off inner cannula.
• Reinsert it and lock it in place.
• Connect ventilator to patient.

is being emptied.) With an in-line thermometer held as close to the patient connector as possible, check the temperature of the air delivered to the patient. The delivered air temperature should be close to body temperature.

Change the tubing and humidifier every 24 to 48 hours, or as specified by hospital policy, to reduce the risk of bacterial contamination.

Monitoring a newborn or young child receiving mechanical ventilation differs somewhat from monitoring an adult or older child. (See also *Pediatric Considerations*, page 307.)

Care of the patient
Be sure to maintain a patent airway. Check the airway regularly to make sure the tape or securing device hasn't loosened or allowed the tube to slip out of position. This is especially important in the patient whose airway is connected to the heavy ventilator tubing, which may pull on the tube. (Don't routinely retape an endotracheal tube—each time the tube is retaped, it moves and creates more trauma to the vocal cords.) Place the tube in a central position in the patient's mouth, away from the oral mucosa in the corners of the mouth and the lips; retape it only if the tape is soiled or loose, allowing the tube to move. Provide mouth care as needed.

Also, suction only as needed, not routinely. Remember—suctioning carries risks. Because patients with neuromuscular disease usually produce less secretions than those with chronic

• Remove 4" x 4" dressing around tracheostomy.
• Clean peristomal skin with mixture of ½ hydrogen peroxide and ½ normal saline or other solution, as ordered.
• Record peristomal skin condition.
• Place new 4" x 4" dressing around tracheostomy.
• Change tracheostomy tapes only if another person can help. This can be the patient if he's able.
• Explain danger of outer cannula coming out. Describe what to do: immediately replace with sterile tracheostomy and tie securely, notify doctor, and assess respiratory status.

Troubleshooting ventilator problems
• While giving routine respiratory care, family member will learn how long patient can tolerate being off ventilator. Tell family member that if this isn't enough time to troubleshoot the ventilator problem, he should call respiratory therapist, doctor, or ambulance service immediately.

• If there's time to troubleshoot, family member should identify possible causes of respiratory distress or ventilator alarm going off. Explain how to deal with these problems:
  For an obstructed tracheostomy—
1. Preoxygenate patient using handheld resuscitation bag.
2. Irrigate with normal saline solution if necessary.
3. Suction patient.
4. Connect patient to ventilator and assess respiratory status.
5. If patient is still in distress, dial emergency phone number to arrange transportation to nearest hospital.
  Water in tubing—
1. Disconnect tubing from ventilator.
2. Empty water from tubing.
  Improper cuff pressure—
1. Inflate cuff with appropriate amount of pressure. (Explain importance of cuff inflation.)
2. During next visit to doctor and respiratory therapist, report problems and solutions.

---

lung disease, they'll probably require less suctioning. Indications for suctioning in the ventilated patient include increasing peak inspiratory pressure, rhonchi, loud crackles, and decreased breath sounds. Optimally, suctioning should be done after administration of respiratory therapy, such as inhaled bronchodilators or chest physiotherapy, and after administration of pain medication in the surgical patient. (See also Chapter 12.)

If your patient is alert, he may become frustrated by his inability to communicate freely during mechanical ventilation. An endotracheal or tracheostomy tube makes speech impossible. The endotracheal tube passes through the vocal cords, maintaining them in an open position and preventing speech because the vocal cords can't open and close. Never ask a patient with an endotracheal tube to move his mouth to allow you to lip-read. This will reflexively abduct and adduct the vocal cords around the tube and can cause significant cord edema. However, a patient with a tracheostomy tube may move his lips because the tube is below the vocal cords.

A magic slate, letter board, or pen and paper help solve the communication problem. For best legibility, especially for an elderly patient, a dark blue felt-tipped marker on yellow paper provides the best contrast and is easiest to read; a felt-tipped marker requires less pressure on the paper.

Nutrition can pose a serious problem in a ventilated patient. The patient with

Home Care Discharge Guidelines for Ventilator-Dependent Patients

Goal	Actions
Patient and family will be suitable candidates for home care discharge.	• Do baseline nursing assessment (body systems, blood pressure, pulse, apical heart rate, respirations, and intake and output). Note family's normal schedule (work hours, sleep patterns, mealtimes, and so forth). • Health care team should discuss home care with patient and family. Questions to consider: Are family members willing to provide home care? Are they capable of doing so? Is their home conducive to such care? • While assessing patient's home and family, note such things as family interactions and availability of transportation. • Social worker should do complete psychosocial history and assess patient's financial status and medical insurance coverage.
Patient and family will understand what home care involves.	• Describe patient's home care needs, including medications and feedings. Introduce patient and family to home health agency's nursing supervisor and visiting nurse. • Nursing supervisor should describe all services patient will receive. Patient and family should know fees for home health service and extent of insurance coverage; 24-hour phone number of home health agency; person to contact when assigned home care nurse isn't on duty.
Patient and family will learn how respiratory care is administered at home.	• Discuss equipment, including tracheostomy tube and ventilator. Also explain the need for suction and oxygen if appropriate. • Introduce patient and family to representative of medical equipment company that provides home ventilators. He'll explain equipment and company services. • Demonstrate specific respiratory care procedures (see *Patient and Family Teaching before Discharge* on pages 308 and 309). Then assess and document ability of patient and family members to perform them.
Family will learn what to do in case of emergency.	• Review steps to take when patient is in respiratory distress, such as using hand-held resuscitation bag and dialing emergency phone number to report that home ventilator patient needs immediate transportation to nearest facility. • To prepare for power failure, social worker should notify power company and fire department that ventilator patient is in house. Place patient's name on hospital's list of people to be contacted in emergencies such as power failures. Make sure patient and family know how long batteries can run ventilator and suction equipment. (Home ventilator should have emergency battery capable of providing power for at least 24 hours.) Emphasize need to use hand-held resuscitation bag in prolonged emergency.

Home Care Discharge Guidelines for Ventilator-Dependent Patients *(continued)*

Goal	Actions
Patient and family will be given appropriate discharge instructions.	• Make sure discharge instruction sheet includes names and phone numbers of appropriate community services, times of follow-up appointments, emergency phone numbers, and special instructions.
For 4 days before discharge, patient will use home ventilator in hospital, and his condition will remain stable.	• After consulting with hospital respiratory therapist and critical care clinical specialist, doctor will order patient's home ventilator. Hospital respiratory therapist should check ventilator for safety, then place patient on it in presence of primary nurse and home care respiratory therapist. Hospital respiratory therapist should record patient's response to ventilator after 8 hours, then daily.
Patient will be transported home safely.	• When arranging for transportation, health care team should consider these questions: —What will be power source for ventilator during trip? It may be an outlet in emergency vehicle or a battery. —Does emergency vehicle have suction equipment and hand-held resuscitation bag? —Who should accompany patient? Usually, home care respiratory therapist and emergency medical technicians ride with patient; visiting nurse meets him at home. —Will insurance pay for trip?
Follow-up will be done on post-discharge care.	• Within 24 hours of discharge, call family and visiting nurse. • Review initial written report from visiting nurse and home care respiratory therapist. • Depending on circumstances, doctor may make follow-up home visits, or patient may come to office or clinic. If patient will visit doctor, arrange for appropriate transportation.

chronic lung disease may have preexisting malnutrition because eating tires him and may cause significant shortness of breath. Trauma and surgical patients require high caloric intake for tissue repair; consequently, a standard replacement diet may be inadequate.

Nutritional requirements must be considered early in the course of the patient's illness and during ventilation. Otherwise, inadequate muscle mass may delay weaning. If the patient has an intact, functioning GI tract (evidenced by normal bowel sounds), high calorie-per-ounce tube feedings may be the preferred nutritional choice. If more precise nutritional control is needed, and trauma or surgery has disrupted the patient's GI tract, I.V. hyperalimentation with supplemental intralipid infusions may be used.

Also make sure your patient is adequately hydrated. Besides maintaining intravascular volume, blood pressure, and cardiac output, adequate hydration helps maintain the fluidity of tracheobronchial secretions. Avoid overhydration, which can cause pulmonary edema and impair gas exchange. Monitor the patient's input and output as well as daily

Flowsheet to Monitor Home Ventilation

This sample flowsheet, designed for home use, helps maintain optimum ventilator function. It also allows documentation of respiratory care.

PATIENT NAME MICHAEL ROBINSON

1. Patient can breathe on his own? (Yes) No
O₂ delivery days TUESDAY, THURSDAY, SATURDAY

1987 DATE	8/26		8/26	8/26
TIME	10 A.	2 P.	6 P.	10 P.
2. O₂ source checked	2200		2000	1850
3. O₂ recorded	30%		29%	30%
4. Alarm checked	✓		✓	—
5. Inspiratory pressure	40		42	36
6. High-pressure alarm	✓		✓	—
7. Tidal volume set	900		900	900
8. Humidifier/water	FULL		ok	OK
9. Temperature	99°		98°	99°
10. Tubing water	EMPTY		empty	OK
11. Respiratory rate	12		11	12
12. Resuscitation bag	✓	↓	✓	✓
1. Tracheostomy	✓ *	—	—	NO
2. Respiratory treatments	PT. AERO	PT. AERO	pt. aero	
3. Breath sounds checked	✓ OK	✓ OK	✓	
4. Suctioning	✓ OK	✓ OK	✓	
5. Tubing changed	—	BY RT	—	↓

✓ checked
— not checked or done
*refer to

M. Whitford, RN
M. Whitford, RN
L. Jacobs, RN
Mary Robinson, wife

weights to assess his fluid status. In some patients, invasive monitoring with a central venous pressure or Swan-Ganz catheter may be necessary for precise hemodynamic measurements.

Because of the ventilated patient's limited mobility and activity, active or passive range-of-motion exercises should be performed to maintain strength and joint mobility of all extremities as soon as his physical condition allows. Family members can help assist with these exercises.

Skin breakdown commonly accompanies impaired mobility. Besides causing discomfort and unsightliness, decubitus ulcers can tax the patient's immune system, compromising immune functions in other body areas. This is especially dangerous in the patient with an artificial airway because the airway provides a direct route for bacteria to enter the lungs. To minimize decubitus ulcer formation, turn the patient every 2 hours, keep sheets wrinkle-free, and provide a flotation mattress or Clinitron therapy bed to minimize pressure. The Roto Rest bed, another option, turns slowly, moving the immobilized patient with it and maintaining gentle continuous motion. This helps maintain skin integrity by decreasing pressure and also allows for better lung ventilation and perfusion by changing the focus of gravitational pull as the patient and bed rotate. Promptly change wet sheets caused by incontinence or massive diaphoresis and dry the skin thoroughly.

Because many ventilated patients are in critical care units, which are active 24 hours a day, their sleep patterns may be disrupted. Sleep disturbance can contribute to intensive care unit psychosis and can be physically exhausting, posing a particular problem when preparing the patient for weaning. Whenever possible, schedule activities to allow uninterrupted hours at night for sleep. A bedtime routine that includes a backrub, subdued lighting, and limited visitors can help relax the patient and encourage rest. Posi-

tioning the patient's bed so that he can see a window will provide him with environmental cues for sleep.

Finally, consider the psychological implications of mechanical ventilation. Some patients develop an altered body image that is integrated with the machine and are therefore reluctant to give the machine up even if they can successfully breathe on their own. Many patients experience anxiety about their care and dependence on the machine. Others become overly demanding, to mask their feelings of powerlessness and helplessness about being unable to breathe on their own. Keeping these problems in mind can allow you to intervene promptly with appropriate reassurances and limit-setting.

The patient who is overly anxious about the critical care experience needs constant reassurance about the progress of his condition. Let him know that he won't be abandoned and that a caregiver will respond promptly whenever he rings the call bell. However, to prevent him from using the call bell constantly, tell him when you will return. Let him know if you have to care for another patient and about some of your other responsibilities, such as reviewing laboratory and X-ray reports so that you can provide the best care for him. Be sure to explain every procedure before proceeding. Never do anything when he's not paying attention.

An anxious patient may bite on the endotracheal tube. Don't try to prevent this with an oral airway—it can easily make the patient vomit, risking aspiration—even with a cuffed endotracheal tube in place. Try talking to the patient to determine the source of his anxiety. Guided imagery may help the patient "leave" the critical care setting to get a break from constant sensory stimulation. A small, portable tape recorder with headphones and tapes of his choice also can provide an escape. If the patient's anxiety is uncontrolled and impairs his ventilation, sleep, or care, he may need anxiolytic medi-

Care of Ventilated Patients on Neuromuscular Blocking Agents

Long-acting neuromuscular blocking agents, such as pancuronium (Pavulon), are used for patient management when the patient is extraordinarily restless—so much so that mechanical ventilation is almost impossible.

Patients who may require neuromuscular blocking agents
• Multiple trauma patients with head injury
• Seizure disorder patients, if the seizure movements disrupt ventilation
• Traumatic brain injury patients (used in conjunction with powerful barbiturates to control intracranial pressure)
• Patients with cerebral edema after metabolic insult, as seen in Reye's syndrome (used in conjunction with powerful barbiturates to control intracranial pressure)

Special clinical considerations
• Whenever pharmacological paralysis is instituted, it should be done on a full-time basis. Intermittent paralysis and movement can exacerbate the patient's anxiety and restlessness, and make mechanical ventilation even more difficult. It can also cause huge increases in intracranial pressure. The commitment should be made to use the paralytic, and the order should be written to allow more medication to be

given as needed as soon as movement is detected.
• Often, assisting the ventilator is the first indication that the drug is wearing off and that more should be administered. Medications like morphine and diazepam (Valium) should be administered routinely with a paralytic drug to provide pain relief, mood alteration, and amnesia of the episode.
• The caregiver must never forget that although the patient is unable to move, his mentation is unaffected by the neuromuscular blocking agent and his ability to feel pain and any body manipulations may actually be sharpened because of his inability to respond.
• The patient should be allowed to emerge from the medications once a day to allow for a full neurologic assessment (unless it is determined that the stimulation from emergence may dangerously spike the intracranial pressure).
• All clinical considerations of the mechanically ventilated patient also apply to ventilated patients receiving neuromuscular blocking agents. This includes meticulous bedside care. Especially important is maintaining continuous communication with the patient, explaining all procedures, and paying particular attention to body alignment and comfort measures.

cation. The confused patient may require soft arm restraints to remind him not to remove the endotracheal tube.

Sometimes you'll find it necessary to administer neuromuscular blocking agents to accomplish mechanical ventilation. For an overview of the care required by these patients, see *Care of Ventilated Patients on Neuromuscular Blocking Agents.*

Patients who are medically stable but dependent on mechanical venti-

lation can be discharged and maintained at home on mechanical ventilation. Candidates for home ventilation include patients with neuromuscular disease and those with chronic lung disease in the absence of other major system complications (see *Patient and Family Teaching before Discharge*, pages 308 and 309; *Home Care Discharge Guidelines for Ventilator-De-*

pendent Patients, pages 310 and 311; and *Flowsheet to Monitor Home Ventilation,* page 312).

Complications

• *Barotrauma.* Barotrauma refers to the effects of pressure on the lung tissue. Damage can occur from high ventilatory pressures, high PEEP, or both. Long exposure time and high pressure increase the risk of barotrauma. Each patient has a different threshold, depending on the underlying lung condition. For example, a patient with necrotizing pneumonia and fragile lung tissue has a much higher risk than a patient with normal, healthy lungs who is being ventilated for mechanical reasons. Barotrauma most commonly presents as a pneumothorax but also may present as subcutaneous emphysema. Barotrauma can eventually result in chronic loss of lung function and, in newborns, may lead to a chronic obstructive disorder called bronchopulmonary dysplasia.

• *Pulmonary oxygen toxicity.* Cellular changes occur in lung tissue exposed to high levels of inspired oxygen for a prolonged time. Lung tissue oxidizes, which may lead to decreasing compliance. The FIO_2 and duration of therapy required to cause pulmonary oxygen toxicity is variable from patient to patient. An FIO_2 of 1.0 causes damage much earlier; an FIO_2 below 0.4 is considered safe.

• *Decreased venous return.* Positive-pressure ventilation increases mean intrathoracic pressures. This can decrease the effectiveness of the thoracic pump and retard venous return. If the venous return decrease is significant, cardiac output and blood pressure will drop. To detect this problem early, monitor blood pressure (and any other hemodynamic values available) when the patient is placed on the ventilator and when ventilator changes in rate or pressure occur, such as with the addition of PEEP.

• *Increased antidiuretic hormone (ADH) production.* Positive pressure transmitted to intrathoracic structures from the lungs may cause intravascular baroreceptors to incorrectly sense a decrease in total body fluid volume when positive pressure decreases venous return and blood pressure. Therefore, ADH production will increase; urine output may drop; and dependent edema may develop. Diuretics may be needed to combat this problem.

Weaning from mechanical ventilation

Description

Weaning is the gradual discontinuance of mechanical ventilatory support, usually accomplished by one of two methods: the conventional method and intermittent mandatory ventilation (IMV).

With the conventional method, which was used widely until the early 1970s, the patient is removed from total ventilatory support and expected to breathe spontaneously with supplemental oxygen from a T-tube or tracheostomy collar. When weaning begins, the patient usually breathes on his own for 5 to 10 minutes/hour. This time is increased gradually, as tolerated. Although much less popular today, this method is appropriate for some patients, such as those ventilated to produce pharmacologic paralysis for a procedure. Once the drug wears off, the patient doesn't require a long weaning period because the need for ventilation has been eliminated. He can be connected to a T-piece and monitored, then extubated. Patients ventilated postoperatively for a short period until anesthetic effects have worn off also can be weaned conventionally.

IMV, or synchronized IMV (SIMV), allows the patient to take spontaneous breaths between a preset number of ventilator breaths per minute. Since its introduction in the early 1970s, IMV has gained popularity. Because weaning should be considered when mechanical

Criteria for Weaning

Discontinuing mechanical ventilation shouldn't be done on a hit-or-miss basis. Certain prognostic values can indicate whether the patient is a good candidate for the weaning process. While not all patients who meet these criteria will be weaned successfully, and not all patients who are weaned successfully meet these criteria, they offer you a place to start to evaluate your patient.

Subjective criteria
• Has the patient recovered from the immediate effects of anesthesia or any other depressant drugs?
• Is he alert?
• Does he have neurologic deficits?
• Are laryngeal reflexes intact?

Objective criteria
• Tidal volume spontaneously greater than 6 ml/kg
• Vital capacity spontaneously greater than 15 ml/kg
• Acceptable blood gas values (normal for the patient)
• Inspiratory force greater than 25 cmH$_2$O
• Compliance greater than 30 ml/cmH$_2$O
• Stable circulation

---

ventilation begins, many patients now are ventilated with IMV/SIMV from the start because spontaneous breaths help maintain respiratory muscle tone.

When a patient is ready for weaning with IMV or SIMV, the number of ventilator breaths is gradually decreased over a period of days. As these decrease, the patient is expected to increase spontaneous respirations, replacing the ventilation no longer provided by the machine. Instead of ordering specific rates, some doctors write such orders as "40% IMV," meaning that the machine should be set to provide 40% of the patient's total minute ventilation. IMV or SIMV is most appropriate for patients who've

been ventilated for a period of days, weeks, or months, and who have developed respiratory muscle atrophy and a strong psychological dependence on the machine. It may take a week or longer to wean them slowly by IMV or SIMV, decreasing the mechanical support by one breath every 1 or 2 days.

Purpose
To allow the patient to resume spontaneous respirations while keeping mechanical support readily available

Procedure
Before weaning
• Assess the patient's overall status. (See *Criteria for Weaning.*) Make sure he is adequately nourished and has sufficient muscle mass to maintain spontaneous respirations.
• Assess his psychological status, and determine his dependence level on the machine.
• Thoroughly explain the purpose of weaning, and gauge his reaction to the prospect of weaning.
• If possible, make sure he gets adequate sleep before any decrease in mechanical support.

Conventional method
• Check the doctor's order for a weaning schedule.
• Explain the procedure to the patient. Allow him to express his fears, and reassure him that you'll be present to monitor his progress.
• Establish a means of providing high-flow humidified oxygen via a T-tube or tracheostomy collar.
• Place the patient in semi-Fowler's or high Fowler's position as his condition allows.
• Record baseline measurements of respiratory rate, vital capacity (VC), tidal volume (TV), negative inspiratory force (NIF), heart rate and rhythm (from an EKG strip), and blood pressure.
• Remove the ventilator tubing from the endotracheal tube and attach the

T-tube (attach a tracheostomy collar to the tracheostomy).
• Turn off the ventilator.
• During periods when the patient breathes on his own, monitor his vital signs and heart rhythm, checking for tachycardia and extrasystole, and assess his general condition (such as restlessness, skin color, presence of diaphoresis). Be alert to any of his complaints. If possible, monitor O_2 saturation with an oximeter and check for decreasing O_2 saturation.
• At the end of a predetermined interval, obtain a blood specimen for ABG analysis and repeat the specific measurements done at the start of weaning.
• If the patient tires, reconnect him to the ventilator; if he's comfortable and stable, wait until ABG results are available. If these results are acceptable, the patient may continue to breathe on his own until he tires (check with the doctor and hospital policy for specific instructions).
• If the patient's condition deteriorates during weaning, reconnect him to the ventilator. (See *When to Discontinue Weaning*.)
• As the patient's tolerance for weaning improves, gradually increase his time off the ventilator, as ordered, until he breathes on his own all the time.

Intermittent mandatory ventilation
• Check the doctor's order.
• Explain the procedure to the patient.
• If necessary, change the ventilator mode to IMV or SIMV.
• Set the rate as ordered.
• Monitor the patient as during conventional weaning. (Although monitoring is as important with IMV or SIMV as with the conventional method, it can be less intensive because IMV allows more gradual weaning, which eliminates sudden stress on and adjustments by the patient.)
• Periodically check vital signs and spirometry results (VC, NIF, and TV).
• Obtain a blood specimen for ABG analysis after a predetermined time interval.

When to Discontinue Weaning

Weaning should be discontinued when any of the following occur:
• A rise in systolic blood pressure of 20 mm Hg or a rise in diastolic blood pressure of 10 mm Hg
• An increase in respiratory rate of 10 breaths/minute or a respiratory rate greater than 30 breaths/minute
• A change in heart rate of 20 beats/minute or a heart rate greater than 120 beats/minute
• The onset of dysrhythmias
• Fatigue, as indicated by increased labored breathing
• Arterial blood gas measurements should also be monitored, but remember that CO_2 is the main respiratory stimulus. The $Paco_2$ may have to *rise* in order to stimulate breathing.

• Continue to decrease the rate (usually one breath at a time) as ordered, to decrease the patient's mechanical ventilatory support and allow him to gradually take over the work of breathing.

Clinical considerations
Weaning may be the most complicated aspect of care for the patient on a mechanical ventilator. Keep in mind that weaning parameters are simply *guidelines* to help predict which patients can be successfully weaned; don't assume that they apply to all patients. A patient may be stable clinically, yet not meet weaning criteria. If his condition is otherwise stable, weaning can still begin (with a doctor's order) with careful monitoring. Some patients still don't meet weaning criteria even after they've been weaned and discharged. This occurs most commonly in patients with chronic obstructive pulmonary disease and neuromuscular disorders whose baseline measure-

ments of respiratory rate, VC, NIF, heart rate and rhythm, and blood pressure are abnormal from the start.

Measure weaning criteria in every mechanically ventilated patient, even if you don't think the patient is ready for weaning. In some patients, especially those with reversible neuromuscular disease, respiratory function often returns before other gross motor functions. Monitoring weaning criteria in such patients may permit weaning to begin earlier, decreasing ventilatory support time.

Some patients can breathe adequately without ventilatory support during the day because of constant sensory stimulation, but need ventilatory support at night when the environment becomes quiet and they need to sleep. Plan weaning to allow a period of uninterrupted sleep; this may mean weaning during the day, with full mechanical support during the night for a week or more.

Patients being weaned may need more aggressive pulmonary hygiene because their breaths are shallower than the ones the ventilator provides.

Make sure they're adequately hydrated to keep secretions loose and to prevent inspissation and mucus plugging.

The most common problem associated with weaning is fatigue. This is most likely to occur in patients after a long period of ventilatory support. Monitor for increased use of accessory respiratory muscles, increased respiratory rate with decreased TV, and poor patient posture (such as slumping in the bed or chair).

If respiratory distress progresses, check for cardiac dysrhythmias (hypoxemia is most commonly associated with premature ventricular contractions), tachycardia, and increased or decreased blood pressure. In a patient in distress who's decompensating, expect ABG measurements to show increased $PaCO_2$, decreased pH, and decreased PaO_2 levels.

Complications
The most serious complication of weaning is respiratory failure with cardiopulmonary arrest. However, careful monitoring and assessment can prevent this complication.

Selected References

Burton, G.G., and Hodgkin, J.E., eds. *Respiratory Care: A Guide to Clinical Practice,* 2nd ed. Philadelphia: J.B. Lippincott Co., 1984.

Carroll, P.F. "Caring for Ventilator Patients," *Nursing86* 16(2):34-39, February 1986.

Carroll, P.F. "Home Care for the Ventilator Patient: A Checklist You Can Use," *Nursing87* 17(10):82-83, October 1987.

Caring for the Critically Ill Patient. Springhouse, Pa.: Springhouse Corp., 1986.

Ensuring Intensive Care. Nursing Photobook series. Springhouse, Pa.: Springhouse Corp., 1983.

McPherson, S.P. *Respiratory Therapy Equipment,* 3rd ed. St. Louis: C.V. Mosby Co., 1984.

Procedures. Nurse's Reference Library. Springhouse, Pa.: Springhouse Corp., 1983.

Respiratory Disorders. Nurse's Clinical Library. Springhouse, Pa.: Springhouse Corp., 1984.

Spearman, C.B., and Sanders, H.G., Jr. "The New Generation of Mechanical Ventilators," *Respiratory Care* 32(6):403-18, June 1987.

White, K.D., and Perez, P.W. "Your Ventilator Patient *Can* Go Home Again," *Nursing86* 16(12):54-56, December 1986.

14 THORACIC SURGERY AND CHEST TUBES

Introduction

Thoracic surgery can be as conservative as a small incision to allow chest tube placement or as radical as a pneumonectomy. In any case, careful patient assessment and teaching are the keys to successful treatment. Preoperatively, the patient's respiratory function must be evaluated to determine if he can tolerate the stress of surgery and potential loss of lung tissue. His respiratory system must be assessed regularly to allow early detection of complications or deterioration in his condition.

Patient teaching is especially important because thoracic surgery may arouse more fear than many other operations. However, preoperative teaching can help alleviate fear and make the postoperative period smoother for both the patient and caregiver.

When chest surgery involves the pleural space, the patient will have one or two chest tubes inserted and connected to a closed chest drainage system. Chest tubes also may be warranted for chest trauma victims with a pneumothorax or hemothorax. These patients require careful assessment and care to prevent or detect possible life-threatening complications. Caregivers must be familiar with the equipment used.

Thanks to safer, simpler equipment and techniques, autotransfusion—the collection, filtration, and reinfusion of a patient's own blood; used in patients with chest trauma and chest surgery —

has become a widely accepted procedure in emergency departments, trauma centers, and postoperative units. Autotransfusion plays an important part in nonemergency and emergency surgery. This procedure is used more often today because it prevents the transmission of acquired immunodeficiency syndrome and other diseases.

Thoracic surgery

Indications
A patient may undergo a thoracic surgical procedure after:
• spontaneous pneumothorax
• chest trauma (such as from a motor vehicle accident, gunshot wound, or stabbing)
• various disorders, including lung cancer, noncancerous growths, and lung abscess
• localized structural abnormalities, such as blebs and bronchiectasis.

Preoperative care
Preoperative evaluation
When deciding whether surgical treatment for a respiratory disorder is warranted, the doctor assesses the patient's history and physical findings to determine the surgical risk factors. Gathering information during preoperative assessment can also help predict which postoperative problems are probable.

With trauma patients, thorough preoperative assessment isn't always possible. In these cases, the decision to operate must be based on the patient's pre-

Common Risk Factors for Thoracic Surgery

History
- Cigarette smoking
- Myocardial infarction
- Chronic obstructive pulmonary disease (COPD)
- Over age 60

Physical findings
- More than 20% overweight
- Gross malnutrition
- Limited diaphragmatic excursion
- Barrel chest (indicating COPD)
- Dyspnea on exertion
- Orthopnea
- Dependent edema

Pulmonary function studies
- Forced expiratory volume in the 1st second (FEV_1) below 70% of predicted value
- Vital capacity below 20 ml/kg (10 ml/lb)
- FEV_1/FVC less than 70%
- Pao_2 below 70 mm Hg on room air
- $Paco_2$ above 45 mm Hg

senting condition. Before elective surgery, appropriate diagnostic procedures—such as X-rays, computed tomography, bronchography, and pulmonary function studies—also may be performed to aid in assessing the surgical risk. (See *Common Risk Factors for Thoracic Surgery*.)

The results of renal, cardiovascular, and other tests also will be considered. Keep in mind that requirements for surgery are more stringent in the patient undergoing pneumonectomy because the entire lung is removed.

Preoperative therapy
Preoperative care is designed to improve the patient's condition and decrease the surgical risk as much as possible.

If your patient smokes cigarettes, advise him to stop smoking. Ciliary movement may improve as soon as 4 weeks after smoking cessation; this helps the patient clear secretions during the postoperative period. Also, the resulting decrease in carbon monoxide can improve blood oxygen-carrying capacity.

If the patient has a history of chronic lung disease or secretion retention, 48 hours of intensive preoperative respiratory therapy may help. Such a program may include:
- I.V. aminophylline to maximize bronchodilation (be sure to measure peak and trough blood drug levels to ensure that therapeutic levels are reached)
- inhaled bronchodilators, such as metaproterenol or isoetharine, given four times daily before chest physiotherapy (these sympathomimetic drugs use a different pathway than aminophylline to achieve bronchodilation)
- chest physiotherapy four times daily (for maximal effectiveness, this should be done approximately 30 minutes after administration of an inhaled bronchodilator to allow for maximal bronchodilation and, therefore, maximal secretion movement)
- proper deep-breathing and coughing techniques, with ample practice time.

Preoperative teaching
Preoperative teaching can prove crucial to the success of thoracic surgery. Effective preoperative teaching addresses the patient's fears about surgery and the likelihood of being in the intensive care unit (ICU) and requiring mechanical ventilatory support. When providing preoperative teaching, be sure to assess the patient's level of anxiety and his ability to assimilate information. An exceptionally anxious patient who uses denial as a defense mechanism may benefit more by going to the door of the ICU rather than taking a full tour, as most patients do.

Whenever possible, include the patient's spouse or partner in the teaching process. This person can reinforce your teaching; knowledge of the postoperative routine also can help diminish that person's anxiety. Be sure to document all preoperative teaching, especially if the patient will be transferred to a different unit postoperatively.

For more information about preoperative teaching, see *Thoracic Surgery: Patient-Teaching Checklist*.

Surgical procedures
Exploratory thoracotomy
In this procedure, the chest is opened and the thorax explored. After the surgeon makes the incision (usually posterolaterally), he spreads the ribs and enters the pleura. This procedure is done to confirm a suspected diagnosis, to allow for direct examination of tissue, and to diagnose the cause of bleeding from trauma. Postoperatively, expect chest tubes connected to underwater drainage.

Pneumonectomy
This surgery involves removal of the entire lung after ligation of the pulmonary artery, pulmonary vein, and mainstem bronchus. The phrenic nerve on the operative side is crushed to paralyze the diaphragm and to allow it to rise in the chest and help fill the empty thoracic space.

This procedure is indicated for patients with lung cancer or a severely traumatized lung. Postoperatively, the patient probably won't have chest tubes because no lung remains to reexpand. Fluid collecting in the space will consolidate and prevent mediastinal shift.

Lobectomy
This procedure involves removal of one lobe of a lung. The incision's location depends on the lobe removed.

This procedure is indicated for patients with diseases confined to one lobe, with the remaining lobes capable of expanding and filling the space. Such diseases include isolated tumors, cysts, bronchiectasis, emphysematous blebs or bullae with repeated pneumothorax, abscess, tuberculosis, and localized lung injury. Postoperatively, the patient may need one or two chest tubes connected to underwater drainage. If he needs two

Thoracic Surgery: Patient-Teaching Checklist

Your preoperative teaching plan for a patient scheduled for thoracic surgery should include the following, if appropriate:
• Review of the surgeon's explanation of the procedure
• Location where the patient will wake up (recovery room or ICU)
• Endotracheal tube placement, preventing the patient from speaking
• Possible use and purpose of ventilator or T-tube
• Oxygen administration (type)
• Location of dressings
• Explanation of chest tubes and drainage device
• Use of cardiac monitor in immediate postoperative period
• Positioning
• Turning, coughing, and deep-breathing methods
• Proper incisional splinting for coughing
• Other chest physiotherapy techniques
• Incentive spirometry technique
• Availability of pain medication
• Frequency of vital sign measurement and general assessment
• Presence of I.V. lines
• Possible invasive arterial or venous monitoring
• Possible stored blood transfusions or autotransfusion (addressing, in particular, concerns about acquired immunodeficiency syndrome transmission by blood transfusion, as necessary)
• Importance of range-of-motion and leg exercises
• Likelihood that the patient will be out of bed the evening of the day of surgery, unless he's on ventilatory support
• Dietary restrictions and expected dietary progression
• Visiting policies
  Modify the teaching plan according to the procedure, the patient's comprehension level, and his preoperative condition.

chest tubes, one will be anterior and superior to drain air; the other will be dependent to drain fluid.

Segmental resection

This procedure involves removal of one or more lobe segments. Less radical than lobectomy, this procedure attempts to preserve as much lung function as possible. Usually a long procedure because careful intraoperative dissection is necessary, it's indicated for patients with bronchiectasis, abscess, cysts, metastatic carcinoma, blebs, and tuberculosis. Postoperatively, the patient will need a chest tube connected to underwater drainage. Air leaks may be more common from the segmental surface, and the lung may take longer to expand.

Wedge resection

This surgery involves removal of a well-defined diseased area (usually near the lung surface) without regard to anatomical demarcation. The resected area is sutured off before removal. Lung function is usually minimally disrupted. The procedure is indicated when a biopsy is necessary and for patients with well-localized benign and metastatic tumors or localized inflammatory disease. Expect chest tube(s) and underwater drainage postoperatively.

Decortication

This surgery involves stripping a thick, fibrinous membrane that can develop over the visceral pleura with empyema. It's indicated in patients with chronic empyema. Chest tubes and underwater drainage are used postoperatively. If lung expansion has been restricted for a prolonged period, reexpansion may be difficult.

Thoracoplasty

This surgery involves removal of ribs or rib portions to decrease the size of the thoracic cavity and thereby reduce the risk of mediastinal shift. Formerly the basic surgical treatment for tuberculosis, it's now performed infrequently, when the lung fails to

reexpand after resectional surgery. Because it's an extrapleural procedure, it doesn't require chest tubes postoperatively.

Postoperative care

The intensity of postoperative care usually depends on the procedure performed, the length of anesthesia time, and the patient's preoperative condition.

Monitoring

For all patients, check vital signs regularly in the immediate postoperative period. Usually, you'll record measurements every 15 minutes for the first 2 hours, then every hour until they are stable. If much blood has drained through the chest tube, check for a rapid pulse, an early sign of hypovolemia; later, blood pressure may decrease. An increasing respiratory rate may indicate a decreasing tidal volume from atelectasis, external lung compression from fluid or air in the pleural space, or restricted chest movement from pain.

When listening to breath sounds, be especially alert for signs of decreased ventilation, which may stem from atelectasis or fluid accumulation in the pleural space on the affected side.

Monitor chest tube drainage when checking vital signs. (See "Closed chest drainage," page 329, for more information.)

Monitor arterial blood gas (ABG) measurements according to the patient's condition and the extent of surgery. A patient on a ventilator will need ABG analysis more frequently than a patient who is ambulatory shortly after surgery and can cough well on his own. ABG analysis is indicated for an unexplained increase in pulse and respiratory rate, when dysrhythmias appear without intracardiac catheters, or when any other marked change occurs in the patient's condition.

In any patient receiving oxygen at an FIO_2 of 0.40 or greater, draw a sample for ABG analysis at least once a day, as ordered, to determine his continued need for supplemental oxygen.

Check results of a postoperative chest X-ray to confirm proper placement of chest tubes and any other tubes, such as an endotracheal tube or central venous pressure catheter.

Positioning

Change the patient's position frequently after surgery, taking into account the effects of gravity. Blood flow to the dependent lung will be increased but ventilation will be compromised. Changing the patient's position from back to side and then to the opposite side every 2 hours permits improved distribution of ventilation and perfusion. Some surgeons allow the pneumonectomy patient to be positioned on his back or on the operative side only, because they believe that lying on the unaffected side can compromise ventilation of the only lung available for gas exchange. Be sure to check doctor's orders or your institution's procedure manual for positioning after pneumonectomy. As ordered, place the patient in semi-Fowler's to high Fowler's position to maximize diaphragmatic excursion.

If the patient develops postoperative atelectasis or pneumonia, periodically assist him (if permitted) to the postural drainage position for the affected lung segment at times other than those scheduled for therapy. Monitor his condition to ensure that he can tolerate this position. Be especially cautious if the patient is in a head-down position. (See Chapter 10.)

Respiratory therapy

The intensity of respiratory therapy depends on the patient's condition and his ability to function independently.

Incentive spirometry provides feedback to the patient while he takes deep breaths. Optimally, the patient should use the incentive spirometer to take 10 breaths every waking hour. The initial postoperative goal should be set at 60% to 75% of his preoperative inspiratory volume, with gradual increases as he's able to take deeper breaths.

In some hospitals, chest physiotherapy percussion is routine for the postoperative thoracic surgery patient; in others, it's used only if atelectasis or pneumonia develops. When percussion is warranted, never percuss directly over the incision or chest tubes.

The patient may be afraid to cough because he's apprehensive about the pain and fears that coughing could disrupt sutures. Provide gentle reassurance and teach him that coughing helps keep his lungs clear. Provide adequate splinting to minimize pain. The patient with a lateral incision can place a pillow under his arm on the affected side, then bend his arm and place the pillow against his side, holding his arm so that it looks like a chicken wing over the pillow. This way, the elbow creates the force that keeps the pillow against the chest wall. If the patient can't adequately splint his side when coughing, you can splint his affected side by giving him a bear hug from the inoperative side. Reach your arms around the patient and hold the pillow in place, with your hands pulling the pillow down over the incision.

If the patient can't cough, suctioning may be indicated. Observe and document the character and amount of the suctioned secretions. Secretions may be blood-tinged for the first few days after surgery. Green or yellow secretions indicate infection and warrant temperature monitoring and, as ordered, chest X-ray and possible white blood cell count and sputum culture. Aerosol therapy may be indicated if the patient has underlying lung disease or bronchospasm. The most commonly used inhaled bronchodilators are such sympathomimetic drugs as metaproterenol (Alupent) and isoetharine (Bronkosol).

Pain management

Adequate pain relief promotes patient cooperation with postoperative care and allows him to take the deep breaths necessary to prevent atelectasis and pneumonia. Administer narcotic analgesics, as ordered, every 3 to 4 hours during the first 48 to 72 hours after surgery. If pain isn't adequately managed, the patient won't be able to breathe effectively or move around in and out of bed. Schedule respiratory therapy, coughing, and deep-breathing sessions approximately 30 to 60 minutes after narcotic doses. Anesthetic intercostal nerve blocks are used sometimes to provide local pain relief without the risk of narcotic sedation. However, these blocks require multiple needle punctures, which increase the risk of pneumothorax. Also, they must be repeated once or twice daily to be effective.

Other medications

Depending on the reason for surgery, antibiotics may be ordered routinely. For example, such surgical problems as massive empyema and abscesses warrant immediate postoperative antibiotics. Any postoperative patient who develops a fever, redness, and induration around the incision or a change in sputum color also may need antibiotics.

Aminophylline may be indicated if the patient has a history of chronic obstructive pulmonary disease (COPD) or develops bronchospasm postoperatively.

Mobilization

While the patient is in bed, passive and active range-of-motion (ROM) exercises must be performed to maintain blood flow and joint mobility. Give special attention to prevent deep vein thrombus formation, to exercising the legs, and to the arm on the operative side. Because this arm is positioned away from the body during surgery, it will be stiff. Full ROM exercises help decrease stiffness and allow the patient to regain full function. To allow for full arm rotation, perform ROM exercises with the patient sitting on the edge of the bed or, if ordered, standing.

Patient ambulation should begin as soon as possible after surgery, as the patient's condition allows.

Wound care

Maintain sterile technique at all times when providing wound care. Initially, observe the dressings surrounding the chest tube and over the incision site for bleeding. Report any bleeding to the doctor.

Make sure the dressing over the chest tube insertion site remains airtight. Follow hospital policy regarding the initial dressing change and intervals for subsequent care (for more information on dressings, see "Chest tube insertion," page 326). Observe the incision for evidence of healing, redness, induration, drainage, and odor. Document your findings and report abnormal findings to the doctor.

Chest tubes

Monitor chest tubes for patency and drainage. They should remain unclamped until removal is planned; then the clamped tube can alert you to how the patient will tolerate tube removal. Monitor the chest tube drainage device for type and amount of drainage and check for air leaks.

Nutrition and hydration

Proper nutrition proves crucial to good wound healing and provides energy for recuperation. A patient who is malnourished preoperatively, especially one with cancer, may need special supplements and possibly total parenteral nutrition. Because most patients are anorexic after surgery, provide foods that have a high calorie–per–volume ratio, such as milk shakes and eggnog.

Monitor the patient's fluid status carefully, observing and documenting intake and output for the first 48 to 72 hours postoperatively. Expect a pneumonectomy patient to have decreased pulmonary vascular resistance from the loss of one lung's pulmonary vascular bed. Pulmonary edema may occur with volume overload. Check for decreased compliance (in ventilated patients), crackles on auscultation, increasing respiratory rate, and decreasing tidal volume. Diuretics also may be necessary if volume overload occurs.

Adequate hydration helps maintain the fluidity of pulmonary secretions, making them easier to expectorate.

Psychological considerations

After thoracic surgery, be sure to keep the patient informed about his condition and progress. If the diagnosis of cancer was made, the patient probably will experience a grief reaction and will need time to cope with the diagnosis. Encourage him to verbalize his feelings; if appropriate, include oncology team members in his care. Also, include his spouse or partner in his care whenever possible, to minimize feelings of isolation and helplessness.

Complications

The main surgical complications resulting from open-chest surgery are bleeding and persistent air leakage.

Bleeding

Bleeding is demonstrated by significant bloody drainage in the collection chamber of the chest-tube collection device within 24 hours of surgery. The doctor may want to monitor the drainage progression and, if it slows down, let the bleeding stop on its own. To boost coagulation, he may order transfusions, such as fresh frozen plasma. Instead, however, he may decide a return to the operating room is necessary. A sudden gush of bright red blood indicates arterial bleeding; call the doctor immediately. He may open the chest in the unit and clamp the offending vessel if the patient is exsanguinating and an operating room is not available. Prepare for rapid volume replacement.

Bleeding is most likely to occur in trauma patients (because of the likelihood of multiple small-vessel damage), malnourished patients with decreased circulating clotting factors, and patients with liver disease and decreased clotting factor production.

Persistent air leakage

A persistent air leak appears as a continuous bubbling in the water-seal chamber of the chest drainage device. The leak may be a small bubbling or a large rush of air that compromises ventilation. In any case, the doctor has several options. He may choose to watch the patient for several days to see if the leak resolves on its own, to remove the patient from mechanical ventilation to decrease pressure on the lung tissue, or to reoperate to suture the lung tissue.

Monitor the patient's respiratory rate, excursion, and breath sounds. One Pleur-evac model has a patient air leak meter that lets you monitor the magnitude of airflow out of the chest tube. (See *Anatomy of a Pleur-evac*, pages 334 and 335.) If the leak changes significantly, monitor ABG measurements to ensure adequate ventilation.

Persistent air leaks are more likely in trauma patients, who may have multiple tiny holes in the parenchyma, and in patients with friable tissue, which may not hold sutures well. Patients undergoing segmental resection also may be more likely to develop air leaks because of the fine dissection necessary during the procedure.

Respiratory failure

Respiratory failure is most likely in patients with borderline preoperative respiratory function and in malnourished, elderly patients with little energy reserve.

This complication is characterized by increasing respiratory distress with an increasing respiratory rate, decreasing tidal volume, increasing heart rate, diaphoresis, restlessness, and confusion. ABG measurements initially show an increased $PaCO_2$ level with a subsequent decrease in PaO_2 level. Treatment is mechanical ventilation.

Atelectasis

Atelectasis occurs most commonly in the patient who's overweight, immobile, and reluctant to breathe deeply and cough.

The patient will develop decreased breath sounds in dependent areas and may have an increased respiratory rate. Treatment involves an aggressive program of coughing, deep breathing, spirometry, and chest physiotherapy. An intercostal nerve block may help decrease pain and allow for easier deep breathing.

Pneumonia

Pneumonia commonly occurs after atelectasis has developed in a lung segment. With decreased ventilation, normal secretions pool and may become colonized with bacteria. Patients at risk for pneumonia include those who are at risk for atelectasis. Patients with decreased immune function and those who've been intubated also are at risk (endotracheal tubes serve as a passageway for bacteria to enter the lung).

The patient develops a fever, decreased breath sounds, or adventitious sounds (such as crackles and rhonchi) in the affected area. An infiltrate appears on chest X-ray. Treatment resembles that used to treat atelectasis, with an aggressive pulmonary hygiene regimen and the addition of sputum culturing and antibiotics.

Mediastinal shift

A mediastinal shift may occur after pneumonectomy. Monitor the location of the patient's trachea to determine if it is midline or if it has shifted toward the operative side. If you note a deviation, notify the doctor.

Discharge and home care

Before the patient goes home, make sure to include these patient-teaching points:
• Take only showers, not baths, until the doctor allows you to take baths. Check the incision for redness or drainage, and notify the doctor if present.
• Continue to breathe deeply and cough several times a day. If the hospital uses disposable incentive spirometers, take one home and continue to use it several times a day, especially if you're taking narcotic medication to relieve pain, because this can depress respirations.
• Be sure to take medications as prescribed by the doctor. Medications usually include pain medication, such as Tylenol with or without codeine. (Pulmonary drugs and antibiotics may be ordered as indicated by the patient's history or complications.)

Note: Oxygen is rarely used at home after thoracic surgery, because patients who are ill enough to require oxygen at home are not usually surgical candidates.
• Be sure to maintain a generous fluid intake at home (unless you have a heart or kidney disorder). Stop smoking and discourage smoking by others living in the house.
• Make and keep follow-up appointments with the thoracic surgeon and your family doctor shortly after discharge. If the diagnosis was lung cancer, an appointment will be scheduled with an oncologist and arrangements made for follow-up chemotherapy or radiation therapy, if needed. Call the doctor immediately if you develop severe shortness of breath, sudden difficulty swallowing, sharp chest pain, or if you cough up blood.

Evaluate the patient's knowledge of these discharge instructions. If possible, include his spouse or partner in teaching sessions.

Chest tube insertion

Description

The pleural space normally contains a thin layer of lubricating fluid that allows frictionless lung movement during respiration. Excess fluid, air, or both in this space alters intrapleural pressure and causes partial or complete lung collapse.

Chest tube insertion is indicated for patients with pneumothorax, hemothorax, empyema, pleural effusion, and chylothorax. Performed by a doctor or physician's assistant with a nurse assisting, this procedure requires sterile technique. The insertion site varies, depending on the patient's condition and the doctor's judgment. For a pneumothorax, the usual site is the anterior chest on the midclavicular line, at the second or third intercostal space, because air rises to the top of the intrapleural space. For a hemothorax or pleural effusion, the tube is placed lower in the chest, on the midaxillary line at the fourth to sixth intercostal space, because fluid settles to lower levels of the intrapleural space. For removal of both air and fluid, a chest tube is inserted into both a high and a low site.

After insertion, the chest tube is connected to a thoracic drainage system that provides for drainage of air or fluid out of the pleural space and prevents backflow into that space, thereby promoting lung reexpansion.

Purpose
• To drain air, blood, fluid, or pus from the pleural space
• To reestablish atmospheric and intrathoracic pressure gradients
• To allow complete lung reexpansion

Procedure
• Explain the procedure to the patient and answer his questions. Reassure him that it will help him breathe more easily.
• Record baseline vital signs.
• Gather the necessary equipment: a chest tube insertion tray, a chest tube (if it's not included in the tray), a local anesthetic (usually lidocaine) with needles and syringes, an antiseptic (usually povidone-iodine), sterile suture mate-

rial, petrolatum gauze, dressing sponges and tapes, and sterile gloves. Place the equipment in the patient's room.
• Set up the thoracic drainage system so that it's ready for use, and place it next to the patient's bed so that it will be below chest level to facilitate drainage.
• Administer any ordered medications—usually an analgesic, and, for some patients, a tranquilizer or sedative.
• Position the patient in semi-Fowler's to high Fowler's position for tube insertion into the second or third intercostal space; or in high Fowler's position for tube insertion into the fourth or sixth intercostal space, if the patient's condition permits this position.
• Assist in preparing the patient's skin with povidone-iodine solution.
• Drape the area with sterile towels.
• The doctor will anesthetize the skin area where he plans to insert the tube. Help the patient hold still while the doctor makes a skin incision (directly over the rib) and inserts the tube. He then dissects up and over the rib in an angular pattern much like a Z-track injection technique. This allows the hole to seal when the tube is removed.
• Reassure the patient that the considerable pressure he feels as the doctor advances the tube through the muscle and pleura will last only a short time.
• After insertion, immediately connect the chest tube to the thoracic drainage system or momentarily clamp the tube close to the patient's chest until it can be connected to the drainage system.
• The doctor may then suture the tube to the chest wall to minimize the risk of displacement.
• Petrolatum gauze is then wrapped around the insertion site, and a dry, sterile occlusive dressing is applied.
• Tape all tube connections securely to prevent separation.
• Tape the dressings, covering them completely. Make sure the dressing is airtight so that air can't be drawn into the pleural space around the insertion site.

• Tape the chest tube to the patient's chest distal to the insertion site to help prevent accidental tube dislodgment.

• Coil the drainage tubing and secure it to the bed linen with tape and a safety pin, providing enough slack for the patient to move and turn. This prevents the drainage tubing from kinking or dropping to the floor, which would impair drainage into the drainage bottle, and also helps prevent accidental tube dislodgment.

• Immediately after the chest tube is inserted and all connections are made, instruct the patient to take a deep breath, hold it momentarily, and slowly exhale to assist drainage of the pleural space and lung reexpansion.

• After tube insertion, a portable chest X-ray is taken to check tube position.

• Take the patient's vital signs every 15 minutes for the first hour, then every hour for 2 hours or as ordered. Auscultate his lungs at least every 4 hours to assess air exchange in the affected lung. Diminished or absent breath sounds indicate that the lung hasn't reexpanded.

Clinical considerations

Despite analgesia and anesthetization of the insertion site, chest tube insertion is still painful (mainly because it's hard to anesthetize the pleura adequately). So be sure to provide emotional support throughout the procedure.

Place rubber-tipped clamps or special tubing clamps at the bedside to clamp the chest tube in case of bottle breakage, cracking of a commercially prepared system, or tubing disconnection. You may wrap a piece of petrolatum gauze around the chest tube at the insertion site to make an airtight seal.

If the chest tube comes out or becomes dislodged, take immediate action. Call for help and ask whoever responds to notify the patient's doctor at once. Replace the patient's oxygen mask. Tell him that you know he's having trouble breathing and that you've called for his doctor. Obtain sterile petrolatum gauze and place it over the chest tube insertion site to form an airtight seal. Apply firm pressure with your hand. Have another nurse reassess the patient's vital signs and make sure that an I.V. site is available for administration of an antiarrhythmic or vasopressor, if needed. As you maintain pressure, have someone obtain supplies that the doctor may need: a chest tube, a chest tube insertion tray or suture tray, sterile gloves and towels, antiseptic skin solution, a local anesthetic, silk suture (if it's not in the tray), and an arterial blood gas (ABG) kit.

When the doctor arrives, describe the patient's condition to him. As he inserts the new chest tube, assist as necessary, maintaining a sterile field. Monitor the patient's vital signs, staying especially alert for an irregular pulse rate and falling blood pressure.

Once the tube is in place, continue to monitor the patient's vital signs and check to see that he's breathing more easily. Call the radiology department for a stat portable chest X-ray to confirm the tube's position. Draw a blood specimen for ABG analysis 30 to 45 minutes after the new tube is inserted, if the patient's condition has deteriorated. Make sure the doctor gets both the X-ray and ABG results at once. He may need to reposition the chest tube if the X-ray shows incomplete reexpansion of the middle and lower lung lobes. He also may want to reassess ABG levels if the patient remains hypoxic despite insertion of the new tube.

Reassure the patient that his breathing will become easier. Remember, he's probably exhausted and frightened. Make him as comfortable as possible, and answer his and his family's questions.

In some cases, the patient does well after the chest tube is dislodged, and reinsertion is unnecessary. Instead, a dressing is applied and the patient is monitored carefully. In many cases, however, the doctor must insert a new tube without delay to allow the patient to breathe more easily.

With some patients, chest tube dislodgment leads to collapse of the affected lung from lack of negative pressure in the pleural space; the PaO_2 level then falls drastically while the $PaCO_2$ level rises. Bleeding also may occur. These problems can lead to dysrhythmias, shock, and cardiopulmonary arrest. The longer the chest tube remains dislodged, the more serious the patient's condition is.

If a chest tube dressing must be replaced, wrap the chest tube with petrolatum gauze where the skin meets the chest tube. Then cover the petrolatum gauze with gauze pads that contain a slit designed for tracheostomy dressings; the slit in the tracheostomy dressing is placed around the chest tube. Next, cover with 4″ x 4″ gauze squares and an occlusive tape dressing.

Monitor the chest tube for patency and drainage. It should remain unclamped until removal is planned; then it will be clamped to test how well the patient will tolerate tube removal. Monitor the chest tube drainage device for air leaks and for type and amount of drainage. (See "Closed chest drainage" below.)

Complications
- Bleeding from intercostal blood vessels at the tube insertion site
- Pulmonary laceration
- Tube mistakenly placed in the lung instead of the pleural space
- Persistent pneumothorax from improper tube position

Closed chest drainage
(thoracic drainage, underwater seal drainage)

Description
Because negative pressure within the pleural cavity exerts a suction force that keeps the lungs expanded, chest trauma that disrupts this pressure may cause lung collapse. Consequently, after chest trauma, one or more chest tubes may be inserted surgically, then connected to a closed chest drainage system.

Closed chest drainage uses gravity and sometimes suction to restore negative pressure and remove any material collected in the pleural cavity. An underwater seal in the drainage system allows air and fluid to escape from the pleural cavity but prevents air from reentering.

Types of thoracic drainage systems include the one-bottle, two-bottle, and three-bottle systems, as well as commercially prepared systems, such as the Pleur-evac, Thora-Drain III, and Argyle systems. A popular commercial unit, the Pleur-evac is described in *Anatomy of a Pleur-evac*, pages 334 and 335. The other commercial units, although similar to the Pleur-evac, usually have one or more distinguishing features. The Thora-Drain III system has a replaceable collection chamber. When the chamber fills with drainage, you simply change it—without replacing the entire system. The Argyle Double Seal unit has a fourth chamber, an additional water seal that's vented to the atmosphere to prevent possible pressure buildup.

The one-bottle and two-bottle systems are primarily gravity systems, whereas the three-bottle and commercially prepared systems also provide for suction, which may be applied through a specifically regulated suction machine or by addition of a suction-control bottle or chamber. A one-way valve that can be used for chest drainage in an emergency also is available. (See *Heimlich Flutter Valve*, page 330.)

Purpose
- To remove accumulated air, fluids (blood, pus, chyle, serous fluids, gastric juice), or solids (blood clots) from the pleural cavity
- To restore negative pressure in the pleural cavity
- To reexpand a partially or totally collapsed lung

Heimlich Flutter Valve

During World War I, military medical personnel created makeshift one-way valves to apply to chest tubes under combat conditions, which made the traditional three-bottle system impractical. Similar devices were improvised during World War II. In the 1960s, Dr. Henry Heimlich introduced a small plastic portable one-way valve for chest drainage (Heimlich is better known as the originator of the abdominal thrust that has saved the lives of many choking victims). The Heimlich valve was used extensively during the Vietnam War, when it proved to be a lifesaving device.

Today, many communities have sophisticated emergency trauma teams that can rush to the scene of an accident by ambulance or helicopter. The Heimlich valve, vital for these teams, allows safe chest drainage during transport.

The device consists of a flutter valve, essentially a length of rubber tubing flattened at one end. The valve lets air or fluid pass in one direction only, preventing it from reentering the chest. A plastic cylinder encases the valve, primarily to protect it from external compression and occlusion. If the cylinder should crack or break during transport, the flutter valve still works.

When using a Heimlich valve, be sure to maintain sterile conditions. Connect the proximal blue end of the valve to the chest tube. Make sure the connection is airtight, then tape it to prevent it from dislodging. In an emergency, you may leave the distal end open if only air is being evacuated. However, because this may compromise sterility, it's better to connect the distal end to some sort of drainage bag (a sterile glove will do nicely), especially when blood is draining. The drainage bag must be vented so that air exiting the chest won't get trapped in the drainage bag.

In some hospitals, the Heimlich valve is used in treating spontaneous pneumothorax. Because only air is draining, the small portable device allows more freedom of movement.

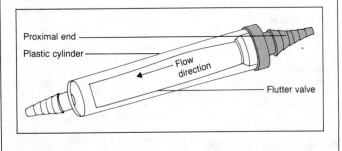

Proximal end
Plastic cylinder
Flow direction
Flutter valve

Procedure
• Explain the procedure to the patient, and wash your hands.
• Maintain sterile technique throughout the entire procedure when making a change in the system or altering any connections, to avoid introducing pathogens into the pleural space.

To set up the Pleur-evac, Thora-Drain III, and Argyle systems
• Assemble the necessary equipment. Read the manufacturers' instructions for other equipment needed and assembly directions. Usually, the system requires only a 50-ml catheter-tip syringe (for the Argyle system), sterile distilled water or normal sterile saline

solution (depending on hospital policy), two rubber-tipped Kelly clamps, and adhesive tape, besides the packaged unit.

• Open the packaged unit and place it on the floor in the rack supplied by the manufacturer to avoid accidentally knocking it over or dislodging the components. After it's prepared, it may be hung from the side of the patient's bed.

• Remove the plastic connector from the short tube attached to the water-seal chamber. Using a 50-ml catheter-tip syringe, instill sterile distilled water or normal saline solution into the water-seal chamber until it reaches the 2-cm mark. Replace the plastic connector. For the Argyle system, fill both water-seal chambers and replace the plastic connector. With the Thora-Drain III system, you can pour the fluid directly into the chambers. A syringe isn't necessary.

• If suction is ordered, remove the cap (muffler, atmospheric vent cover) on the suction-control chamber to open the vent. Next, if necessary, using the syringe, instill sterile distilled water or normal saline solution to the 20-cm mark or the ordered level and recap the suction-control chamber.

• Clamp the chest tube with the padded Kelly clamps and, if necessary, take the protective cover off the distal end of the tube.

• Using the long tube, connect the chest tube to the closed drainage collection chamber. Maintain sterile technique when making this connection. Secure the connection with tape.

• Connect the short tube on the drainage system to the suction source.

• Remove the padded Kelly clamps, and tape the junction of the latex tubing and the chest tube to secure it.

• Turn on the suction device. Mild, continuous bubbling should begin in the suction chamber, indicating that the correct suction level has been reached. Keep the bubbling as low as

possible. A vigorously bubbling drainage system may be surprisingly loud and could disturb the patient and hasten fluid evaporation; it's also unnecessary unless the patient has a large pleural air leak. Keep in mind that vigorous bubbling doesn't mean increased suction. The amount of water in the suction-control chamber determines the amount of negativity in the pleural space.

To set up any bottle system
• Fill the water-seal bottle with approximately 300 ml of sterile distilled water. Put a stopper on the bottle, and make sure that the long straw (water-seal straw) is submerged approximately ¾″ (2 cm) to create the water seal.

• If you're using a suction-control bottle, add sterile distilled water to this bottle until the long straw is submerged to the ordered length. If you're using a drainage collection bottle, no special preparation is needed; this bottle has a rubber stopper with two short straws already in place.

• Place the bottle(s) in a rack on the floor beside the patient's bed to avoid spills or breakage.

• Keep the bottle(s) below the level of the patient's chest to avoid introducing liquid into the pleural space.

• Use the clear plastic tubing to make the necessary connections, including suction, if ordered. Attach the tubing to the patient's chest tube, securely taping all connections. Turn on the suction, as ordered. (See *Underwater Seal Drainage Systems*, pages 332 and 333, for illustrations and further explanation of the bottle system.)

• Place a strip of adhesive tape vertically on the drainage collection bottle; the fluid level should be recorded here at the end of each shift. In the one-bottle or the two-bottle system (when the second bottle's used as the suction-control bottle), mark the original fluid level.

Underwater Seal Drainage Systems

The *one-bottle system*, below left, is the simplest underwater seal drainage system. The drainage tubing leads to a single 2-liter bottle that serves as both a collection container and a water seal. The bottle has a rubber stopper with two holes in which glass straws can be placed. The short straw acts as an air vent to equalize pressure between the air space of the bottle and the atmosphere. The long straw is attached to tubing leading to the patient for drainage.

The bottle is filled with about 300 ml of sterile water; the long straw rests about ¾" (2 cm) below water level, which rises with inhalation and falls with expiration. This creates a water seal that prevents air from reentering the chest while allowing expulsion of drainage. However, because water and drainage share the same bottle, a continuous fluid increase eventually reduces the system's effectiveness by creating resistance to further drainage.

In the *two-bottle system*, below right, liquid drainage falls through a short straw into the collection bottle and air flows beyond into the water-seal bottle. The bottle's stopper has two holes. One hole holds a long submerged

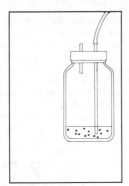

One-bottle system

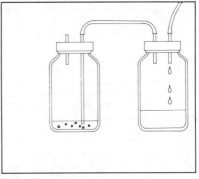

Two-bottle system

Clinical considerations

When caring for the patient with a closed-chest underwater-seal drainage system:

• Check the water-seal chamber for bubbling. Bubbles here indicate entry of air. This is expected if the patient has a pneumothorax (because air is being drained from the pleural cavity). However, if the patient doesn't have a pneumothorax, bubbling could indicate a leak in the tubing between the pleural cavity and the unit, or even a crack in the unit itself. Bubbling that begins or

ends suddenly is always important and requires immediate intervention. (See *Troubleshooting Chest Drainage Systems*, pages 336 and 337.)

• As the patient breathes, check for fluctuation in fluid line of the water-seal straw in the bottle system or the water-seal chamber of a commercially prepared system. Normal fluctuations of 2" to 4" (5 to 10 cm) reflect pressure changes in the pleural space during respiration. With spontaneous breathing, the water level increases with inspiration and decreases with expiration. With mechanical ventilation, the opposite oc-

straw that creates the water seal; a second hole holds a short straw, which further functions as the air vent. This set-up keeps the water seal at a fixed level, allowing more accurate observation of the volume and type of drainage. However, this system sometimes doesn't supply sufficient suction. If suction is ordered and you're using a suction source with built-in controls, make the connection at the vent stem of the water-seal bottle. Remember, some two-bottle systems don't have a separate collection bottle. In such systems, the second bottle serves as the vacuum-control bottle and the first bottle as both the water-seal and drainage collection bottle.

The *three-bottle system*, illustrated below, adds a suction control bottle between the water seal and suction source. This additional bottle has a long straw in it with the upper end open to the atmosphere, providing another site where air can enter, and the lower end submerged under sterile saline solution. The approximate amount of suction that can be exerted on the drainage system depends on the depth of a submerged control straw.

Commercial chest drainage units duplicate or modify the bottle systems.

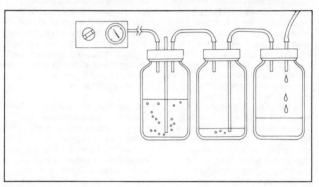

Three-bottle system

curs—the water level decreases with inspiration and increases with expiration. With a suction system, the fluid line in the water-seal straw should remain constant. To check for fluctuation, momentarily disconnect the suction system so that the air vent opens and observe for fluctuation.

• Make sure the water in the suction-control chamber bubbles gently. You may want to turn down the suction so that bubbles disappear momentarily, then slowly turn it back up until the bubbles begin to reappear.

• Check the water level in the water-seal chamber or bottle every 8 hours. If necessary, using aseptic technique, carefully add sterile distilled water or normal saline solution, as appropriate, until water reaches the 2-cm level indicated on the water-seal chamber of a commercially prepared system.

• Mark the drainage level in the collection chamber or bottle with the date and time when the collection begins and then every 8 hours, or more often if a large amount of drainage exists. Keep in mind how much drainage to expect. If you don't know how much to expect, check

Anatomy of a Pleur-evac

A one-piece, disposable, molded plastic unit, the Pleur-evac consists of three chambers that duplicate the classic three-bottle system (see illustration). Special features include a positive-pressure relief valve that prevents possible pressure buildup in the pleural space; a high negativity relief valve; and a high negativity float valve, which maintains the water seal even with high negative intrathoracic pressures.

Collection chamber
The Pleur-evac's drainage collection chamber, located on the right, has three calibrated columns showing how much drainage has been collected. When the first column fills, it overflows into the second, which eventually overflows into the third; together, the columns have a capacity of approximately 2,500 ml. On the right of each calibrated column, you may mark the drainage level with the date and time.

By using resealable diaphragms on the back of the collection chamber, you can withdraw a drainage sample for analysis without disrupting the system. Remember to clean the diaphragm with an antiseptic solution (such as povidone-iodine) before puncturing it to obtain the sample.

A high negativity relief valve located over the collection chamber on the back of the unit permits venting of excess negative pressure (indicated by a rising water level in the water-seal chamber), which can occur with chest tube milking and stripping and increased respiratory effort.

Water-seal chamber
The unit's middle compartment is the water-seal chamber. The stan-dard water-seal level (2 cmH$_2$O) is marked at the bottom of this chamber. With a higher water-seal level, more pressure would be needed to push air through the water. (For the same reason, you can blow bubbles through a straw in a quarter-filled glass of water more easily than through a full glass.)

At the top of the water-seal chamber, you'll find a positive-pressure relief valve. This relief valve vents excess pressure into the atmosphere, preventing pressure buildup. The risk of pneumothorax is minimized if the tubing between the Pleur-evac and the pleural space is patent. (The water-seal chamber also has a special float valve at the top that maintains the water seal even in the event of high negative intrapleural pressure, such as from the deep breath taken with vigorous coughing, especially during endotracheal suctioning.)

Suction-control chamber
Located on the left, the suction-control chamber has a clearly marked water-level line. You may fill it to various suction levels, according to doctor's orders or hospital policy. A rubber diaphragm on the back of this chamber allows you to add water to replace what's been lost through evaporation or to remove water if the chamber's overfilled. Remember that increased bubbling in the chamber causes the water to evaporate faster; as the water level drops, the amount of suction transmitted to the pleural cavity decreases.

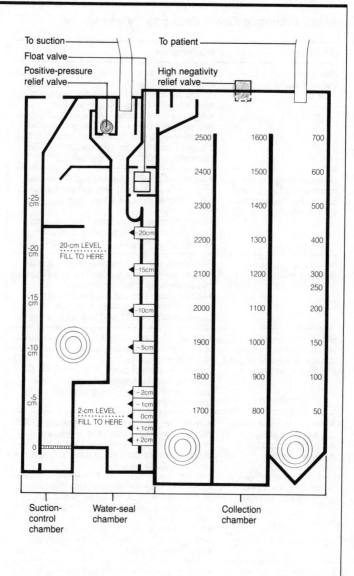

Troubleshooting Chest Drainage Systems

Situation	Intervention
Patient rolls over onto drainage tubing, causing obstruction.	• If only air is being drained, coil tubing and pin it to drawsheet. If fluid is being drained, keep tubing straight. Leave enough room for patient to move in bed, but keep tubing in sight. • Assess patient to determine whether air or fluid has reaccumulated in pleural cavity. Auscultate for decreased breath sounds, and percuss for dullness (indicating fluid accumulation) or hyper-resonance (indicating air accumulation).
Dependent loops in tubing trap draining fluid, possibly causing fluid accumulation in pleural cavity.	• Make sure unit is below chest level. If necessary, raise bed (keeping side rails up) and put unit on floor to increase gravity drainage. Keep tubing straight. • Monitor patient for decreased breath sounds, indicating possible pleural fluid accumulation. Percuss for dullness.
No drainage appears in collection chamber.	• If blood or fluid is being drained, suspect clot or other obstruction in tubing. If permitted, gently milk tubing to try to expel obstruction. • Monitor patient for compression of lung tissue by accumulated pleural fluid. Auscultate for decreased breath sounds, and percuss for dullness.
Substantial increase in bloody drainage indicates possible active bleeding or drainage of old blood.	• Monitor vital signs. Check for increased pulse rate and decreased blood pressure, possibly indicating acute blood loss. • Measure drainage every 15 to 30 minutes to see if it occurs continuously or in just a single gush caused by patient changing position or by postural drainage.
Water in water-seal chamber fluctuates, rising during inspiration and falling during expiration.	• None. This reflects normal pressure changes in pleural cavity during respiration. It indicates pneumothorax has been drained and chest tube possibly could be removed (if there is no substantial fluid drainage).
No bubbling occurs in suction-control chamber.	• Check tubing from suction-control chamber back to suction regulator. Tubing should be free of obstructions, and all connections should be tight. • Make sure wall suction is turned on. Increase suction slowly until you see gentle bubbling in suction-control chamber.
Loud, vigorous bubbling occurs in suction-control chamber.	• Turn down suction source until bubbling stops in suction-control chamber. Then gradually increase until bubbling is just visible.

Troubleshooting Chest Drainage Systems (continued)

Situation	Intervention
Evaporation causes water level in suction-control chamber to drop below desired level (20 cmH$_2$O).	• Add water or saline solution, using syringe and needle through resealable diaphragm on back of suction-control chamber.
Patient returns from special procedure. Chest drainage unit is placed on bed between patient's legs. Patient complains of difficulty breathing.	• Reposition unit to allow for proper gravity drainage, and raise head of bed. • Perform a quick respiratory assessment, and take vital signs. Improper positioning of unit may have disrupted water seal, allowing air to accumulate in pleural cavity. Check unit to make sure water-seal and suction chambers contain adequate water. • Inform person who put unit on bed that unit should always be positioned below chest tube insertion site.
As bed is lowered, unit gets caught under bed. Tubing comes apart on floor and becomes contaminated, allowing air to be drawn into pleural space through disconnected tubing.	• Open sealed jar of sterile water or saline solution for irrigation (this should be kept at patient's bedside). • Insert uncontaminated end of chest tube into jar to level of 2 to 4 cm, creating emergency water seal while another caregiver sets up new unit.

the report from the previous shift and the patient's chart; you also can check the X-ray reports.

• Periodically note the character, consistency, and amount of drainage in the collection chamber or bottle.

• Check the water level in the suction-control chamber or bottle periodically. Detach the chamber or bottle from the suction source; when bubbling stops, observe the water level. If necessary, add sterile distilled water to bring the level to the 20-cm line, or as ordered.

• Make sure the connections between chest tube and drainage tubing and between suction tubing and short latex tubing are tight and wrapped with adhesive tape.

• Check dressing to make sure it's clean, dry, intact, covered with adhesive tape, and airtight. Don't remove the dressing unless the chest tube has moved or fluid is leaking around the insertion site and soiling the dressing. If you suspect a leak beneath the dressing or an infection at the insertion site, remove the dressing and assess further if policy permits.

• Periodically check to make sure the unit's air vent isn't occluded. Occlusion results in pressure buildup that could lead to a tension pneumothorax. (Some commercial drainage systems, such as Pleur-evac, have pressure-relief valves to prevent pressure buildup.)

• Coil the unit's tubing and secure it to the edge of the bed with a rubber band or tape and a safety pin. Avoid creating dependent loops, kinks, or pressure on the tubing, as these may interfere with chest drainage.

• Avoid lifting drainage bottles above the patient's chest, as this may cause backflow of fluid into the pleural space.

• Make sure two rubber-tipped clamps are at the bedside. Use these to clamp the chest tube if a bottle breaks or a commercial unit cracks, or to locate air leaks.

• Encourage the patient to cough frequently and breathe deeply to help drain the pleural space and expand the lungs.

• Instruct the patient to sit upright for optimal lung expansion and to splint the chest tube insertion site while coughing, to minimize pain.

• Check the patient's respiratory rate and quality, and percuss and auscultate his lungs periodically to assess air exchange in the affected lung. If the chest tube is used to drain fluid, listen for a dull percussion note, indicating fluid accumulation in the chest. (Use chest X-rays as a guide to the appropriate area to percuss.) A dull percussion note could mean that all fluid hasn't drained yet. Some fluid may be loculated—walled off in a chest region that the tube can't reach. Or the patient may need to change his position to promote gravity drainage. If he had a pneumothorax, listen for a distinctly hollow percussion note that could mean air has accumulated again in the pleural cavity.

• When you auscultate, remember that decreased breath sounds may indicate air or fluid between your stethoscope and the lung. If you have trouble hearing breath sounds (the bubbling sounds from the unit can be transmitted to the patient's chest), turn off the suction to the unit for a minute or two.

• Notify the doctor at once if the patient develops cyanosis; rapid, shallow breathing; subcutaneous emphysema; chest pain; or excessive bleeding.

• Tell the patient to report any breathing difficulty immediately.

• Stripping and milking of chest tubes, especially stripping, can be hazardous. (Milking is considered gentle.) Both techniques involve manually compressing the drainage tubing between the chest tube and the unit, then releasing it. This creates suction through the tube back to the pleural space. Negative pressures as high as -350 cmH$_2$O may occur with stripping.

• If hospital policy permits, consider stripping or milking a chest tube only when you detect fresh bleeding with visible clots in the tubing and a dramatic decrease in drainage. Even then, use caution, especially if the patient has weak, friable lung tissue. The high negative pressure can suck lung tissue into the chest tube's drainage holes, rupture alveoli, and cause a pleural air leak. (If the unit is draining air only, stripping and milking aren't necessary because an obstruction from a blood clot can't occur.)

• Encourage active or passive range-of-motion exercises of the arm on the affected side if the patient has been splinting that arm. (Usually, the thoracotomy patient splints his arm to relieve discomfort.)

• Give ordered pain medication to increase patient comfort and to make deep breathing, coughing, and range-of-motion exercises easier.

• Remind the ambulatory patient to keep the bottles below chest level and to be careful not to disconnect the tubing because this will disrupt the water seal. With a suction system, the patient must stay within the range of the tubing length attached to a wall outlet or portable pump.

• Instruct staff and visitors to avoid touching the equipment to prevent complications from separated connections and bottle misplacement or breakage.

• If the drainage collection bottle or chamber fills, replace the bottle or the commercial unit. To do this, double-clamp the tube close to the insertion site (use two clamps facing in opposite directions), exchange the bottle or system, remove the clamps, and retape the bottle connection. Never leave the tubes clamped for more than a minute or two to prevent a tension pneumo-

thorax, which may occur when clamping stops air and fluid from escaping.
• To replace the drainage chamber in the Thora-Drain III, obtain a Thora-Drain III replacement chamber and remove it from its sterile package. (*Note:* If required by hospital policy, double-clamp the chest tube close to the insertion site before replacing the chamber.)

Then twist the collection chamber to the left to loosen it. Remove the replacement chamber's cap. Position the chamber in the empty space, and turn it to the left; lock it in place by turning it to the right. (If you clamped the chest tube, remove the clamps now.)

Next, replace the filled collection chamber's cap. Note the drainage amount, color, and consistency before discarding it, and document your findings. To reduce the suction level in the Thora-Drain III, first discontinue the suction. Then, remove the suction chamber, rotating it to the left. Adjust the fluid level and replace the chamber, snapping it in place to the right. Reconnect the suction.
• If a bottle breaks or a commercial unit cracks, clamp the chest tube with two rubber-tipped clamps kept at the bedside. Place the clamps close to each other near the insertion site, facing in opposite directions to provide a more complete seal. Stay with the patient and observe for altered respirations while another staff member brings replacement equipment. If the patient develops respiratory distress, unclamp the chest tube and continue to monitor respiratory status (rate, quality, and depth of respirations and breath sounds). Submerge the tube's distal end in a container of sterile normal saline solution or sterile distilled water, if available, to create a temporary water seal while you replace the bottle.

Complications
The most serious complication of chest tube drainage is tension pneumothorax—air under pressure within the pleural cavity. In this life-threatening complication, pressure that's gen-

erated compresses the soft tissues within the chest—not only the lungs but also the heart and great vessels. The entire mediastinum may be compressed if enough pressure builds within the pleural cavity, severely impairing venous return. As a result, the patient's cardiac output and blood pressure drop quickly.

The patient most likely to develop tension pneumothorax is one with a closed pneumothorax who's receiving positive-pressure mechanical ventilation. Positive pressure forces air into the pleural cavity on the affected side. The pneumothorax size, determined by the amount of air between the pleurae, can increase dramatically within minutes.

The following may indicate a developing tension pneumothorax:
• Repeated soundings of the high-pressure alarm, if the patient is on a ventilator. Also, the manometer on the front of the ventilator will register high pressure and won't return to the zero baseline at the end of exhalation.
• The affected chest side will look inflated and won't move up and down with respiration; it is hyperresonant on percussion.
• If the tension pneumothorax is severe enough to cause a mediastinal shift away from the affected side, you may detect it by palpating the trachea above the sternum. From its normal midline position directly above the sternum, the trachea shifts away from the affected side.
• On auscultation, you won't detect breath sounds on the affected side. (This occurs with any tension pneumothorax, not just one that is severe enough to cause mediastinal shift.)

If the patient develops any of these signs of tension pneumothorax, check the drainage tubing immediately to make sure that it's patent all the way from the chest to the unit. If the problem can't be corrected quickly, be prepared to assist the doctor with needle thoracostomy or insertion of another chest tube. Monitor the patient's vital signs frequently, checking for decreased blood pressure and a rapid, thready pulse. If necessary, call a code.

To prevent tension pneumothorax, be meticulous about keeping drainage tubing obstruction-free. If an air leak has been documented, don't clamp the chest tube and drainage tubing (except momentarily to assess the source of an air leak).

Chest tube removal

Description

Chest tube removal usually is performed by a doctor with a nurse assisting. Because prolonged intubation invites infection along the chest tube tract, the tube is removed when air or fluid drainage stops and the tube is no longer needed. Once a chest X-ray confirms full lung expansion, the tube is clamped with large, smooth, rubber-tipped clamps for up to 24 hours before removal. This allows time to observe the patient for signs of respiratory distress, an indication that air or fluid is collecting in the pleural space. A chest X-ray usually is taken about 2 hours after clamping; if the patient develops respiratory distress or the X-ray reveals recurrent pneumothorax, the tube clamps should be removed immediately. A chest X-ray is taken again after chest tube removal to confirm full lung expansion.

Chest tube removal is contraindicated when an X-ray shows incomplete lung expansion or when clamping induces respiratory distress.

Purpose

To remove a chest tube from the pleural space without introducing air or infectious microorganisms

Procedure

• Assess the depth and quality of the patient's respirations, and obtain baseline vital signs.

• Explain the procedure to the patient. Administer an analgesic, as ordered, 30 minutes before tube removal.

• Assemble all supplies at the patient's bedside—sterile gloves, sterile petrolatum gauze, sterile 4″ x 4″ gauze sponges, 2″ to 3″ (5 to 7.5 cm) wide adhesive or nonallergenic tape, and a linen-saver pad, as well as dressing removal supplies and, if indicated, a suture removal kit.

• Cut three 6″ (15-cm) strips of adhesive tape (or nonallergenic tape, if patient is allergic to adhesive). Open the sterile packages and create a sterile field. Maintaining sterile technique, drop the sterile petrolatum gauze on a sterile gauze sponge for use as an airtight dressing.

• Place the patient in semi-Fowler's position or on his unaffected side.

• Place the linen-saver pad under the patient's affected side to protect linen from drainage and to provide a place to put the chest tube after removal.

• Put on sterile gloves and remove the chest tube dressings, taking care not to dislodge the chest tube. Discard soiled dressings in the waterproof trash bag.

• The doctor puts on sterile gloves, then holds the chest tube in place with sterile forceps and cuts the suture anchoring the tube.

• Make sure that the chest tube is clamped securely; then instruct the patient to inhale fully, hold his breath, and grunt (Valsalva's maneuver). This causes slight exhalation against a closed glottis, which increases intrapulmonary pressure and prevents air from being sucked into the pleural space during tube removal.

• The doctor picks up the airtight dressing, then removes the chest tube and immediately covers the insertion site with the dressing.

• Secure the dressing with tape strips. Be sure to cover the dressing completely with the tape to make it as airtight as possible.

• Properly dispose of the chest tube, soiled gloves, and equipment, according to hospital policy.

• Take vital signs, as ordered, and assess the depth and quality of the patient's respirations.

• For the first few hours after chest tube removal, check the dressing site for sounds of air leakage and observe the patient closely for evidence of complications, such as recurrent pneumothorax, or subcutaneous emphysema. Signs and symptoms of pneumothorax include dyspnea, chest pain, tachycardia, cyanosis, restlessness, and absent breath sounds in the affected area. Pneumothorax may result from an ineffective seal at the chest tube insertion site or from the underlying disease. Subcutaneous emphysema is indicated by a crackling sound when you palpate the area around the wound. It results from a poor seal at the insertion site.

Clinical considerations
If the doctor requests culturing of the chest tube, he'll hold it as you obtain a swab specimen from inside the tube.

Complications
Recurrent pneumothorax, subcutaneous emphysema, or infection may result from chest tube removal.

Autotransfusion

Description
Autotransfusion is the collection, filtration, and reinfusion of the patient's own blood. Currently used primarily in patients with chest wounds or during or after chest surgery, autotransfusion is indicated when at least 2 or 3 units of blood can be salvaged.

Relative contraindications include malignant tumors; intrathoracic, pulmonary, or systemic infection or infestation; coagulopathies; enteric contamination; and excessive hemolysis. It's also contraindicated when a topical antibiotic not suitable for I.V. infusion, such as povidone-iodine, was used at the site. However, the doctor must weigh the risk of the potential contraindication against the likelihood of death from exsanguination.

Autotransfusion may be ordered instead of a stored blood transfusion because it:

• eliminates the risk of transfusion reaction

• eliminates the risk of transmission of such diseases as hepatitis and acquired immunodeficiency syndrome

• prevents recipient hypothermia because the blood is already warm

• avoids hypokalemia, hypocalcemia, and acidosis commonly associated with stored blood

• improves oxygen delivery to the tissues

• helps conserve banked blood.

Purpose
To replace blood loss immediately with compatible blood

Procedure
The procedure described below is used with Pleur-evac ATS, a widely used system made by the Deknatel Division of Pfizer Hospital Products Group, Inc.

• Set up the underwater seal drainage system for the Pleur-evac. Note that, with the ATS unit, a small latex tube connects the collection chamber to one side of the ATS bag, and the traditional 6′ latex patient tube is connected to the other side of the ATS bag with color-coded connectors.

• Connect the 6′ tubing to the chest tube, maintaining sterile technique.

• Make sure all connections are tight.

• Open all white tubing clamps.

• Observe the unit to ensure that blood from the chest cavity is flowing into the ATS collection bag.

• If ordered by the doctor, add citrate phosphate dextrose or heparin as an anticoagulant, using an 18G (or smaller) needle and injecting it through the small rubber diaphragm on the top of the ATS bag.

• When the bag is almost full, prepare the next bag by removing it from its packaging and closing the white tubing clamps. Remove the red and blue protective caps from the tubing on top of the new ATS bag.

• Before removing the initial bag for reinfusion, release any excess negative pressure in the system by depressing the button on the top of the high negativity relief valve, located at the top of the Pleur-evac collection chamber.

• Close the white clamp on the patient tubing and the two white clamps on top of the ATS bag.

• Disconnect the tubes from the top of the ATS bag, maintaining sterile technique.

• Attach the patient tubing with the red connector to the corresponding red connector on the new ATS bag.

• Connect the two blue tubing connectors, allowing the ATS bag to communicate with the Pleur-evac collection chamber.

• Open all the clamps, ensure airtight connections, and watch for blood to drain into the new ATS bag.

• Connect the blue (male) and red (female) connectors at the end of the tubes on the top of the original (full) ATS bag to make a closed loop.

• Spread and disconnect the metal support arms from the metal ATS bag stand, and remove the initial stand and bag by disconnecting them at the foot on the base of the Pleur-evac collection chamber.

• Attach the new ATS stand and bag by hooking the loop on the bottom of the metal stand around the foot on the base of the Pleur-evac collection chamber. Spread the metal support arms at the top of the metal stand.

• To reinfuse, slide the ATS bag off the metal stand and invert the bag.

• Remove the blue protective cap from the spike port now at the top of the ATS bag.

• Insert a microaggregate filter into the port, using a constant twisting motion.

• Prime the filter by gently squeezing the ATS bag. Continue squeezing until the filter is saturated with blood and the drip chamber is half full.

• Close the clamp on the reinfusion line, and remove residual air from the ATS bag.

• Invert the bag so that the latex tubing loop is at the top. Suspend the bag from an I.V. pole.

• Flush the tubing to remove all air, and infuse the blood according to hospital transfusion policy.

Note: For other autotransfusion procedures, consult the manufacturer's instructions.

Clinical considerations

Be sure to maintain sterile technique when changing an ATS bag and handling connectors, to prevent infection.

Check tubing clamps before disconnecting tubing to prevent air entry into the system and subsequent pneumothorax.

A microaggregate filter is recommended for use during blood reinfusion; a new filter should be used with each ATS bag.

Blood collected and stored for more than 4 hours should not be reinfused. Monitor the amount of blood collected and reinfused on appropriate intake and output flowsheets. Reinfuse bloody drainage only; if you detect any other material in the tubing or ATS bag, discard the drainage and don't use it for reinfusion. Never add blood collected via the ATS system to the donor blood supply; this blood can't be stored.

Use of anticoagulants remains controversial; some doctors believe that thoracic blood lacks fibrinogen and therefore won't clot. Anticoagulants should be added to the ATS bag only on the specific order of the doctor.

Complications

Autotransfusion can lead to air and particulate embolism; be especially cautious if no anticoagulants are used. To minimize the risk, check the entire system for air leaks before reinfusion. Always use in-line microaggregate filters. The doctor may consider administering corticosteroids when massive autotransfusion is performed.

Hemolysis may occur, usually from turbulent blood flow and high vacuum pressures. If a suction tip is used to remove blood into the ATS unit, keep it at the bottom of a pool of blood to minimize blood-air contact and try to limit suction pressure to 15 mm Hg. Other factors increasing the risk of hemolysis include acidosis, dehydration, and shock.

Thrombocytopenia with associated bleeding can occur if the patient receives more than 4,000 ml of blood via autotransfusion. (However, this complication is less common than with banked blood transfusions because some platelets remain viable). Transfusion of fresh platelets or fresh frozen plasma may be necessary.

Sepsis can occur if proper aseptic technique isn't followed during the entire autotransfusion procedure. Besides using meticulous technique, use in-line filters that can trap particulate contaminants. Don't use blood that may have been contaminated with enteric or infected pulmonary secretions. Administer broad-spectrum antibiotics, as ordered.

Selected References

Burton, G.G., and Hodgkin, J.E., eds. *Respiratory Care: A Guide to Clinical Practice*, 2nd ed. Philadelphia: J.B. Lippincott Co., 1984.

Carroll, P.F. "The Ins and Outs of Chest Drainage Systems," *Nursing86* 16(12):26-33, December 1986.

Emergency Care Handbook. Springhouse, Pa.: Springhouse Corp., 1986.

1987 Nursing Photobook Annual. Nursing Photobook series. Springhouse, Pa.: Springhouse Corp., 1987.

Phipps, W.J., et al. *Medical-Surgical Nursing: Concepts and Clinical Practice*, 3rd ed. St. Louis: C.V. Mosby Co., 1986.

Procedures. Nurse's Reference Library. Springhouse, Pa.: Springhouse Corp., 1983.

Quinn, A. "Thora-Drain III: Closed Chest Drainage Made Simpler and Safer," *Nursing86* 16(9):46-51, September 1986.

Respiratory Emergencies. NursingNow series. Springhouse, Pa.: Springhouse Corp., 1984.

Shapiro, B.A., et al. *Clinical Applications of Respiratory Care.* Chicago: Year Book Medical Pubs., 1985.

Thompson, J.M., et al. *Clinical Nursing.* St. Louis: C.V. Mosby Co., 1985.

White, R.C. "Action Stat! Dislodged Chest Tube," *Nursing85* 15(12):25, December 1985.

15 RESPIRATORY DRUG THERAPY

Introduction

This chapter covers many drugs used to alleviate the symptoms or to correct the cause of ventilatory dysfunction in patients with acute or chronic respiratory disease. In most cases, drugs have been classified according to their clinical use. Keep in mind that many of these drugs can be used for nonrespiratory indications.

Note: Many drugs used to treat other diseases may adversely influence ventilatory function. See Appendix 5 for a summary of these adverse effects.

Bronchodilators

Currently, three pharmacologically distinct classes of compounds are used as bronchodilators; each has a distinct mechanism of action.

Sympathomimetics (adrenergics)

These agents mimic or induce the release of naturally occurring sympathetic agonists: norepinephrine (found in sympathetic nerve terminals) or epinephrine (found in the adrenal medulla). The physiologic effects of sympathetic activation depend on the degree and site of stimulation.

Because neurochemists can synthesize compounds with relative target organ specificity, receptor subtypes in the sympathetic nervous system have been identified. Stimulation of alpha receptors in capillary blood vessels, the uterus, and sphincter muscles causes smooth muscle contraction, resulting in increased blood pressure, and uterine and sphincter contraction. Beta receptors fall into two groups: beta$_1$ receptors, located in the heart, which cause an increased heart rate (chronotropic effect) and increased force of contraction (inotropic effect) when stimulated; and beta$_2$ receptors, located primarily in the bronchi, skeletal muscles, blood vessels, and uterus, which are largely inhibitory. When activated, they cause bronchodilation, vasodilation, and uterine relaxation. Many beta$_2$ agonists can produce adverse effects because they excite beta$_1$ receptors (producing tachycardia).

albuterol
Proventil, Proventil Syrup, Ventolin

Mechanism of action
Relaxes bronchial smooth muscle by acting on beta$_2$-adrenergic receptors.

Respiratory indications and dosage
• To prevent and treat bronchospasm in patients with reversible obstructive airway disease—
Adults and children over age 13: 1 to 2 inhalations q 4 to 6 hours. Each metered dose delivers 90 mcg of albuterol. More frequent administration or a greater number of inhalations is not recommended. For oral tablets, 2 to 4 mg t.i.d. or q.i.d. Maximum dosage is 8 mg q.i.d.
Children age 6 to 13: 2 mg (1 teaspoonful) t.i.d. or q.i.d.

Children age 2 to 5: 0.1 mg/kg t.i.d., not to exceed 2 mg (1 teaspoonful) t.i.d. or q.i.d.

Adults over age 65: 2 mg t.i.d. or q.i.d.

• To prevent exercise-induced asthma—*Adults:* 2 inhalations 15 minutes before exercise.

Adverse reactions

CNS: tremor, nervousness, dizziness, insomnia, headache.

CV: tachycardia, palpitations, hypertension.

EENT: drying and irritation of nose and throat (with inhaled form).

GI: heartburn, nausea, vomiting.

Other: muscle cramps.

Interactions

Propranolol and other beta blockers: blocked bronchodilating effect of albuterol. Monitor patient carefully.

Clinical considerations

• Use cautiously in patients with cardiovascular disorders, including coronary insufficiency and hypertension; in patients with hyperthyroidism or diabetes mellitus; and in patients who are usually responsive to adrenergics. Cardiac arrest can occur.

• Warn patient about the possibility of paradoxical bronchospasm. If this occurs, the drug should be discontinued immediately.

• Patients may use tablets and aerosol concomitantly. Monitor closely for toxicity.

• Albuterol reportedly produces less cardiac stimulation than other sympathomimetics, especially isoproterenol.

• Elderly patients usually require a lower dose.

• Teach patient how to administer metered dose correctly. Have him shake container; exhale through nose; administer aerosol while inhaling deeply on mouthpiece of inhaler; and hold breath for a few seconds, then exhale slowly. Tell him to allow 2 minutes between inhalations.

• Pleasant-tasting syrup may be taken by children as young as age 2. Preparation contains no alcohol or sugar. Store drug in light-resistant container.

ephedrine sulfate

Mechanism of action

A direct- and indirect-acting sympathomimetic that stimulates alpha- and beta-adrenergic receptors.

Respiratory indications and dosage

• Bronchodilator or nasal decongestant—

Adults: 12.5 to 50 mg P.O. b.i.d., t.i.d., or q.i.d. Maximum dosage is 400 mg/day in six to eight divided doses.

Children: 2 to 3 mg/kg P.O. daily in four to six divided doses.

Adverse reactions

CNS: insomnia, nervousness, dizziness, headache, muscle weakness, sweating, euphoria, confusion, delirium.

CV: palpitations, tachycardia, hypertension.

EENT: dryness of nose and throat.

GI: nausea, vomiting, anorexia.

GU: urinary retention, painful urination from visceral sphincter spasm.

Interactions

Monoamine oxidase (MAO) inhibitors and tricyclic antidepressants: When given with sympathomimetics may cause severe hypertension (hypertensive crisis). Don't use together.

Methyldopa: may inhibit ephedrine's effect. Give together cautiously.

Clinical considerations

• Drug is contraindicated in patients with porphyria, severe coronary artery disease, cardiac dysrhythmias, narrow-angle glaucoma, and psychoneurosis; and in patients receiving MAO inhibitors. Use with caution in elderly patients and in patients with hypertension, hyperthyroidism, nervousness or excitability, cardiovascular disease, or prostatic hypertrophy.

• Give I.V. injection slowly.
• Check for signs of hypoxia, hypercapnia, and acidosis, which may reduce effectiveness or increase the incidence of adverse reactions. These conditions must be identified and corrected before or during ephedrine administration.
• Effectiveness decreases after 2 to 3 weeks, possibly necessitating increased dosage. Although tolerance develops, drug is not known to cause addiction.
• To prevent insomnia, avoid giving within 2 hours before bedtime.
• Warn patient not to take over-the-counter drugs containing ephedrine without doctor's approval.

epinephrine
Inhalants: Bronkaid Mist, Primatene Mist

epinephrine bitartrate
Adrenaline, Sus-Phrine

Mechanism of action
Stimulates alpha- and beta-adrenergic receptors within the sympathetic nervous system.

Respiratory indications and dosage
• Bronchospasm, hypersensitivity reactions, and anaphylaxis—
Adults: 0.1 to 0.5 ml (1:1,000) S.C. or I.M. Repeat q 10 to 15 minutes, p.r.n. Or 0.1 to 0.25 ml (1:1,000) I.V.
Children: 0.01 ml/kg (1:1,000) S.C. Repeat q 20 minutes to 4 hours, p.r.n. Or 0.005 ml/kg (1:200, Sus-Phrine). Repeat q 8 to 12 hours, p.r.n.
• Acute asthmatic attacks (inhalation)—
Adults and children: 1 or 2 inhalations of 1:100 or 2.25% racemic q 1 to 5 minutes until relief is obtained; 0.2 mg/dose is usual content.

Adverse reactions
CNS: nervousness, tremor, euphoria, anxiety, cold extremities, vertigo, headache, sweating, cerebral hemorrhage, disorientation, agitation; in patients with Parkinson's disease, the drug increases rigidity and tremor.
CV: palpitations, widened pulse pressure, hypertension, tachycardia, ventricular fibrillation, cerebrovascular accident, anginal pain, EKG changes (including decreased T-wave amplitude).
Metabolic: hyperglycemia, glycosuria.
Other: pulmonary edema, dyspnea, pallor.

Interactions
Tricyclic antidepressants: severe hypertension (hypertensive crisis). Don't give together.
Propranolol: vasoconstriction and reflex bradycardia. Monitor patient carefully.

Clinical considerations
• Drug is contraindicated in patients with narrow-angle glaucoma, shock (except anaphylactic shock), organic brain damage, cardiac dilation, and coronary insufficiency; during general anesthesia with halogenated hydrocarbons or cyclopropane; and in patients in labor (may delay second stage). Use with extreme caution in patients with longstanding bronchial asthma and emphysema who have developed degenerative heart disease. Use with caution in elderly patients and in patients with hyperthyroidism, angina, hypertension, psychoneurosis, and diabetes.
• Don't mix with alkaline solutions. Use dextrose 5% in water (D_5W), normal saline solution, or a combination of D_5W and normal saline solution. Mix just before use.
• Epinephrine is destroyed rapidly by oxidizing agents, such as iodine, chromates, nitrates, nitrites, oxygen, and salts of easily reducible metals (for example, iron).
• Epinephrine solutions deteriorate after 24 hours. Discard after that time or before if solution is discolored or contains precipitate. Keep solution in light-resistant container and don't remove before use.

• Massage site after injection to counteract possible vasoconstriction. Repeated local injection can cause necrosis at site (from vasoconstriction).

• Avoid I.M. administration of oil injection into buttocks. Gas gangrene may occur because epinephrine reduces oxygen tension of the tissues, encouraging growth of contaminating organisms.

• This drug may widen pulse pressure.

• In case of a sharp blood pressure rise, rapid-acting vasodilators, such as nitrites or alpha-adrenergic blocking agents, can be given to counteract the marked pressor effect of large epinephrine doses.

• Observe patient closely for adverse reactions. If these develop, dosage may need to be adjusted or the drug discontinued.

• If patient has acute hypersensitivity reactions, teach him how to inject epinephrine.

• Ephinephrine is the drug of choice in emergency treatment of acute anaphylactic reactions, including anaphylactic shock. (See Chapter 12 for epinephrine administration through the endotracheal route.)

isoetharine hydrochloride 1%
Belta-Z Solution, Bronkosol

isoetharine mesylate
Bronkometer

Mechanism of action
Relaxes bronchial smooth muscle by acting on beta$_2$-adrenergic receptors.

Respiratory indications and dosage
• Bronchial asthma and reversible bronchospasm that may occur with bronchitis and emphysema—
Adults: Hydrochloride: Administered by hand nebulizer, 3 to 7 inhalations (undiluted); by oxygen aerosolization, 0.5 ml, diluted 1:3 in normal saline solution; by IPPB, 0.5 ml, diluted 1:3 in normal saline solution.
Adults: Mesylate: 1 to 2 inhalations. Occasionally, more may be required.

Adverse reactions
CNS: tremor, headache, dizziness, excitement.
CV: palpitations, increased heart rate.
GI: nausea, vomiting.

Interactions
Propranolol and other beta blockers: blocked bronchodilating effect of isoetharine. Monitor patient carefully if used together.

Clinical considerations
(See Chapter 11 for information on how to administer the aerosol form of this drug.)
• Use cautiously in patients with hyperthyroidism, hypertension and coronary disease, and in those with sensitivity to sympathomimetics.
• Excessive use can lead to decreased effectiveness.
• Monitor for severe paradoxical bronchoconstriction after excessive use. Discontinue immediately if bronchoconstriction occurs.
• Although isoetharine has minimal effects on the heart, it should be used cautiously in patients receiving general anesthetics that sensitize the myocardium to sympathomimetic drugs.
• Instruct patient in the use of aerosol and mouthpiece.
• Because drug oxidizes when diluted with water, pink sputum resembling hemotysis may appear after inhalation of isoetharine solution. Tell patient not to be concerned.

isoproterenol hydrochloride
Isuprel, Proternol (tabs)
Inhalants: Norisodrine, Vapo-Iso

isoproterenol sulfate
Iso-Autohaler, Luf-Iso Inhalation
Medihaler-Iso, Norisodrine

Mechanism of action
Relaxes bronchial smooth muscle by acting on beta$_2$-adrenergic receptors. As a cardiac stimulant, acts on beta$_1$-adrenergic receptors in the heart.

Respiratory indications and dosage
• Bronchial asthma and reversible bronchospasm (hydrochloride)—
Adults: 10 to 20 mg. S.L. q 6 to 8 hours.
Children: 5 to 10 mg S.L. q 6 to 8 hours. Not recommended for children under age 6.
• Bronchospasm (sulfate)—
Adults and children: For acute dyspneic episodes, 1 inhalation initially. May repeat if needed after 2 to 5 minutes. Maintenance dose is 1 to 2 inhalations four to six times/day. May repeat once more 10 minutes after second dose. Not more than 3 doses should be administered for each attack.

Adverse reactions
CNS: headache, mild tremor, weakness, dizziness, anxiety, insomnia.
CV: palpitations, tachycardia, anginal pain; blood pressure may be elevated and then fall.
GI: nausea, vomiting.
Metabolic: hyperglycemia.
Other: sweating, facial flushing, bronchial edema, inflammation.

Interactions
Propranolol and other beta blockers: blocked bronchodilating effect of isoproterenol. Monitor patient carefully if used together.

Clinical considerations
• Drug is contraindicated in tachycardia caused by digitalis intoxication; in preexisting dysrhythmias, especially tachycardia, because drug's chronotropic effect on the heart may aggravate such disorders; and in recent myocardial infarction. Use cautiously in coronary insufficiency, diabetes, and hyperthyroidism.
• If heart rate exceeds 110 beats/minute, decrease infusion rate or temporarily stop infusion, if ordered. Doses sufficient to increase the heart rate to more than 130 beats/minute may induce ventricular dysrhythmias.
• If precordial distress or anginal pain occurs, stop drug immediately.

• Oral and sublingual tablets are absorbed poorly and erratically.
• Teach patient how to take sublingual tablet properly. Tell him to hold tablet under tongue until it dissolves and is absorbed and not to swallow saliva until that time. Prolonged use of sublingual tablets can cause tooth decay. Instruct patient to rinse mouth with water between doses; this also helps prevent oropharynx dryness.
• If possible, don't give at bedtime because drug interrupts sleep patterns.
• This drug may cause slight systolic blood pressure rise and slight to marked drop in diastolic blood pressure.
• Use a microdrip or infusion pump to regulate infusion flow rate.
• Observe patient closely for adverse reactions. Dosage may need to be adjusted or the drug discontinued.
• Teach patient to perform oral inhalation correctly. Give the following instructions for using a metered-dose nebulizer:
—Clear nasal passages and throat.
—Breathe out, expelling as much air from lungs as possible.
—Place mouthpiece well into mouth as dose from nebulizer is released, and inhale deeply.
—Hold breath for several seconds, remove mouthpiece, and exhale slowly.
• Instructions for metered powder nebulizer are the same, except that deep inhalation isn't necessary.
• Patient may develop tolerance to this drug. Warn against overuse.
• Warn patient using oral inhalant that drug may turn sputum and saliva pink.
• Drug may aggravate ventilation perfusion abnormalities; although it eases breathing, it may cause arterial oxygen tension to fall paradoxically.
• Discard inhalation solution if it is discolored or contains precipitate.

metaproterenol sulfate
Alupent, Metaprel

Mechanism of action
Relaxes bronchial smooth muscle by acting on beta$_2$-adrenergic receptors.

Respiratory indications and dosage
• Acute episodes of bronchial asthma—
Adults and children: 2 to 3 inhalations. Should not repeat inhalations more often than q 4 hours. Should not exceed 12 inhalations daily.
• Bronchial asthma and reversible bronchospasm—
Adults: 20 mg P.O. q 6 to 8 hours.
Children over age 9 or over 27 kg: 20 mg P.O. q 6 to 8 hours (0.4 mg to 0.9 mg/kg/dose t.i.d.).
Children age 6 to 9 or under 27 kg: 10 mg P.O. q 6 to 8 hours (0.4 mg to 0.9 mg/kg/dose t.i.d.).

Not recommended for children under age 6.

Adverse reactions
CNS: nervousness, weakness, drowsiness, tremor.
CV: tachycardia, hypertension, palpitations; cardiac arrest with excessive use.
GI: vomiting, nausea, bad taste in mouth.
Other: paradoxical bronchiolar constriction with excessive use.

Interactions
Propranolol and other beta blockers: blocked bronchodilating effect of metaproterenol. Monitor patient carefully if used together.

Clinical considerations
• Drug is contraindicated in patients with tachycardia or dysrhythmias associated with tachycardia. Use with caution in patients with hypertension, coronary artery disease, hyperthyroidism, and diabetes.
• Safe use of inhalant in children under age 12 has not been established.
• Teach patient how to administer metered dose correctly. Have him shake container, exhale through nose, administer aerosol while inhaling deeply on mouthpiece of inhaler, hold breath for a few seconds, then exhale slowly. Allow 2 minutes between inhalations. Store drug in light-resistant container.

• Metaproterenol inhalations should precede steroid inhalations (when prescribed) by 10 to 15 minutes to maximize therapy.
• Warn patient about the possibility of paradoxical bronchospasm. If this occurs, the drug should be discontinued immediately.
• Patients may use tablets and aerosol concomitantly. Monitor closely for toxicity.
• Metaproterenol reportedly produces less cardiac stimulation than other sympathomimetics, especially isoproterenol.
• Inhalant solution can be administered by IPPB diluted in normal saline solution or via a hand nebulizer at full strength.
• Tell patient to notify doctor if no response occurs. Warn against changing dose without calling doctor.

terbutaline sulfate
Brethaire, Brethine, Bricanyl

Mechanism of action
Relaxes bronchial smooth muscle by acting on beta$_2$-adrenergic receptors.

Respiratory indications and dosage
• Relief of bronchospasm in patients with reversible obstructive airway disease—
Adults and children over age 11: 2 inhalations separated by a 60-second interval, repeated q 4 to 6 hours. May also administer 2.5 to 5 mg P.O. q 8 hours or 0.25 mg S.C.

Adverse reactions
CNS: nervousness, tremors, headache, drowsiness, sweating.
CV: palpitations, increased heart rate.
EENT: drying and irritation of nose and throat (with inhaled form).
GI: vomiting, nausea.

Interactions
MAO inhibitors: possible severe hypertension (hypertensive crisis). Don't use together.

Propranolol and other beta blockers: blocked bronchodilating effects of terbutaline.

Clinical considerations
• Use cautiously in patients with diabetes, hypertension, hyperthyroidism, severe cardiac disease, and cardiac dysrhythmias.
• Protect injection from light. Don't use if discolored.
• Make sure patient and his family understand why drug is necessary.
• Give S.C. injections in lateral deltoid area.
• Tolerance may develop with prolonged use.
• Warn patient about the possibility of paradoxical bronchospasm. If this occurs, the drug should be discontinued immediately.
• Patient may use tablets and aerosol concomitantly. Monitor closely for toxicity.
• Teach patient how to administer metered dose correctly. Have him shake container, exhale through nose, administer aerosol while inhaling deeply on mouthpiece of inhaler, hold breath for a few seconds, then exhale slowly.

Anticholinergics
The parasympathetic innervation of the respiratory system controls secretory functions and regulation of muscle tone. Vagal stimulation increases airway secretions and bronchiolar constriction by activating muscarinic cholinergic receptors.

Anticholinergics have been used infrequently in respiratory disorders because they can cause systemic and local adverse reactions (including tachycardia and increased viscosity of bronchial secretions). Recently, local administration of atropine sulfate (by inhalation) and the development of a poorly absorbed quaternary derivative (ipratropium) have been reintroduced as treatments for chronic lung disorders.

atropine sulfate
Dey-Dose

Mechanism of action
Produces bronchodilation by blocking muscarinic receptors on bronchial smooth muscle. Additional benefits may come from blockade of acetylcholic-induced release of mast cell mediators.

Respiratory indications and dosage
• Prevention and short-term treatment of bronchial spasm associated with chronic obstructive lung disease, bronchitis, and chronic bronchial asthma—
Adults: 0.025 mg/kg diluted with 3 to 5 ml normal saline solution given by nebulizer t.i.d. or q.i.d. Do not exceed 2.5 mg/dose.
Children: 0.05 mg/kg diluted in normal saline solution and given by nebulizer t.i.d. or q.i.d. Do not exceed 2.5 mg/dose.

Adverse reactions
CNS: headache, mental confusion.
CV: tachycardia with palpitations, bradycardia.
EENT: mydriasis, slight blurring of near vision, dry nose, dry mouth, viscous secretions.
Other: dry or flushed skin, speech disturbance, dysphagia.

Clinical considerations
• Drug is contraindicated in patients with glaucoma, adhesions (synechiae) between iris and lens of eye, prostatic hypertrophy, and hypersensitivity.
• Systemic absorption can occur, but the extent is highly variable and unpredictable. Monitor patient closely for adverse reactions.
• Adverse reactions are more common in children and tend to be dose-related.
• Inhalation of doses greater than 5 mg can cause central nervous system (CNS) stimulation and mental disturbances.
• Overdose can be treated with respiratory assistance and physostigmine.

• Drug may increase the viscosity of respiratory secretions, possibly causing airway obstruction.

ipratropium bromide
Atrovent

Mechanism of action
A quaternary ammonium derivative of atropine that acts locally to inhibit muscarinic cholinergic receptors on bronchial smooth muscle and large airways of the respiratory tract, causing bronchodilation.

Respiratory indications and dosage
• Maintenance treatment of bronchospasm, chronic obstructive pulmonary disease, chronic bronchitis—
Adults and children over age 12: 2 inhalations (36 mcg) q.i.d. Patients may take additional inhalations as required, but should not exceed 12 inhalations/day.

Adverse reactions
CNS: sleepiness, dizziness, nervousness, headache.
CV: slight decrease in pulse rate, palpitations.
EENT: dry mouth, bad taste in mouth, throat irritation, visual disturbances (blurred vision, decreased accommodation).
GI: nausea, distress.
Other: rash.

Clinical considerations
• Drug is contraindicated in patients with hypersensitivity to atropine or its derivatives.
• Ipratropium is absorbed poorly from the lungs and GI tract. Few systemic adverse reactions occur.
• Drug has caused isolated cases of airway obstruction from increased sputum viscosity and decreased mucociliary clearance.
• Use with caution in patients with narrow-angle glaucoma.
• Temporary blurred vision may result if compound is sprayed into the eyes.

Methylxanthines
Methylxanthines (or xanthine derivatives) are categorized pharmacologically as CNS stimulants. Their use in respiratory therapy derives from their bronchodilatory effects; they are also mild diuretics and cardiac stimulants and may directly stimulate the brain's medullary respiratory centers.

The mechanism through which they exert their effect is complex and not completely understood. In the respiratory tract's smooth muscle, they appear to alter intracellular calcium availability through a direct effect on sarcoplasmic reticulum, and they increase cyclic adenosine monophosphate (AMP) (an important mediator in cellular calcium transport) by inhibiting phosphodiesterase. However, at therapeutic concentrations, their effect appears to stem more from inhibition of adenosine receptors, substances that probably act as regulatory autocoids.

aminophylline or theophylline ethylenediamine
Aminophyllin, Corophyllin, Phyllocontin, Somophyllin-DF

Mechanism of action
Acts directly on airway smooth muscle to produce bronchodilation.

Respiratory indications and dosage
• Acute and chronic bronchial asthma and bronchospasm; also used for Cheyne-Stokes respiration—
Adults: For oral route, 500 mg immediately; then 250 to 500 mg q 6 to 8 hours. Maintenance dose is 0.3 to 0.9 mg/kg I.V. hourly by continuous infusion, 500 mg by suppository, or q 6 to 8 hours by retention enema.
Children: For oral route, 7.5 mg/kg immediately; then 3 to 6 mg/kg q 6 to 8 hours. For I.V. administration, inject slowly—minimum time, 4 minutes; don't exceed 25 mg/minute infusion rate. Loading dose is 5.6 mg/kg over 30 minutes. For children under age 9, maintenance dose is 1 mg/kg/hour.

Adverse reactions

CNS: restlessness, dizziness, headache, insomnia, light-headedness, convulsions, muscle twitching.

CV: palpitations, sinus tachycardia, extrasystole, flushing, marked hypotension, increased respiratory rate.

GI: nausea, vomiting, anorexia, bitter aftertaste, dyspepsia, heavy feeling in stomach, diarrhea.

Skin: urtcaria.

Local: irritation (with rectal suppositories).

Interactions

Alkali-sensitive drugs: reduced activity. Don't add to I.V. fluids containing aminophylline.

Beta-adrenergic blockers: antagonized effects. Propranolol and nadolol, especially, may cause bronchospasm in sensitive patients. Use together cautiously.

Troleandomycin, erythromycin, cimetidine: decreased hepatic clearance of theophylline; elevated theophylline levels. Monitor for signs of toxicity.

Barbiturates, phenytoin: enhanced metabolism and decreased theophylline blood levels. Monitor for decreased aminophylline effect.

Clinical considerations

• Drug is contraindicated in patients with hypersensitivity to xanthine compounds (such as caffeine and theobromine) and in those with preexisting cardiac dysrhythmias, especially tachydysrhythmias. Use cautiously in young children; in elderly patients with congestive heart failure or other cardiac or circulatory impairment, cor pulmonale, or hepatic disease; in patients with active peptic ulcer, because drug may increase volume and acidity of gastric secretions; and in patients with hyperthyroidism or diabetes mellitus.

• Individuals metabolize xanthines at different rates. Adjust dose by monitoring response, tolerance, pulmonary function, and theophylline blood levels. Therapeutic level is 10 to 20 mcg/ml; toxicity may occur at levels over 20 mcg/ml.

• Plasma clearance may decrease in patients with congestive heart failure, hepatic dysfunction, or pulmonary edema. Smokers show accelerated clearance. Dose must be adjusted.

• I.V. administration can cause burning; dilute with dextrose in water solution.

• Monitor vital signs; measure and record intake and output. Expected clinical effects include improved quality of pulse and respiration.

• Warn elderly patients that drug may cause dizziness, a common adverse reaction at the start of therapy.

• GI symptoms may be relieved by taking the oral drug with a full glass of water at meals, although food in the stomach delays absorption. Enteric-coated tablets may also delay and impair absorption. Antacids reportedly do not reduce GI adverse reactions.

• Suppositories are absorbed slowly and erratically; retention enemas may be absorbed more rapidly. Rectally administered preparations can be given if the patient can't take the drug orally. Schedule dose after evacuation, if possible; dose may be retained better if given before a meal. Advise patient to remain recumbent 15 to 20 minutes after insertion.

• Question patient closely about other drugs used. Warn that over-the-counter remedies may contain ephedrine in combination with theophylline salts; excessive CNS stimulation may result. Tell him to check with the doctor or pharmacist before taking any other medications.

• Before giving loading dose, check that patient has not had recent theophylline therapy.

• Teach patient about home care and dosage schedule. Some patients may require a round-the-clock dosage schedule.

• Warn patient with allergies that exposure to allergens may exacerbate bronchospasm.

dyphylline
Air-Tabs, Brophylline, Dilin, Dilor, Dyflex, Dylline, Emfabid, Lufyllin, Protophylline

Mechanism of action
Acts directly on airway smooth muscle to produce bronchodilation.

Respiratory indications and dosage
• Relief of acute and chronic bronchial asthma and reversible bronchospasm associated with chronic bronchitis and emphysema—
Adults: 200 to 800 mg P.O. q 6 hours; or 250 to 500 mg I.M. injected slowly at 6-hour intervals.
Children over age 6: 4 to 7 mg/kg P.O. daily in divided doses.

Adverse reactions
CNS: restlessness, dizziness, headache, insomnia, light-headedness, convulsions, muscle twitching.
CV: palpitations, sinus tachycardia, extrasystoles, flushing, marked hypotension, increased respiratory rate.
GI: nausea, vomiting, anorexia, bitter aftertaste, dyspepsia, heavy feeling in stomach.
Skin: urticaria.

Interactions
Alkali-sensitive drugs: reduced activity. Don't add to I.V. fluids containing aminophylline.
Beta-adrenergic blockers: antagonism. Propranolol and nadolol, especially, may cause bronchospasm in sensitive patients. Use together cautiously.
Troleandomycin, erythromycin, cimetidine: decreased hepatic clearance of theophylline; elevated theophylline levels. Monitor for signs of toxicity.
Barbiturates, phenytoin: enhanced metabolism and decreased theophylline blood levels. Monitor for decreased theophylline effect.

Clinical considerations
• Drug is contraindicated in patients with hypersensitivity to xanthine compounds (caffeine, theobromine) and preexisting cardiac dysrhythmias, especially tachycardia. Use cautiously in young children; elderly patients with congestive heart failure, impaired cardiac or circulatory function, cor pulmonale, or renal or hepatic disease; and in patients with peptic ulcer, hyperthyroidism, or diabetes mellitus.
• I.V. use is not recommended.
• Dyphylline is metabolized faster than theophylline; dosage intervals may have to be decreased to ensure continual therapeutic effect. Higher daily doses may be needed.
• Dose should be decreased in patients with renal insufficiency.
• Monitor vital signs; measure and record intake and output. Expected clinical effects include improved quality of pulse and respiration.
• Warn elderly patients of dizziness, a common adverse reaction.
• Gastric irritation may be relieved by taking oral drug after meals. Tell patient that there is no evidence that suggests that antacids reduce this GI irritation. Drug may produce less gastric discomfort than theophylline.
• Discard dyphylline ampule if precipitate appears. Protect from light.
• Question patient closely about other drugs used. Warn that over-the-counter remedies may contain ephedrine in combination with theophylline salts; excessive CNS stimulation may result. Tell him to check with the doctor or pharmacist before taking any other medications.
• Teach patient about home care and dosage schedule.

oxtriphylline
Choledyl, Theophylline Choline

Mechanism of action
Acts directly on airway smooth muscle to produce bronchodilation.

Respiratory indications and dosage
• To relieve acute bronchial asthma and reversible bronchospasm associated with

chronic bronchitis and emphysema—
Adults and children over age 12: 200 mg P.O. q 6 hours.
Children age 2 to 12: 4 mg/kg P.O. q 6 hours. Increase as needed to maintain therapeutic theophylline levels (10 to 20 mcg/ml).

Adverse reactions
CNS: restlessness, dizziness, headache, insomnia, light-headedness, convulsions, muscle twitching.
CV: palpitations, sinus tachycardia, extrasystole, flushing, marked hypotension, increased respiratory rate.
GI: nausea, vomiting, anorexia, bitter aftertaste, dyspepsia, heavy feeling in stomach.
Skin: urticaria.

Interactions
Erythromycin, troleandomycin cimetidine: decreased hepatic clearance of theophylline, increased plasma level. Monitor for signs of toxicity.
Barbiturates, phenytoin: enhanced metabolism and decreased theophylline blood levels. Monitor for decreased effect.
Beta-adrenergic blockers: antagonism. Propranolol and nadolol, especially, may cause bronchospasms in sensitive patients. Use together cautiously.

Clinical considerations
• Drug is contraindicated in patients with a hypersensitivity to xanthines (such as caffeine and theobromine) or preexisting cardiac dysrhythmias, especially tachydysrhythmias.
• Tell patient to report GI distress, palpitations, irritability, restlessness, nervousness, or insomnia; these may indicate excessive CNS stimulation.
• Administer drug after meals and at bedtime.
• Store at 59° to 86° F. (15° to 30° C.). Protect elixir from light; protect tablets from moisture.
• Drug is equivalent to 64% anhydrous theophylline.

• Monitor therapy carefully.
• Combination products that contain ephedrine are not recommended; excessive CNS stimulation (nervousness, tremors, akathisia) may result.

theophylline
Immediate-release tablets and capsules: Bronkodyl, Elixophyllin, Slo-Phyllin, Somophyllin-T
Immediate-release liquids: Accurbron, Aerolate, Aquaphyllin, Asmalix, Bronkodyl, Elixicon, Elixomin, Elixophyllin, Lanophyllin, Lixolin, Slo-Phyllin, Theolair, Theolixir, Theon, Theophyl
Timed-release capsules: Aerolate, Bronkodyl S-R, Elixophyllin SR, Lodrane, Slo-bid, Slow-Phyllin, Somophyllin-CRT, Theo-24, Theobid, Theobid Jr., Theobron SR, Theo-Dur Sprinkle, Theophyl SR, Theospan-SR, Theovent
Timed-release tablets: Constant-T Duraphyl, LABID, Quibron-T/SR, Respbid, Sustaire, Theo-Dur, Theolair-SR, Theo-Time, Uniphyl

theophylline sodium glycinate
Acet-AM, Synophylate

Mechanism of action
Acts directly on airway smooth muscle to produce bronchodilation.

Respiratory indications and dosage
• Prophylaxis and symptomatic relief of bronchial asthma, bronchospasm of chronic bronchitis and emphysema—
Adults: 6 mg/kg P.O. followed by 2 to 3 mg/kg q 4 hours for two doses. Maintenance dose is 1 to 3 mg/kg q 8 to 12 hours.
Children age 9 to 16: 6 mg/kg P.O. followed by 3 mg/kg q 4 hours for three doses. Maintenance dose is 3 mg/kg q 6 hours.
Children age 6 months to 9 years: 6 mg/kg P.O. followed by 4 mg/kg q 4 hours for three doses. Maintenance

dose is 4 mg/kg q 6 hours. Most oral timed-release forms are given q 8 to 12 hours. Several products, however, may be given q 24 hours.

• Symptomatic relief of bronchial asthma, pulmonary emphysema, and chronic bronchitis—

Adults: 330 to 660 mg (sodium glycinate) P.O. q 6 to 8 hours, after meals.

Children over age 12: 220 to 330 mg (sodium glycinate) P.O. q 6 to 8 hours.

Children age 6 to 12: 330 mg (sodium glycinate) P.O. q 6 to 8 hours.

Children age 3 to 6: 110 to 165 mg (sodium glycinate) P.O. q 6 to 8 hours.

Children age 1 to 3: 55 to 110 mg (sodium glycinate) P.O. q 6 to 8 hours.

Adverse reactions

CNS: restlessness, dizziness, headache, insomnia, light-headedness, convulsions, muscle twitching.

CV: palpitations, sinus tachycardia, extrasystoles, flushing, marked hypotension, increased respiratory rate.

GI: nausea, vomiting, anorexia, bitter aftertaste, dyspepsia, heavy feeling in stomach, diarrhea.

Skin: urticaria.

Interactions

Erythromycin, troleandomycin, cimetidine: decreased hepatic clearance of theophylline; increased plasma levels. Monitor for signs of toxicity.

Barbiturates, phenytoin: enhanced metabolism and decreased theophylline blood levels. Monitor for decreased effect.

Beta-adrenergic blockers: antagonism. Propranolol and nadolol, especially, may cause bronchospasms in sensitive patients. Use together cautiously.

Clinical considerations

• Drug is contraindicated in patients with hypersensitivity to xanthine compounds (such as caffeine and theobromine) and in patients with preexisting cardiac dysrhythmias, especially tachydysrhythmias. Use cautiously in young children; in elderly patients with congestive heart failure or other circulatory impairment, cor pulmonale, or renal or hepatic disease; and in patients with peptic ulcer, hyperthyroidism, or diabetes mellitus.

• Individuals metabolize xanthines at different rates; determine proper dose by monitoring response, tolerance, pulmonary function, and theophylline plasma levels. Therapeutic level is 10 to 20 mcg/ml.

• Monitor vital signs; measure and record intake and output. Expected clinical effects include improved quality of pulse and respiration.

• Warn elderly patients of dizziness, a common adverse reaction at start of therapy.

• GI symptoms may be relieved by taking oral drug with full glass of water after meals, although food in stomach delays drug absorption.

• Question patient closely about other drugs used. Warn that over-the-counter remedies may contain ephedrine in combination with theophylline salts; excessive CNS stimulation may result. Tell him to check with the doctor or pharmacist before taking any other medications.

• Teach patient about home care and dosage schedule.

• Daily dosage may need to be decreased in patients with congestive heart failure or hepatic disease or in elderly patients, because metabolism and excretion may be decreased. Monitor carefully, using blood levels, observation, physical assessment, and interview. Give drug round-the-clock, using sustained-release product at bedtime.

• Drug dosage may need to be increased in smokers because smoking causes faster drug metabolism.

• Be careful not to confuse sustained-release dosage forms with standard-release dosage forms.

• Warn patient not to dissolve, crush, or chew slow-release products. Small children unable to swallow these can ingest (without chewing) the contents of bead-filled capsules sprinkled over soft food.
• Warn patients not to exceed prescribed dosages. (Some may want to take extra "breathing pills.")

Corticosteroids

Used to treat chronic pulmonary diseases, corticosteroids are potent anti-inflammatory agents. Because long-term administration can produce serious adverse reactions, corticosteroids aren't typically used if a patient can be controlled with other drugs.

Corticosteroids may be used in acute emergency situations (such as status asthmaticus). However, because of their delayed onset of action, they're used more commonly as adjuncts to other, more aggressive, bronchodilator therapy. In an acute emergency, they can be used to inhibit the inflammatory response (such as edema and capillary dilation). Long-term therapy can provide prophylaxis against inflammation by inhibiting inflammatory cell function.

beclomethasone dipropionate
Beclovent, Vanceril

Mechanism of action
Decreases inflammation by stabilizing leukocyte lysosomal membranes, inhibiting macrophage accumulation in inflamed areas, and reducing capillary wall permeability.

Respiratory indications and dosage
• Steroid-dependent asthma—
Adults: 2 to 4 inhalations t.i.d. or q.i.d. Maximum dosage is 20 inhalations/day.

Children age 6 to 12: 1 to 2 inhalations t.i.d. or q.i.d. Maximum dosage is 10 inhalations/day.

Adverse reactions
EENT: hoarseness, fungal infections of mouth and throat.
GI: dry mouth.

Clinical considerations
• Drug is contraindicated in patients with status asthmaticus. Do not use for asthma controlled solely by bronchodilators or other noncorticosteroids or for nonasthmatic bronchial diseases.
• Oral glucocorticoid therapy should be tapered slowly. Acute adrenal insufficiency and death have occurred in asthmatic patients who changed abruptly from oral corticosteroids to beclomethasone.
• During times of stress (such as trauma, surgery, or infection), systemic corticosteroids may be needed to prevent adrenal insufficiency in previously steroid-dependent patients.
• Instruct patient to carry a card indicating his need for supplemental systemic glucocorticoids during stress.
• Patients requiring bronchodilator should use it several minutes before taking beclomethasone.
• Instruct patient to allow 1 minute to elapse before taking subsequent puffs of medication and to hold breath for a few seconds to enhance drug action.
• Inform patient that beclomethasone doesn't provide relief for an acute asthma attack.
• Instruct patient to contact doctor if he notices a decreased response. Dose may have to be adjusted. Patient shouldn't exceed recommended dose on his own.
• Check mucous membranes frequently for signs of fungal infection.
• Oral fungal infections can be prevented by following inhalations with a glass of water.
• Tell patient to keep inhaler clean and unobstructed by washing it with warm water and drying thoroughly.

hydrocortisone
Cortef, Hydrocortone

hydrocortisone sodium phosphate
Hydrocortone Phosphate

hydrocortisone sodium succinate
A-HydroCort, S-Cortilean, Solu-Cortef

Mechanism of action
Decreases inflammation, mainly by stabilizing leukocyte lysosomal membranes. Also, suppresses the immune response; stimulates bone marrow; and influences protein, fat, and carbohydrate metabolism.

Respiratory indications and dosage
• Adjunctive treatment of acute respiratory distress—
Adults: 5 to 30 mg P.O. b.i.d., t.i.d., or q.i.d. (as much as 80 mg P.O. q.i.d. may be given in acute situations); or initially, 100 to 250 mg (succinate) I.M. or I.V., then 50 to 100 mg I.M., as indicated; or 15 to 240 mg (phosphate) I.M. or I.V. q 12 hours.
Children: 0.16 to 1 mg/kg (phosphate or succinate) I.M. or I.V. b.i.d. or t.i.d.

Adverse reactions
Most adverse reactions are dose- or duration-dependent.
CNS: euphoria, insomnia, psychotic behavior, pseudotumor cerebri.
CV: congestive heart failure, hypertension, edema.
EENT: cataracts, glaucoma.
GI: peptic ulcer, irritation, increased appetite.
Metabolic: possible hypokalemia, hyperglycemia and carbohydrate intolerance, growth suppression in children.
Skin: delayed wound healing, acne, various skin eruptions.
Other: muscle weakness, pancreatitis, hirsutism, susceptibility to infections. Acute adrenal insufficiency may occur with increased stress (such as infection, surgery, or trauma), or abrupt withdrawal after long-term therapy. Withdrawal symptoms include rebound inflammation, fatigue, weakness, arthralgia, fever, dizziness, lethargy, depression, fainting, orthostatic hypotension, dyspnea, anorexia, and hypoglycemia. Sudden withdrawal may be fatal.

Interactions
Barbiturates, phenytoin, rifampin: decreased corticosteroid effect. Corticosteroid dose may need to be increased.
Indomethacin, aspirin: increased risk of GI distress and bleeding. Give together cautiously.

Clinical considerations
• Drug is contraindicated in patients with systemic fungal infections. Use cautiously in patients with GI ulcers or renal disease, hypertension, osteoporosis, varicella, vaccinia, exanthema, diabetes mellitus, Cushing's syndrome, thromboembolic disorders, seizures, myasthenia gravis, metastatic cancer, congestive heart failure, tuberculosis, ocular herpes simplex, hypoalbuminemia, and emotional instability or psychotic tendencies. Use cautiously in children.
• Gradually reduce dosage after long-term therapy. Tell patient not to discontinue drug abruptly or without doctor's consent.
• Always give lowest effective dose.
• Drug has both glucocorticoid and mineralocorticoid effect.
• Monitor patient's weight, blood pressure, and serum electrolyte level.
• Drug may mask or exacerbate infection.
• Instruct patient to carry a card identifying his need for supplemental systemic glucocorticoids during stress.
• Teach patient signs and symptoms of early adrenal insufficiency: fatigue, muscular weakness, joint pain, fever, anorexia, nausea, dyspnea, dizziness, fainting.
• Watch for depression or psychotic episodes, especially in patients receiving high-dose therapy.

• Inspect patient's skin for petechiae. Warn patient about easy bruising.
• Diabetic patients may need increased insulin; monitor blood glucose levels.
• Monitor growth in infants and children on long-term therapy.
• Give I.M. injection deep into gluteal muscle. Avoid subcutaneous injection, as atrophy and sterile abscesses may occur.
• Unless contraindicated, give salt-restricted diet rich in potassium and protein. Potassium supplement may be needed. Watch for additional potassium depletion from diuretics and amphotericin B.
• Give P.O. dose with food when possible.
• Warn patients on long-term therapy about cushingoid symptoms.
• Acetate form not for I.V. use.
• Immunizations may show decreased antibody response.
• Do not confuse Solu-Cortef with Solu-Medrol.
• Injectable forms are not for alternate-day therapy.

prednisone

Colisone, Deltasone, Liquid Pred, Meticorten, Orasone, Prednicen-M, SK-Prednisone, Wojtab

Mechanism of action

Decreases inflammation, mainly by stabilizing leukocyte lysosomal membranes. Also suppresses the immune response, stimulates bone marrow, and influences protein, fat, and carbohydrate metabolism.

Respiratory indications and dosage

• Severe bronchial asthma or chronic obstructive pulmonary disease—
Adults and children: 5 to 10 mg P.O. daily (preferably in a.m.). Individualized dosage is recommended based on severity of disease and patient response. Prednisone is recommended for use only after therapeutic failure of other drugs or as an adjunct to therapy.

Adverse reactions

CNS: euphoria, insomnia, psychotic behavior, pseudotumor cerebri.
CV: congestive heart failure, hypertension, edema.
EENT: cataracts, glaucoma.
GI: peptic ulcer, GI irritation, increased appetite.
Metabolic: possible hypokalemia, hyperglycemia and carbohydrate intolerance, growth suppression in children.
Skin: delayed wound healing, acne, various skin eruptions.
Other: muscle weakness, pancreatitis, hirsutism, susceptibility to infections. Acute adrenal insufficiency may occur with increased stress (such as from infection, surgery, or trauma) or abrupt withdrawal after long-term therapy. Withdrawal symptoms include rebound inflammation, fatigue, weakness, arthralgia, fever, dizziness, lethargy, depression, fainting, orthostatic hypotension, dyspnea, anorexia, and hypoglycemia. Sudden withdrawal may be fatal.

Interactions

Barbiturates, phenytoin, rifampin: decreased corticosteroid effect. Corticosteroid dose may need to be increased.
Indomethacin, aspirin: increased risk of GI distress and bleeding. Give together cautiously.

Clinical considerations

• Drug is contraindicated in patients with systemic fungal infections. Use cautiously in patients with GI ulcers, renal disease, hypertension, osteoporosis, varicella, vaccinia, exanthema, diabetes mellitus, Cushing's syndrome, thromboembolic disorders, seizures, myasthenia gravis, metastatic cancer, congestive heart failure, tuberculosis, ocular herpes simplex, hypoalbuminemia, emotional instability, or psychotic tendencies.
• Gradually reduce dosage after long-term therapy. Tell patient not to dis-

continue drug abruptly or without doctor's consent.
- Always give lowest effective dose.
- Monitor patient's blood pressure, sleep patterns, and serum potassium levels.
- Weigh patient daily; report sudden weight gain to doctor.
- Drug may mask or exacerbate infections. Tell patient to report slow healing.
- Instruct patient to carry a card identifying his need for supplemental systemic glucocorticoids during stress.
- Teach patient about signs and symptoms of early adrenal insufficiency: fatigue, muscular weakness, joint pain, fever, anorexia, nausea, dyspnea, dizziness, and fainting.
- Watch for depression or psychotic episodes, especially in patients receiving high-dose therapy.
- Diabetic patients may need increased insulin; monitor blood glucose levels.
- Monitor growth in infants and children on long-term therapy.
- Give salt-restricted diet rich in potassium and protein. Potassium supplement may be needed.
- Unless contraindicated, give P.O. dose with food when possible, to reduce GI irritation.
- Drug may be used for alternate-day therapy.
- Watch for additional potassium depletion from diuretics and amphotericin B.
- Warn patients on long-term therapy about cushingoid symptoms.
- Immunizations may show decreased antibody response.
- Drug is now available in oral solution form.

triamcinolone acetonide
Azmacort

Mechanism of action
Decreases inflammation by stabilizing leukocyte lysosomal membranes, inhibiting macrophage accumulation in inflamed areas, and reducing capillary wall permeability.

Respiratory indications and dosage
- Steroid-dependent asthma—
Adults: 2 inhalations t.i.d. to q.i.d. Maximum of 16 inhalations daily.
Children age 6 to 12: 1 to 2 inhalations t.i.d. to q.i.d. Maximum dosage is 12 inhalations/day.

Adverse reactions
EENT: hoarseness, fungal infections of mouth and throat.
GI: dry mouth.

Clinical considerations
- Drug is contraindicated in patients with status asthmaticus, with asthma controlled solely by bronchodilators or other noncorticosteroids, or with non-asthmatic bronchial diseases.
- Oral therapy should be tapered slowly.
- Instruct patient to carry a card indicating his need for supplemental systemic glucocorticoids during stress.
- Patient requiring bronchodilator should use it several minutes before receiving triamcinolone.
- Instruct patient to allow 1 minute to elapse before taking another inhalation and to hold his breath for a few seconds to enhance drug action.
- Inform patient that triamcinolone doesn't provide relief for acute asthma attack.
- Instruct patient to contact doctor if he notices a decreased response. Dose may have to be adjusted. Warn patient not to exceed recommended dose on his own.
- Check mucous membranes frequently for signs of fungal infection. Prevent such infections by following inhalations with glass of water.
- Tell patient to keep inhaler clean and unobstructed by washing it with warm water and drying thoroughly after use.

Anti-infectives

The term anti-infective refers to a broad class of drugs used to treat any organism capable of causing infection.

To simplify the discussion of antibiotics, we present these agents in a condensed format, because of their vast number and broad spectrum of use in the treatment of or prophylaxis against bacterial infection. However, we present antituberculars in detail, because of the respiratory implications of tuberculosis. Antifungals, antiprotozoal agents, and antivirals are presented for completeness.

Antibiotics
Antibiotic (antibacterial) agents act through various mechanisms to kill or impede the growth of pathogenic microorganisms. Most are derived from bacteria or fungi and some are totally man-made.

Antibiotics can be divided loosely into two categories:
• bacteriostatic—agents that impede the growth and replication of microorganisms
• bactericidal—agents that kill bacteria.

These effects result from various mechanisms, ranging from disruption of cell wall integrity to interruption of the synthesis or utilization of necessary cellular substituents.

Because most antibiotics in use today have some harmful adverse effects, the therapeutic goal is to administer the proper agent at the lowest concentration required to eliminate the pathogen.

Preferably, antibiotic therapy begins with identification of the offending pathogen, followed by determination of its antibiotic susceptibility. In some cases, antibiotics have additive or synergistic effects: two agents administered simultaneously may eliminate the offending bacteria more effectively. However, although combining antibiotics can improve the chance of a positive clinical response, it may also increase the risk of producing adverse reactions. See *Commonly used antibiotics*, pages 362 to 368, for information on antibiotics used frequently to treat or prevent respiratory infection.

Antituberculars
These anti-infectives combat different types of tuberculosis. Formerly fatal, tuberculosis has been rendered both controllable and curable through medical progress in the last few decades.

Ethambutol, isoniazid, rifampin, and streptomycin are first-line drugs in treating all tuberculosis forms. Isoniazid is also used prophylactically in susceptible persons who have been exposed to tuberculosis.

ethambutol hydrochloride
Etibi, Myambutol

Mechanism of action
Bacteriostatic; interferes with the synthesis of ribonucleic acid (RNA), thus inhibiting protein metabolism.

Respiratory indications and dosage
• Adjunctive treatment in pulmonary tuberculosis—
Adults and children over age 13: As initial treatment for patients who haven't received previous antitubercular therapy, 15 mg/kg P.O. daily as a single dose. For retreatment, 25 mg/kg P.O. daily as a single dose for 60 days with at least one other antitubercular drug; then decrease to 15 mg/kg P.O. daily as a single dose.

Adverse reactions
CNS: headache, dizziness, mental confusion, possible hallucinations, peripheral neuritis (numbness and tingling of extremities).
EENT: optic neuritis (loss of vision and color discrimination, especially red and green).

GI: anorexia, nausea, vomiting, abdominal pain.
Metabolic: elevated uric acid level.
Other: anaphylactoid reactions, fever, malaise, bloody sputum.

Interactions
None significant.

Clinical considerations
• Drug is contraindicated in patients with optic neuritis and in children under age 13. Use cautiously in patients with impaired renal function, cataracts, recurrent eye inflammations, gout, and diabetic retinopathy.
• Dose must be reduced in patients with renal impairment.
• Perform visual acuity and color discrimination tests before and during therapy.
• Monitor serum uric acid level; observe patient for signs and symptoms of gout.
• Reassure patient that visual disturbances will disappear several weeks to months after drug is stopped.

isoniazid (INH)
Hyzyd, Isotamine, Laniazid, Nydrazid, PMS-Isoniazid, Rimifon, Rolazid, Teebaconin

Mechanism of action
Bactericidal; inhibits cell-wall biosynthesis by interfering with lipid and deoxyribonucleic acid (DNA) synthesis.

Respiratory indications and dosage
• Primary treatment against actively growing tubercle bacilli—
Adults: 5 mg/kg P.O. or I.M. daily as a single dose, up to 300 mg/day, continued for 9 months to 2 years.
Children: 10 to 20 mg/kg P.O. or I.M. daily as a single dose, up to 500 mg/day, continued for 18 months to 2 years. Concomitant administration of at least one other effective antitubercular drug is recommended.
• Prophylactic therapy against tubercle bacilli for patients closely exposed

or those with positive skin tests whose chest X-rays and bacteriologic studies are consistent with nonprogressive tuberculous disease—
Adults: 300 mg P.O. daily as a single dose, continued for 1 year.
Children: 10 mg/kg P.O. daily as a single dose, up to 300 mg/day, continued for 1 year.

Adverse reactions
Blood: agranulocytosis, hemolytic anemia, aplastic anemia, eosinophilia, leukopenia, neutropenia, thrombocytopenia, methemoglobinemia, pyridoxine-responsive hypochromic anemia.
CNS: peripheral neuropathy (especially in malnourished patients, alcoholics, diabetic patients, and slow acetylators), usually preceded by paresthesias of hands and feet; psychosis.
GI: nausea, vomiting, epigastric distress, constipation, dry mouth.
Hepatic: hepatitis, occasionally severe and sometimes fatal (especially in elderly patients).
Local: irritation at injection site.
Metabolic: hyperglycemia, metabolic acidosis.
Other: rheumatic syndrome and systemic lupus erythematosus-like syndrome; hypersensitivity (fever, rash, lymphadenopathy, vasculitis).

Interactions
Aluminum-containing antacids and laxatives: may decrease the rate and amount of isoniazid absorbed. Give isoniazid at least 1 hour before antacid or laxative.
Disulfiram: neurologic signs and symptoms, including changes in behavior and coordination, with concomitant isoniazid use. Avoid concomitant use.
Carbamazepine: increased risk of isoniazid hepatotoxicity. Use together with extreme caution.
Coricosteroids: may decrease therapeutic effectiveness. Monitor need for larger isoniazid dose.

Commonly Used Antibiotics

AMINOGLYCOSIDES
Selected drugs and administration routes
- amikacin sulfate (Amikin): I.M., I.V.
- gentamicin sulfate (Garamycin, U-Gencin): I.M., I.V.
- kanamycin sulfate (Anamid, Kantrex): P.O., I.M., I.V.
- netilmicin sulfate (Netromycin): I.M., I.V.
- Streptomycin sulfate: I.M.
- tobramycin sulfate (Nebcin): I.M., I.V.

Mechanism of action
Bactericidal; inhibits protein synthesis by binding directly to the 30S ribosomal subunit.

Cautions and contraindications
Use cautiously in patients with impaired renal function, and in neonates, infants, and elderly patients.

Adverse reactions
CNS: headache, lethargy, neuromuscular blockade.
EENT: ototoxicity (tinnitus, vertigo, hearing loss).
GI: nausea, vomiting, diarrhea.
GU: nephrotoxicity (urinary cells or casts, urine, proteinuria, decreased creatinine clearance, increased blood urea nitrogen [BUN] and serum creatinine levels).
Skin: rash.

Interactions
Amphotericin B, bumetanide, cephalothin, cisplatin, cyclosporine, ethyacrynic acid, furosemide, streptozocin, vancomycin: May increase potential for ototoxicity and/or nephrotoxicity.
Neuromuscular blockers: May enhance neuromuscular blockade.

Clinical considerations
- Obtain specimen for culture and sensitivity before first dose.
- Weigh patient and obtain baseline renal function studies before therapy.
- Monitor renal function (urine output, urine specific gravity, urinalysis, BUN

levels, creatinine levels, creatinine clearance). Notify doctor of any signs of decreasing renal function.
- Keep patient well hydrated to minimize renal tubule irritation.
- Evaluate patient's hearing before and during therapy. Report tinnitus, vertigo, or hearing loss to the doctor.
- Observe for signs of superinfection.

AMINOPENICILLINS
Selected drugs and administration routes
- amoxicillin trihydrate (Amoxican, Amoxil, Larotid): P.O.
- ampicillin (Amcill, Novoampicillin, Principen): P.O., I.M., I.V.
- Bacampicillin hydrochloride (Penglobe, Spectrobid): P.O.
- cyclacillin (Cyclapen-W): P.O.

Mechanism of action
Bactericidal; inhibits bacterial cell-wall synthesis.

Cautions and contraindications
Contraindicated in patients with hypersensitivity to any penicillin or cephalosporin. Use cautiously in patients with infectious mononucleosis.

Adverse reactions
GI: nausea, vomiting, diarrhea, gastritis, stomatitis.
Hematologic: anemia, thrombocytopenia, thrombocytopenic purpura, eosinophilia, neutropenia, leukopenia.
Other: hypersensitivity (erythematous maculopapular rash, urticaria, overgrowth of nonsusceptible organisms).

Interactions
Probenecid: Increases blood penicillin level (commonly used therapeutically for this purpose).
Estrogen-containing oral contraceptives: May decrease contraceptive effectiveness.

Clinical considerations
- Obtain specimen for culture and sensitivity before first dose.

Commonly Used Antibiotics *(continued)*

• Ask patient about any previous reactions he may have had to penicillin; however, keep in mind that a negative history does not preclude future reactions.
• Tell patient to take drug as prescribed, even after he feels better.
• Observe for signs of superinfection.
• Give at least 1 hour before bacteriostatic antibiotics.
• Advise patient to call doctor if rash, fever, or chills develop.
• Check expiration date; do not use any leftovers to treat new illness.

CEPHALOSPORINS
Selected drugs and administration routes
• cefaclor (Ceclor): P.O.
• cefadroxil monohydrate: (Duricef, Ultracef): P.O.
• cefamandole nafate (Mandol): I.M., I.V.
• cefazolin sodium (Ancef, Kefzol): I.M., I.V.
• cefonicid sodium (Monocid): I.M., I.V.
• cefoperazone sodium (Cefobid): I.M., I.V.
• ceforanide (Precef): I.M., I.V.
• cefotaxime sodium (Claforan): I.M., I.V.
• cefotetan sodium (Cefotan): I.M., I.V.
• cefoxitin sodium (Mefoxin): I.M., I.V.
• ceftazidime (Fortaz, Tazicef, Tazidime): I.M., I.V.
• ceftizoxime sodium (Cefizox): I.M., I.V.
• ceftriaxone sodium (Rocephin): I.M., I.V.
• cefuroxime sodium (Zinacef): I.M., I.V.
• cephalexin monohydrate (Keflex, Novolexin): P.O.
• cephalothin sodium (Ceporacin, Keflin): I.M., I.V.
• cephapirin sodium (Cefadyl): I.M., I.V.
• cephradine (Anspor, Velosef): P.O., I.M., I.V.
• moxalactam disodium (Moxam): I.M., I.V.

Mechanism of action
Bactericidal; inhibits bacterial cell-wall synthesis and cell division and growth, may lyse susceptible bacteria. Rapidly dividing bacteria are most susceptible.

Cautions and contraindications
Contraindicated in patients wtih hypersensitivity to cephalosporins. Use cautiously in patients with renal or hepatic impairment, history of GI disease, and penicillin allergy.

Adverse reactions
CNS: dizziness, headache, malaise, vertigo.
GI: nausea, vomiting, diarrhea, abdominal cramps, dyspepsia, tenesmus, pseudomembranous colitis, glossitis.
Hematologic: neutropenia, eosinophilia, leukopenia, anemia.
Hepatic: transient increase in liver enzyme levels.
Skin: rash.
Local: pain, tenderness, induration (I.M.); phlebitis, thrombophlebitis (I.V.).

Interactions
Probenecid: Decreases renal tubular secretion of cephalosporins excreted this way, increasing risk of toxicity.
Anticoagulants and thrombolytic agents: May increase risk of hemorrhage because of interference with vitamin K metabolism (with cefamandole, cefoperazone, or moxalactam).
Anti-inflammatory analgesics, platelet aggregate inhibitors, sulfinpyrazone: Additive inhibition of platelet function, increasing the risk of hemorrhage.
Ethyl alcohol: May cause a "disulfiramlike" reaction (with cefamandole, cefoperazone, cefotetan, or ormoxalactam).

Clinical considerations
• Obtain specimen for culture and sensitivity before first dose.

(continued)

Commonly Used Antibiotics *(continued)*

• Before administering first dose, ask patient if he's had any reaction to previous cephalosporin or penicillin therapy.
• Observe for signs of superinfection.
• Instruct patient to continue taking oral cephalosporins as prescribed, even after he feels better.

ERYTHROMYCINS
Selected drugs and administration routes
• erythromycin base (E-Mycin, Ilotycin, Novorythro): P.O.
• erythromycin estolate (Ilosone, Novorythro): P.O.
• erythromycin ethylsuccinate (E.E.S., Pediamycin): P.O.
• erythromycin glucoptate (Ilotycin): I.V.
• erythromycin lactobionate (Erythrocin): I.V.
• erythromycin stearate (E-Biotic, Erypar, Erythrocin): P.O.

Mechanism of action
May be bactericidal or bacteriostatic. Penetrate bacterial cell membrane and inhibit protein synthesis by binding to ribosomal 50S subunit.

Cautions and contraindications
Use cautiously in patients with impaired hepatic function (especially erythromycin estolate and ethylsuccinate).

Adverse reactions
EENT: hearing loss with increased I.V. doses.
GI: abdominal pain, cramping, nausea, vomiting, diarrhea.
Hepatic: hepatic dysfunction.
Skin: urticaria, rash.
Local: venous irritation, thrombophlebitis after I.V. injection.
Other: overgrowth of nonsusceptible bacteria or fungi.

Interactions
Warfarin: May cause excessive prolongation of prothrombin time, increasing the risk of hemorrhage.

Theophylline: May decrease liver clearance of theophylline.

Clinical considerations
• Obtain specimen for culture and sensitivity before first dose.
• Tell patient to take medication as directed, even after he feels better.
• For best absorption, instruct patient to take drug orally with a full glass of water 1 or 2 hours after meals. Tell him to take coated tablets with meals. Advise him against taking drug with fruit juice and to avoid swallowing chewable tablets whole.
• Note concentration when administering suspension.
• Monitor hepatic function, especially when administering estolate salt.
• Observe for signs of superinfection.

LINOMYCINS
Selected drugs and administration routes
• clindamycin phosphate (Cleocin, Dalacin C): P.O., I.M., I.V.
• lincomycin hydrochloride (Lincocin): P.O., I.M., I.V.

Mechanism of action
Inhibits bacterial protein synthesis by binding to ribosomal 50S subunit. Bacteriostatic, but may be bactericidal in high concentrations or against highly susceptible organisms.

Cautions and contraindications
Use cautiously in patients with a history of GI disease, especially colitis, and in patients with severe renal or hepatic impairment. Use cautiously, if at all, in patients with persistent diarrhea.

Adverse reactions
GI: nausea, vomiting, abdominal pain, diarrhea, pseudomembranous enterocolitis.
Hematologic: leukopenia, eosinophilia, thrombocytopenia.
Hepatic: elevated SGOT, alkaline phosphatase, and bilirubin levels.
Skin: rash, urticaria.

Commonly Used Antibiotics *(continued)*

Local: pain, induration, sterile abscess with I.M. injections; thrombophlebitis, erythema, pain after I.V. administration.
Other: anaphylaxis.

Interactions
Inhalation anesthetics or neuromuscular blockers: May enhance neuromuscular blocking effect.
Antidiarrheals (antiperistaltic or kaolin-containing): Antibiotic-associated pseudomembranous colitis may result in severe diarrhea; antiperistaltic antidiarrheals may delay removal of toxins, whereas kaolin-containing products may decrease drug absorption.

Clinical considerations
• Obtain specimen for culture and sensitivity before first dose.
• Tell patient to report adverse reactions, especially diarrhea.
• Observe for signs of superinfection.
• Monitor laboratory results for evidence of adverse reactions.
• Give medication deep I.M. Rotate sites.
• Check I.V. site for phlebitis and irritation.

EXTENDED-SPECTRUM PENICILLINS
Selected drugs and administration routes
• azlocillin sodium (Azlin): I.V.
• carbenicillin (Geocillin, Geopen, Geopen Oral, Pyopen): P.O., I.M., I.V.
• mezlocillin sodium (Mezlin): I.M., I.V.
• piperacillin sodium (Pipracil): I.M., I.V.
• ticarcillin disodium (Ticar): I.M., I.V.

Mechanism of action
Bactericidal; inhibits bacterial cell-wall synthesis.

Cautions and contraindications
Contraindicated in patients with hypersensitivity to any penicillin or cephalosporin. Use cautiously in hypokalemic or uremic patients and in those with bleeding tendencies.

Adverse reactions
CNS: neuromuscular irritability, headache, dizziness.
GI: nausea, vomiting, diarrhea, abdominal cramps.
Hematologic: bleeding with high doses, neutropenia, eosinophilia, leukopenia, thrombocytopenia.
Metabolic: hypokalemia.
Local: pain at infusion site, vein irritation, phlebitis with I.V. administration; pain, erythema, and induration with I.M injections.
Other: hypersenstivity (fever, rash, chills, pruritus, anaphylaxis).

Interactions
Anticoagulants or thrombolytic agents, nonsteroidal anti-inflammatory analgesics, sulfinpyrazone: May increase hemorrhage risk.
Probenecid: Decreases renal tubular penicillin secretion, increasing and prolonging penicillin concentration.

Clinical considerations
• Obtain specimen for culture and sensitivity before first dose.
• Ask patient about previous reactions to penicillin; however, keep in mind that a negative history does not preclude future reactions.
• Monitor complete blood count (CBC) and serum potassium levels.
• Observe for signs of superinfection.
• Give at least 1 hour before bacteriostatic antibiotics.
• Oral form of carbenicillin cannot be used to treat systemic infections; useful only for urinary tract infections.

NATURAL PENICILLINS
Selected drugs and administration routes
• penicillin G (Crystapen, Pentids, Pfizerpen): P.O., I.M., I.V.
• penicillin V potassium (Novopen VK, V-Cillin K): P.O.

Mechanism of action
Bactericidal; inhibits bacterial cell-wall synthesis.

(continued)

Commonly Used Antibiotics (continued)

Cautions and contraindications
Contraindicated in patients with hypersensitivity to any penicillin or cephalosporin.

Adverse reactions
CNS: hallucinations, confusion, lethargy, twitching, seizures.
GI: epigastric distress, nausea, vomiting, diarrhea.
Hematologic: eosinophilia, hemolytic anemia, leukopenia, thrombocytopenia.
Other: hypersensitivity (rash, urticaria, chills, fever, edema, anaphylaxis), overgrowth of nonsusceptible organisms.

Interactions
Probenecid: Increases blood levels of penicillin (often used therapeutically for this purpose).

Clinical considerations
• Obtain specimen for culture and sensitivity before first dose.
• Ask patient about previous reactions to penicillin; however, keep in mind that a negative history does not preclude future reactions.
• Observe for signs of superinfection.
• Monitor renal and hematologic function test results.
• Give at least 1 hour before bacteriostatic antibiotics.

PENICILLINASE-RESISTANT PENICILLINS
Selected drugs and administration routes
• cloxacillin sodium (Bactopen, Tegopen): P.O.
• dicloxacillin sodium (Dynapen): P.O.
• methicillin sodium (Staphcillin): I.M., I.V.
• nafcillin sodium (Nafcil, Unipen): P.O., I.M., I.V.
• oxacillin sodium (Prostaphlin): P.O., I.M., I.V.

Mechanism of action
Bactericidal; inhibits bacterial cell-wall synthesis. Bacteria resist penicillin by producing enzymes—penicillinases—that break down penicillin. These penicillinase-resistant penicillins resist this enzymatic breakdown.

Cautions and contraindications
Contraindicated in patients wtih hypersensitivity to any penicillin or cephalosporin.

Adverse reactions
GI: nausea, vomiting, diarrhea.
Hematologic: eosinophilia, neutropenia, leukopenia, thrombocytopenia.
Local: thrombophlebitis.
Other: hypersensitivity (rash, fever, chills, anaphylaxis), overgrowth of nonsusceptible organisms.

Interactions
Probenecid: Increases blood levels of penicillin (commonly used therapeutically for this purpose).

Clinical considerations
• Obtain specimen for culture and sensitivity before first dose.
• Ask patient about previous reactions to penicillin; however, keep in mind that a negative history does not preclude future reactions.
• Advise patient to take drug as prescribed, even if he feels better.
• Advise patient to call doctor if rash, fever, or chills develop.
• Observe for signs of superinfection.
• Give at least 1 hour before bacteriostatic antibiotics.

SULFONAMIDES
Selected drugs and administrationtion routes
• co-trimoxazole [sulfamethoxazole-trimethoprim] (Apo-Sulfatrim, Bactrim, Cotrim, Septra): P.O., I.V.
• sulfacytine (Renoquid): P.O.
• sulfadiazine (Microsulfon): P.O.
• sulfamethizole (Thiosulfil): P.O.
• sulfamethoxazole (Gantanol): P.O.
• sulfapyridine: P.O.
• Sulfisoxazole (Gantrisin, Novosoxazole): P.O.

Commonly Used Antibiotics *(continued)*

Mechanism of action
Bacteriostatic; interferes with folic acid biosynthesis, which is essential for bacterial growth.

Cautions and contraindications
Contraindicated in patients with porphyria. Use cautiously and in reduced doses in patients with hepatic or renal function impairment, urinary obstruction, blood dyscrasias, severe allergies, asthma, and glucose-6-phosphate dehydrogenase (G-6PD) deficiency.

Adverse reactions
CNS: headache, depression.
GI: nausea, vomiting, diarrhea, abdominal pain, anorexia, stomatitis.
GU: renal damage (renal colic, oliguria, obstructive anuria, hematuria, proteinuria, crystalluria).
Hematologic: agranulocytosis, aplastic anemia, leukopenia, hemolytic anemia.
Hepatic: functional changes causing jaundice.
Skin: erythema multiforme (Stevens-Johnson syndrome), exfoliative dermatitis, photosensitivity, pruritus.
Other: serum sickness, fever, anaphylaxis.

Interactions
Para-aminobenzoic acid (PABA): May antagonize bacteriostatic effect.
Oral anticoagulants, oral antidiabetic agents: Sulfonamides may increase or prolong effects of these drugs.
Methenamine: May form an insoluble precipitate and increase risk of crystalluria.

Clinical considerations
• Obtain specimen for culture and sensitivity before first dose.
• Advise patient to take drug with a full glass of water and to drink plenty of water throughout the day to prevent crystalluria. Monitor intake and output. Sodium bicarbonate may be given to alkalinize urine. Monitor urine pH.
• Advise patient to continue taking medication as prescribed, even if he feels better.
• Caution patient to avoid direct sunlight and ultraviolet light.
• Monitor urine culture results, urinalysis, and CBC.
• Observe for signs of superinfection.
• Co-trimoxazole is one of the preferred anti-infectives used to treat *Pneumocystis carinii.*

TETRACYCLINES
Selected drugs and administration routes
• demeclocycline hydrochloride (Declomycin): P.O.
• doxycycline hyclate (Vibramycin): P.O., I.V.
• methacycline hydrochloride (Rondomycin): P.O.
• minocycline hydrochloride (Minocin, Vectrin): P.O., I.V.
• oxytetracycline hydrochloride (Terramycin): P.O., I.M., I.V.
• tetracycline hydrochloride (Achromycin V, Panmycin, Sumycin): P.O., I.M., I.V.

Mechanism of action
Bacteriostatic usually; may be bactericidal in high concentrations. Reversibly bind to 30S and 50S ribosomal subunits, inhibiting protein synthesis.

Cautions and contraindications
Use cautiously in patients with renal or hepatic function impairment. During last half of pregnancy and in children under age 8, tetracylines may cause permanent tooth discoloration, enamel defects, and retarded bone growth.

Adverse reactions
EENT: dysphagia, glossitis.
GI: anorexia, nausea, vomiting,

(continued)

Commonly Used Antibiotics (continued)

diarrhea, anogenital lesions.
Hematologic: neutropenia, eosinophilia.
Metabolic: increased BUN levels,
diabetes insipidus syndrome (polyuria, polydipsia, weakness).
Skin: maculopapular and erythematous rash, photosensitivity, increased pigmentation, urticaria.

Interactions
*Antacids, calcium supplements, iron
supplements, magnesium-contain-
ing laxatives:* may impair tetracycline absorption.

Clinical considerations
● Obtain specimen for culture and
sensitivity before first dose.
● Some tetracyclines can be taken with
food or milk (such as doxycycline and
minocycline); others should be taken
on an empty stomach (such as demeclocycline, oxytetracycline, and tetracycline). Advise patient accordingly.
● Tetracyclines may cause false-
positive or false-negative Clinistix or
Tes-Tape readings.
● Observe for signs of superinfection.
● Check expiration date.
● Do not expose to light or heat.

Clinical considerations
● Drug is contraindicated in patients
with acute hepatic disease or isonizid-
associated hepatic damage. Use cautiously in patients with chronic non-iso-
niazid-associated hepatic disease,
seizure disorder (especially those taking
phenytoin), severe renal impairment,
and chronic alcoholism; in elderly patients; and in slow acetylators.
● Monitor hepatic function. Tell patient to notify doctor immediately if
signs or symptoms of hepatic impairment occur (loss of appetite, fatigue,
malaise, jaundice, dark urine).
● Concomitant alcohol intake may be
associated with increased incidence of
isoniazid-related hepatitis. Discourage use.
● Pyridoxine should be given to prevent peripheral neuropathy, especially
in malnourished patients.
● Instruct patient to take this drug exactly as prescribed; warn against discontinuing drug without doctor's
consent.
● Encourage patient to comply fully
with treatment, which may take
months or years.

● Advise patient to take drug with food
if GI irritation occurs.

rifampin
Rifadin, Rimactane, Rofact

Mechanism of action
Bactericidal; inhibits DNA-dependent
RNA polymerase, thus impairing RNA
synthesis.

Respiratory indications and dosage
● Primary treatment in pulmonary tuberculosis—
Adults: 600 mg P.O. daily as a single
dose 1 hour before or 2 hours after
meals.
Children over age 5: 10 to 20 mg/kg
P.O. daily as a single dose, 1 hour
before or 2 hours after meals. Maximum dose is 600 mg/day. Concomitant
administration of other effective antitubercular drugs is recommended.

Adverse reactions
Blood: thrombocytopenia, transient
leukopenia, hemolytic anemia.
CNS: headache, fatigue, drowsiness,
ataxia, dizziness, mental confusion,
generalized numbness.

GI: epigastric distress, anorexia, nausea, vomiting, abdominal pain, diarrhea, flatulence, sore mouth and tongue.
Hepatic: serious hepatotoxicity and transient abnormalities in liver function tests.
Metabolic: hyperuricemia.
Skin: pruritus, urticaria, rash.
Other: influenza-like syndrome.

Interactions
Para-aminosalicylate sodium, ketoconazole: may interfere with rifampin absorption. Give these drugs 8 to 12 hours apart.
Probenecid: may increase rifampin blood levels. Use cautiously.

Clinical considerations
• Drug is contraindicated in patients with clinically active hepatitis.
• Use cautiously in patients with hepatic disease or in those receiving hepatotoxic drugs.
• Monitor hepatic function, hematopoietic studies, and serum uric acid levels.
• Watch closely for signs and symptoms of hepatic impairment (appetite loss, fatigue, malaise, jaundice, dark urine, liver tenderness).
• Warn patient about drowsiness; possible red-orange discoloration of urine, feces, saliva, sweat, sputum, and tears; and possible permanent staining of soft contact lenses.
• Although rifampin isn't considered a teratogen, it may cause hemorrhage in newborns of rifampin-treated women.
• Advise patient to avoid alcoholic beverages while taking drug to avoid risk of hepatotoxicity.
• Give 1 hour before or 2 hours after meals for optimal absorption; however, if GI irritation occurs, patient may take rifampin with meals.
• Drug increases liver enzyme activity; patient may require increased doses of warfarin, corticosteroids, oral contraceptives, and oral hypoglycemics.

• Concomitant treatment with at least one other antitubercular drug is recommended.

streptomycin sulfate
Mechanism of action
Generally bactericidal; aminoglycoside antibiotic that inhibits protein synthesis by binding directly to the 30S ribosomal subunit.

Respiratory indications and dosage
• Primary and adjunctive treatment in tuberculosis—
Adults: With normal renal function, 1 g I.M. daily for 2 to 3 months, then 1 g two or three times a week. Inject deeply into upper outer quadrant of buttocks.
Children: With normal renal function, 20 mg/kg/day in divided doses injected deeply into large muscle mass. Give concurrently with other antitubercular agents (but not with capreomycin) and continue until sputum specimen becomes negative.
  For patients with impaired renal function, initial dose is same as for those with normal renal function. Subsequent doses and frequency determined by renal function study results.

Adverse reactions
EENT: ototoxicity (tinnitus, vertigo, hearing loss).
GU: nephrotoxicity (but not nearly as frequent as with other aminoglycosides).
Skin: exfoliative dermatitis.
Local: pain, irritation, and sterile abscesses at injection site.
Other: hypersensitivity (rash, fever, urticaria, angioneurotic edema).

Interactions
Dimenhydrinate: may mask signs and symptoms of streptomycin-induced ototoxicity. Use together cautiously.
I.V. loop diuretics (such as furosemide): increased ototoxicity. Use cautiously.
Cephalothin: increased nephrotoxicity. Use together cautiously.

Clinical considerations
• Drug is contraindicated in patients with labyrinthine disease. Use cautiously in patients with impaired renal function and in elderly patients.
• Keep patient well hydrated during drug therapy to minimize chemical irritation of renal tubules.
• Evaluate patient's hearing before, during, and 6 months after therapy. Notify doctor if patient complains of tinnitus, roaring noises, or fullness in ears.
• Watch for signs of superinfection (such as continued fever).
• Protect your hands when preparing drug. Drug irritates skin.
• In primary treatment of tuberculosis, streptomycin is discontinued when sputum culture results become negative.

Antifungals and antiprotozoals

Drugs presented in this section are used primarily to treat fungal diseases; however, pentamidine isethionate is an antiprotozoal agent used in the treatment of *Pneumocystis carinii*, a protozoal infection that sometimes occurs in immunocompromised patients.

amphotericin B
Fungizone

Mechanism of action
Probably acts by binding to sterols in the fungal cell membrane, altering cell permeability and allowing leakage of intracellular components.

Respiratory indications and dosage
• Systemic fungal infections (histoplasmosis, coccidioidomycosis, blastomycosis, cryptococcosis, disseminated moniliasis, aspergillosis, phycomycosis)—
Adults and children: Initially, 1 mg in 250 ml of D_5W in water infused over 2 to 4 hours; or 0.25 mg/kg/day by slow infusion over 6 hours. Increase daily dosage gradually as patient tolerance develops, to a maximum of 1 mg/kg/day. Dosage must not exceed 1.5 mg/kg. If drug is discontinued for 1 week or more, administration must resume with initial dose and again increase gradually.

Adverse reactions
Blood: normochromic, normocytic anemia.
CNS: headache, peripheral neuropathy; peripheral nerve pain, paresthesias with intrathecal administration.
GI: anorexia, weight loss, nausea, vomiting, dyspepsia, diarrhea, epigastric cramps.
GU: abnormal renal function with hypokalemia, azotemia, hyposthenuria, renal tubular acidosis, nephrocalcinosis; permanent renal impairment, anuria, oliguria with large doses.
Local: burning, stinging, irritation, tissue damage with extravasation, thrombophlebitis, pain at injection site.
Other: arthralgia, myalgia, muscle weakness secondary to hypokalemia, fever, chills, malaise, generalized pain.

Interactions
Other nephrotoxic antibiotics: may cause additive nephrotoxicity. Administer with extreme caution.

Clinical considerations
• Use cautiously in patients with impaired renal function.
• Use parenterally only in hospitalized patients under close supervision, when diagnosis of potentially fatal fungal infection has been confirmed.
• Monitor vital signs; fever may appear 1 to 2 hours after start of I.V. infusion and should subside within 4 hours after discontinuation.
• Monitor intake and output; report change in urine appearance or volume. Renal damage is usually reversible if drug is stopped with first sign of dysfunction.
• Obtain liver and renal function studies weekly. If blood urea nitrogen (BUN) level exceeds 40 mg/dl or if serum creatinine level exceeds 3 mg/dl, doctor may reduce or stop drug until renal function improves. Monitor

complete blood count weekly. Stop drug if bromsulphalein, alkaline phosphatase, or bilirubin levels rise.
• Monitor serum potassium levels closely. Report any signs or symptoms of hypokalemia. Check calcium and magnesium levels periodically.
• If drug is in dry state, store at 35.6° to 46.4° F. (2° to 8° C.). Protect from light. Drug expires 2 years after manufacture date. Reconstitute with 10 ml sterile water only. Mixing with solutions containing sodium chloride, other electrolytes, or bacteriostatic agents (such as benzyl alcohol) causes precipitation. Don't use if solution contains precipitate or foreign matter.
• Drug appears to be compatible with limited amounts of heparin sodium, hydrocortisone sodium succinate, and methylprednisolone sodium succinate.
• Reconstituted solution remains stable for 1 week under refrigeration or 24 hours at room temperature. It has 24-hour stability in room light.
• An initial test dose may be prescribed: 1 mg is added to 50 to 150 ml of D₅W and infused over 20 to 30 minutes.
• Severity of some adverse reactions can be reduced by premedication with aspirin, antihistamines, antiemetics, or small doses of corticosteroids; addition of phosphate buffer and heparin to the solution; and alternate-day dose schedule. For severe reactions, drug may have to be stopped for varying periods.
• For I.V. infusion, an in-line membrane with a mean pore diameter larger than 1 micron can be used. Infuse very slowly; rapid infusion may result in cardiovascular collapse. Warn patient of discomfort at infusion site and other potential adverse reactions. Advise patient that he may need several months of therapy to ensure adequate response.
• Administer in distal veins. If veins become thrombosed, doctor can change to every-other-day regimen.
• Antibiotics should be given separately; don't mix or piggyback with amphotericin B.

flucytosine (5-FC)
Ancobon, Ancotil

Mechanism of action
Appears to penetrate fungal cells, where it's converted to fluorouracil, a known metabolic antagonist. Causes defective protein synthesis.

Respiratory indications and dosage
• For severe fungal infections caused by susceptible strains of *Candida* (including septicemia, endocarditis, and pulmonary infections) and *Cryptococcus* pulmonary infection—
Adults and children weighing over 50 kg: 50 to 150 mg/kg P.O. daily q 6 hours.
Adults and children weighing under 50 kg: 1.5 to 4.5 g/m² P.O. daily in four divided doses. Severe infection, such as meningitis, may warrant doses up to 250 mg/kg.

Adverse reactions
Blood: anemia, leukopenia, bone marrow depression, thrombocytopenia.
CNS: dizziness, drowsiness, confusion, headache, vertigo.
GI: nausea, vomiting, diarrhea, abdominal bloating.
Hepatic: elevated SGOT and SGPT levels.
Metabolic: elevated serum alkaline phosphatase, BUN, and serum creatinine levels.
Skin: occasional rash.

Interactions
None significant.

Clinical considerations
• Use with extreme caution in patients with impaired hepatic or renal function or bone marrow depression.
• Arrange for hematologic tests and renal and liver function studies before therapy and repeat at frequent intervals thereafter. Before treatment, susceptibility tests should establish that organism is flucytosine-sensitive. Tests should be repeated weekly to monitor drug resistance.

• Capsules can be given over a 15-minute period to reduce nausea, vomiting, and stomach upset.
• Monitor intake and output; report any marked change.
• If possible, serum level assays of drug should be performed regularly to maintain flucytosine at therapeutic level (25 to 120 mcg/ml). Higher serum levels may be toxic.
• Drug is always given in combination with amphotericin B; use may be synergistic.
• Store in light-resistant containers.
• Adequate response may take weeks or months.

ketoconazole
Nizoral

Mechanism of action
Inhibits purine transport and DNA, RNA, and protein synthesis; increases cell-wall permeability, making the fungus more susceptible to osmotic pressure.

Respiratory indications and dosage
• Systemic candidiasis, chronic mucocandidiasis, coccidioidomycosis, histoplasmosis, chromomycosis, and paracoccidioidomycosis—
Adults and children over 40 kg: Initially, 200 mg P.O. daily as a single dose. Dosage may be increased to 400 mg/day in patients who don't respond to lower dosage.
Children under 20 kg: 50 mg (¼ tablet)/day as a single dose.
Children 20 to 40 kg: 100 mg (½ tablet)/day as a single dose.

Adverse reactions
CNS: headache, nervousness, dizziness.
GI: nausea, vomiting, abdominal pain, diarrhea, constipation.
Hepatic: elevated liver enzyme levels, fatal hepatotoxicity.
Skin: itching.
Other: gynecomastia with breast tenderness in males.

Interactions
Antacids, anticholinergics, H_2 blockers: decreased absorption of ketoconazole. Wait at least 2 hours after ketoconazole dose before administering these drugs.
Rifampin, isoniazid: increased ketoconazole metabolism. Monitor for decreased antifungal effect.

Clinical considerations
• Make sure patient understands that treatment should be continued until all clinical and laboratory tests indicate that active fungal infection has subsided. If drug is discontinued too soon, infection will recur. Minimum treatment for candidiasis is 7 to 14 days. Minimum treatment for other systemic fungal infections is 6 months.
• Reassure patient that although nausea commonly occurs early in therapy, it will subside. To minimize nausea, divide the daily dosage into two doses, as ordered. Taking drug with meals also helps to decrease nausea.
• Monitor for elevated liver enzyme levels and persistent nausea, and for unusual fatigue, jaundice, and dark urine or pale stools. These may signal hepatotoxicity.

miconazole
Monistat I.V.

Mechanism of action
Inhibits purine transport and DNA, RNA, and protein synthesis; increases cell-wall permeability, making fungus more susceptible to osmotic pressure.

Respiratory indications and dosage
• Systemic fungal infections (coccidioidomycosis, candidiasis, cryptococcosis, paracoccidioidomycosis)—
Adults: 200 to 3,600 mg/day. Doses may vary with diagnosis and with infective agent. May divide daily dose over 3 infusions, 200 to 1,200 mg/infusion. Dilute in at least 200 ml of normal saline solution. Repeated courses may be needed because of re-

lapse or reinfection.
Children: 20 to 40 mg/kg/day. Do not exceed 15 mg/kg infusion.

Adverse reactions
Blood: transient decreases in hematocrit count, thrombocytopenia.
CNS: dizziness, drowsiness.
GI: nausea, vomiting, diarrhea.
Local: phlebitis at injection site.
Metabolic: transient decrease in serum sodium level.
Skin: pruritic rash.

Interactions
None significant.

Clinical considerations
• Rapid injection of undiluted miconazole may produce dysrhythmias.
• Acute cardiorespiratory arrest may occur with first dose. A doctor should be present when first dose is administered.
• Premedication with antiemetic may diminish nausea and vomiting.
• Avoid administration at mealtime to reduce adverse GI reactions.
• Drug causes fewer and less severe adverse reactions than other antifungals.
• Pruritic rash may persist for weeks after drug is discontinued. Pruritus may be controlled with oral or I.V. diphenhydramine.
• Give I.V. infusion over 30 to 60 minutes.
• Inform patient that adequate response may take weeks or months.
• Monitor levels of hemoglobin, hematocrit, serum electrolytes, and lipids regularly. Transient elevations in serum cholesterol and triglycerides may stem from castor oil vehicle.

pentamidine isethionate
Pentam 300

Mechanism of action
Interferes with biosynthesis of DNA, RNA, phospholipids, and proteins.

Respiratory indications and dosage
• Pneumonia caused by *Pneumocystis carinii—*
Adults and children: 4 mg/kg I.V. or I.M. once daily for 14 days.

Adverse reactions
Blood: leukopenia, thrombocytopenia, anemia.
CNS: confusion, hallucinations.
CV: hypotension, tachycardia.
GI: nausea, anorexia, metallic taste.
GU: elevated serum creatinine level, renal toxicity.
Hepatic: elevated liver enzyme level.
Local: sterile abscess, pain, or induration at injection site.
Skin: rash, facial flushing, pruritus.
Other: fever, hypoglycemia, hypocalcemia.

Interactions
None significant.

Clinical considerations
• With firmly established diagnosis of *P. carinii* pneumonia, no absolute contraindications exist to pentamidine therapy.
• Use cautiously in patients with hypertension, hypotension, hypoglycemia, hypocalcemia, leukopenia, thrombocytopenia, anemia, or hepatic or renal dysfunction.
• Patient should be lying down when receiving the drug because sudden severe hypotension may develop. Monitor blood pressure during administration and several times thereafter until it stabilizes.
• When administering I.V., infuse over 60 minutes to minimize hypotension risk.
• Monitor blood glucose, serum creatinine, and BUN levels daily.
• Pain and induration occur with I.M. injection. Administer by deep I.M. injection.
• In patients with acquired immunodeficiency syndrome (AIDS), pentamidine produces less severe adverse reactions than the alternative treat-

ment, co-trimoxazole.Therefore, pentamidine is the treatment of choice in patients with AIDS.

Antivirals

Many drugs that work against viruses in the laboratory seem ineffective in clinical use. However, amantadine hydrochloride has been proven effective in treating and preventing infections caused by the influenza type A virus; ribavirin effectively treats infections caused by the respiratory syncytial virus (RSV).

amantadine hydrochloride
Symmetrel

Mechanism of action
Interferes with influenza A virus penetration into susceptible cells.

Respiratory indications and dosage
• Prophylaxis or symptomatic treatment of influenza A respiratory tract illnesses—
Adults and children age 10 to 64: 200 mg P.O. daily in a single dose or divided b.i.d.
Adults over age 64: 100 mg P.O. once daily.
Children age 1 to 9: 4.4 to 8.8 mg/kg P.O. daily, divided b.i.d. or t.i.d. Do not exceed 150 mg/day.

Continue treating for 24 to 48 hours after symptoms disappear. Prophylaxis should start immediately after initial exposure and continue for at least 10 days after exposure. May continue prophylactic treatment up to 90 days for repeated or suspected exposure if influenza vaccine is unavailable. If used with influenza vaccine, continue dose for 2 to 3 weeks until protection from vaccine develops.

Adverse reactions
CNS: depression, fatigue, confusion, dizziness, psychosis, hallucinations, anxiety, irritability, ataxia, insomnia, weakness, headache, light-headedness, difficulty concentrating.

CV: peripheral edema, orthostatic hypotension, congestive heart failure.
GI: anorexia, nausea, constipation, vomiting, dry mouth.
GU: urinary retention.
Skin: livedo reticularis with prolonged use.

Interactions
None significant.

Clinical considerations
• Use cautiously in patients with history of epilepsy, congestive heart failure, peripheral edema, hepatic disease, mental illness, eczematoid rash, renal impairment, orthostatic hypotension, or cardiovascular disease, and in elderly patients.
• For best absorption, drug should be taken after meals.
• Instruct patient to report adverse drug reactions to the doctor, especially dizziness, depression, anxiety, nausea, and urinary retention.
• Elderly patients have higher risk of adverse neurological reactions. Taking the drug in two daily doses rather than a single dose may reduce this risk.
• If orthostatic hypotension occurs, instruct patient not to stand or change positions too quickly.
• If insomnia occurs, dose should be taken several hours before bedtime.

ribavirin
Virazole

Mechanism of action
Inhibits viral activity by an unknown mechanism. Thought to inhibit RNA and DNA synthesis by depleting intracellular nucleotide pools.

Respiratory indications and dosage
• Hospitalized infants and young children infected by RSV—
Children: Solution in concentration of 20 mg/ml delivered via Viratek Small Particle Aerosol Generator (SPAG-2). Continue treatment for 12 to 18 hours/day for at least 3 but no more than 7 days.

Adverse reactions
Blood: anemia, reticulocytosis.
CV: cardiac arrest, hypotension.
Respiratory: worsening of respiratory status, bacterial pneumonia, pneumothorax, apnea, ventilator dependence.

Interactions
None significant.

Clinical considerations
• Drug is contraindicated in women who are or may become pregnant during treatment.
• Ribavirin aerosol is indicated only for severe lower respiratory tract infection caused by RSV. Although treatment may begin while awaiting diagnostic test results, RSV infection must eventually be documented.
• Most infants and children with RSV infection don't require treatment because the disease is mild and self-limiting. Infants with such underlying conditions as prematurity or cardiopulmonary disease typically suffer severest form of RSV and benefit most from treatment with ribavirin aerosol.
• This treatment must be accompanied by—not replace—supportive respiratory and fluid management.
• Ribavirin aerosol must be administered by SPAG-2. Don't use any other aerosol-generating device.
• Water used to reconstitute this drug must not contain any antimicrobial agents. Use sterile USP water for injection, not bacteriostatic water.
• Discard solutions placed in SPAG-2 unit at least every 24 hours before adding newly reconstituted solution.
• Store reconstituted solutions at room temperature for 24 hours.

Neuromuscular blockers

Neuromuscular blockers (peripheral muscle relaxants) are used to induce temporary skeletal muscle paralysis for intubation, mechanical ventilation, or surgery. Because these potentially dangerous drugs paralyze muscles essential for airway maintenance and ventilation (tracheal, diaphragmatic, and intercostal muscles), they must be accompanied by ventilatory support. These drugs have no effect on the CNS and don't alter consciousness or pain sensation; therefore, sedatives, analgesics, or anesthetics must be administered. Neuromuscular blockers usually are given only by highly trained and experienced personnel. Acting at the motor end plate of the neuromuscular junction, neuromuscular blockers act in one of two ways. Nondepolarizing (or competitive) blockers bind with acetylcholine (ACH) receptors on the postsynaptic membrane, thus blocking ACH access to its receptor. Depolarizing (or noncompetitive) blockers desensitize the postsynaptic junction to ACH by depolarizing the membrane. The important distinction between these two types of blockers is that the effects of nondepolarizing blockers are pharmacologically reversible.

atracurium besylate
Tracrium

Mechanism of action
Prevents acetylcholine from binding to receptors on the motor end plate, thus blocking depolarization. Nondepolarizing agent.

Respiratory indications and dosage
• Adjunct to general anesthesia to facilitate endotracheal intubation and to provide skeletal muscle relaxation during surgery or mechanical ventilation (dose depends on anesthetic used, individual needs, and response; doses are representative and must be adjusted)—
Adults and children over age 2: 0.4 to 0.5 mg/kg by I.V. bolus. Maintenance dose of 0.08 to 0.10 mg/kg within 20 to 45 minutes of initial dose should be administered during prolonged surgical procedures. Maintenance doses may be

administered q 12 to 25 minutes in patients receiving balanced anesthesic.

Adverse reactions
CV: bradycardia.
Skin: flushing, erythema, pruritus, urticaria.
Other: prolonged dose-related apnea.

Interactions
Aminoglycoside antibiotics (amikacin, gentamicin, kanamycin, neomycin, streptomycin), polymyxin antibiotics (polymyxin B sulfate, colistin), clindamycin, quinidine procainamide, local anesthetics: potentiated neuromuscular blockade, causing increased skeletal muscle relaxation and possible respiratory paralysis. Use cautiously during surgical and postoperative periods.
Lithium, magnesium salts, narcotic analgesics, certain inhalation anesthetics: potentiated neuromuscular blockade, causing increased skeletal muscle relaxation and possible respiratory paralysis. Use with extreme caution and reduce atracurium dose.

Clinical considerations
• Use cautiously in patients with cardiovascular disease, severe electrolyte disorders, and neuromuscular diseases.
• Prior succinylcholine administration doesn't prolong duration of action; however, it quickens atracurium's onset of action and may deepen neuromuscular blockade.
• Atracurium provides conditions for adequate intubation within 2 to 2½ minutes. Duration of effect ranges from 20 to 35 minutes.
• Once spontaneous recovery starts, atracurium-induced neuromuscular blockade may be reversed with concomitant administration of an anticholinesterase agent and an anticholinergic drug.
• Don't administer by I.M. injection.
• Atracurium has a longer duration of action than succinylcholine and a shorter duration of action than d-tubocurarine or pancuronium.

gallamine triethiodide
Flaxedil

Mechanism of action
Prevents acetylcholine from binding to muscle end plate receptors, thus blocking depolarization. Nondepolarizing agent.

Respiratory indications and dosage
• Adjunct to anesthesia to induce skeletal muscle relaxation; facilitate intubation, reduction of fractures and dislocations; assist with mechanical ventilation (dose depends on anesthetic used, individual needs, and response; doses are representative and must be adjusted)—
Adults and children over age 1 month: Initially, 1 mg/kg I.V., to maximum of 100 mg regardless of patient's weight; then 0.5 mg to 1 mg/kg q 30 to 40 minutes.
Children under age 1 month but over 5 kg (11 lb): Initially, 0.25 to 0.75 mg/kg I.V. May give additional doses of 0.1 to 0.5 mg/kg q 30 to 40 minutes.

Adverse reactions
CV: tachycardia.
Other: respiratory paralysis, dose-related prolonged apnea, residual muscle weakness, increased oropharyngeal secretions, allergic or idiosyncratic hypersensitivity reactions.

Interactions
Aminoglycoside antibiotics (amikacin, gentamicin, kanamycin, neomycin, streptomycin), polymyxin antibiotics (polymyxin B sulfate, colistin), clindamycin, quinidine, local anesthetics: potentiated neuromuscular blockade, causing increased skeletal muscle relaxation and possible respiratory paralysis. Use cautiously during surgical and postoperative periods.
Narcotic analgesics and certain inhalational anesthetics: potentiated neuromuscular blockade, causing increased skeletal muscle relaxation and possible respiratory paralysis. Use with extreme caution and reduce gallamine

dose. Azathioprine can reverse or decrease neuromuscular blockade.

Clinical considerations
• Drug is contraindicated in patients with hypersensitivity to iodides, patients with impaired renal function or myasthenia gravis, patients in shock, and patients in whom tachycardia may be hazardous. Use cautiously in elderly or debilitated patients; those with hepatic or pulmonary impairment, respiratory depression, myasthenic syndrome of lung cancer, dehydration, thyroid disorders, collagen diseases, porphyria, or electrolyte disturbances; and in patients undergoing cesarean section.
• Monitor baseline electrolyte levels (electrolyte imbalance can potentiate neuromuscular effects).
• Take vital signs every 15 minutes, especially checking for developing tachycardia. Immediately notify doctor of significant changes.
• Measure intake and output (renal dysfunction prolongs drug's duration of action, because drug is unchanged before excretion).
• Keep airway clear. Have emergency respiratory support equipment (such as endotracheal equipment, ventilator, oxygen, atropine, neostigmine) on hand.
• Determine whether patient has iodide allergy.
• Protect drug from light or excessive heat; use only fresh solutions.
• Do not mix solution with meperidine hydrochloride or barbiturate solutions.
• Give I.V. slowly (over 30 to 90 seconds).
• Do not give without doctor's direct supervision.
• Drug may be preferred in patients with bradycardia.
• Neostigmine or edrophonium may be used to reverse drug's effects.

metocurine iodide
Metubine

Mechanism of action
Prevents acetylcholine from binding to muscle end plate receptors, thus blocking depolarization. Nondepolarizing agent.

Respiratory indications and dosage
• Adjunct to anesthesia to induce skeletal muscle relaxation; facilitate intubation, reduction of fractures, and dislocations (dose depends on anesthetic used, individual needs, and response; doses are representative and must be adjusted. Administer as sustained injection over 30 to 60 seconds)—
Adults: Given with cyclopropane, 2 to 4 mg I.V. (2.68 mg average). Given with ether, 1.5 to 3 mg I.V. (2.1 mg average). Given with nitrous oxide, 4 to 7 mg I.V. (4.79 mg average); supplemental injections of 0.5 to 1 mg given in 25 to 90 minutes, repeated p.r.n.

Adverse reactions
CV: hypotension secondary to histamine release, ganglionic blockade with rapid dose or overdose.
Other: dose-related prolonged apnea, residual muscle weakness, increased oropharyngeal secretions, allergic or idiosyncratic hypersensitivity reactions, bronchospasm.

Interactions
Aminoglycoside antibiotics (amikacin, gentamicin, kanamycin, neomycin, streptomycin), polymyxin antibiotics (polymyxin B sulfate, colistin), clindamycin, quinidine, local anesthetics: potentiated neuromuscular blockade, leading to increased skeletal muscle relaxation and possible respiratory paralysis. Use cautiously during surgical and postoperative periods.
Narcotic analgesics: potentiated neuromuscular blockade, leading to increased skeletal muscle relaxation and possible respiratory paralysis. Use with extreme caution, and reduce metocurine iodide dose.

Clinical considerations
• Drug is contraindicated in patients with hypersensitivity to iodide and in

patients with asthma, atrophy, or other conditions that might be jeopardized by histamine release. Use cautiously in elderly or debilitated patients and in patients with renal, hepatic, or pulmonary impairment; respiratory depression; myasthenia gravis; myasthenic syndrome of lung cancer; dehydration; thyroid disorders; collagen diseases; porphyria; electrolyte disturbances; hyperthermia; and, in large doses, cesarean section.

• Neostigmine and edrophonium may be used to reverse metocurine's effects.

• A 1-mg dose is the therapeutic equivalent of 3 mg tubocurarine chloride.

• Monitor baseline electrolyte levels and vital signs, especially respiration. Electrolyte imbalance, especially potassium, calcium, and magnesium, can potentiate neuromuscular effects.

• Measure intake and output (renal dysfunction prolongs drug's duration of action, because drug is mainly unchanged before excretion).

• Keep airway clear. Have emergency respiratory support (such as endotracheal equipment, ventilator, oxygen, atropine, edrophonium, epinephrine, and neostigmine) on hand.

• Determine whether patient has iodide allergy.

pancuronium bromide
Pavulon

Mechanism of action
Nondepolarizing agent; prevents acetylcholine from binding to muscle end plate receptors, thus blocking depolarization.

Respiratory indications and dosage
• Adjunct to anesthesia to induce skeletal muscle relaxation; facilitate intubation; assist with mechanical ventilation (dose depends on anesthetic used, individual needs, and response; doses are representative and must be adjusted)—
Adults: Initially, 0.04 to 0.1 mg/kg I.V.; then 0.01 mg/kg q 30 to 60 minutes.

Children over age 10: Initially, 0.04 to 0.1 mg/kg I.V., then ⅕ initial dose q 30 to 60 minutes.

Adverse reactions
CV: tachycardia, increased blood pressure.
Local: burning sensation.
Other: excessive sweating and salivation, prolonged dose-related apnea, residual muscle weakness, allergic or idiosyncratic hypersensitivity reaction.

Interactions
Aminoglycoside antibiotics (amikacin, gentamicin, kanamycin, neomycin, streptomycin), polymyxin antibiotics (polymyxin B sulfate, colistin), clindamycin, lincomycin, quinidine, quinine, magnesium salts; local anesthetics: potentiated neuromuscular blockade, causing increased skeletal muscle relaxation and possible respiratory paralysis. Use cautiously during surgical and postoperative periods.
Lithium, narcotic analgesics: potentiated neuromuscular blockade, causing increased skeletal muscle relaxation and possible respiratory paralysis. Use with extreme caution and reduce pancuronium dose. Theophylline and azathioprine may antagonize drug effects.

Clinical considerations
• Drug is contraindicated in patients with hypersensitivity to bromides and preexisting tachycardia, and in those for whom even a minor heart rate increase is undesirable. Use cautiously in elderly or debilitated patients and in patients with renal, hepatic, or pulmonary impairment; respiratory depression; myasthenia gravis; myasthenic syndrome of lung cancer; dehydration; thyroid disorders; collagen diseases; porphyria; electrolyte disturbances; hyperthermia; toxemic states; and, in large doses, cesarean section.

• Drug causes no histamine release or hypotension.

• A 1-mg dose is the approximate therapeutic equivalent of 5 mg tubocurarine chloride.

• Monitor baseline electrolyte levels (electrolyte imbalance can potentiate neuromuscular effects) and vital signs (check respiration and heart rate closely).

• Measure intake and output (renal dysfunction may prolong drug's duration of action, because 25% of drug is unchanged before excretion).

• Have emergency respiratory support (such as endotracheal equipment, ventilator, oxygen, atropine, and neostigmine) on hand.

• Allow succinylcholine effects to subside before giving pancuronium.

• Store in refrigerator. Do not store in plastic containers or syringes; however, plastic syringes may be used for administration.

• Do not mix with barbiturate solutions; use only fresh solutions.

• Do not give without doctor's direct supervision.

• Neostigmine or edrophonium may be used to reverse drug effects.

succinylcholine chloride
Anectine, Anectine Flo-Pack Powder

Mechanism of action
Depolarizing agent; prolongs depolarization of muscle end plate.

Respiratory indications and dosage
• Adjunct to anesthesia to induce skeletal muscle relaxation; drug of choice to facilitate intubation and assist with mechanical ventilation or orthopedic manipulations (dose depends on anesthetic used, individual needs, and response; doses are representative and must be adjusted)—
Adults: 25 to 75 mg I.V., then 2.5 mg/minute p.r.n., or 2.5 mg/kg I.M. up to maximum of 150 mg I.M. in deltoid muscle.
Children: 1 to 2 mg/kg I.M. or I.V. Maximum I.M. dose is 150 mg. (Children may be less sensitive than adults to succinylcholine.)

Adverse reactions
CV: bradycardia, tachycardia, hypertension, hypotension, dysrhythmias.
EENT: increased intraocular pressure.
Other: prolonged respiratory depression, apnea, malignant hyperthermia, muscle fasciculation, postoperative muscle pain, myoglobinemia, excessive salivation, allergic or idiosyncratic hypersensitivity reaction.

Interactions
Aminoglycoside antibiotics (amikacin, gentamicin, kanamycin, neomycin, streptomycin), polymyxin antibiotics (polymyxin B sulfate, colistin), echothiophate, local anesthetics, beta-adrenergic blocking agents, furosemide, quinidine, procainamide, oxytocin, certain inhalation anesthetics: potentiated neuromuscular blockade, causing increased skeletal muscle relaxation and possible respiratory paralysis. Use cautiously during surgical and postoperative periods.
Narcotic analgesics, methotrimeprazine: potentiated neuromuscular blockade, causing increased skeletal muscle relaxation and possible respiratory paralysis. Use with extreme caution.
MAO inhibitors, lithium, cyclophosphamide: prolonged apnea. Use with caution.
Magnesium sulfate (parenteral): potentiated neuromuscular blockade, increased skeletal muscle relaxation, and possible respiratory paralysis. Use with caution, preferably with reduced doses.
Cardiac glycosides: possible cardiac dysrhythmias. Use together cautiously.
Diazepam: possible reduced duration of succinylcholine blockade.

Clinical considerations
• Drug is contraindicated in patients with abnormally low plasma pseudo-

cholinesterase levels. Use with caution in patients with personal or family history of malignant hypertension or hyperthermia; in patients with hepatic, renal, or pulmonary impairment; in patients with respiratory depression, severe burns or trauma, electrolyte imbalances, hyperkalemia, paraplegia, spinal neuraxis injury, degenerative or dystrophic neuromuscular disease, myasthenia gravis, myasthenic syndrome of lung cancer, dehydration, thyroid disorders, collagen disease, porphyria, fractures, muscle spasms, glaucoma, eye surgery or penetrating eye wounds, pheochromocytoma, cesarean section (with large doses); in patients receiving quinidine or digitalis therapy; and in elderly or debilitated patients.

• Succinylcholine is the drug of choice for short procedures (less than 3 minutes) and orthopedic manipulations; use cautiously in patients with fractures or dislocations.

• Duration of action can be prolonged to 20 minutes by continuous I.V. infusion or single-dose administration, along with hexafluorenium bromide administration.

• Repeated or continuous infusions of succinylcholine alone is not advised; may cause reduced response or prolonged apnea.

• Monitor baseline electrolyte levels and vital signs (check respiration every 5 to 10 minutes during infusion).

• Keep airway clear. Have emergency respiratory support (such as endotracheal equipment, ventilator, oxygen, atropine, and neostigmine) on hand.

• Reassure patient that postoperative stiffness is normal and will soon subside.

• Store injectable form in refrigerator. Store powder form at room temperature, closed tightly. Use immediately after reconstitution. Discard after 24 hours. Do not mix with alkaline solutions (thiopental, sodium bicarbonate, barbiturates).

• Give test dose (10 mg I.M. or I.V.) after patient has been anesthetized. Normal response (no respiratory depression or transient depression lasting less than 5 minutes) indicates that drug may be given. Do not give if patient develops respiratory paralysis sufficient to permit endotracheal intubation. (Recovery within 30 to 60 minutes.)

• Do not give without doctor's direct supervision.

• Give deep I.M., preferably high into the deltoid muscle.

tubocurarine chloride
Tubarine

Mechanism of action
Nondepolarizing agent; prevents acetylcholine from binding to the receptors on the muscle end plate, thus blocking depolarization.

Respiratory indications and dosage
• Adjunct to anesthesia to induce skeletal muscle relaxation; facilitate intubation, orthopedic manipulations (dose depends on anesthetic used, individual needs, and response; doses listed are representative and must be adjusted)—
Adults: 1 unit/kg or 0.15 mg/kg I.V. slowly over 60 to 90 seconds. Average initial dose is 40 to 60 units I.V. May give 20 to 30 units in 3 to 5 minutes. For longer procedures, give 20 units p.r.n.
Children: 1 unit/kg or 0.15 mg/kg.

• Assist with mechanical ventilation—
Adults and children: Initially, 0.0165 mg/kg I.V. (average dose is 1 mg or 7 units), then adjust subsequent doses to patient's response.

Adverse reactions
CV: hypotension, circulatory depression.
Other: profound and prolonged muscle relaxation, respiratory depression to the point of apnea, hypersensitivity, idiosyncrasy, residual muscle weakness, bronchospasm.

Interactions

Aminoglycoside antibiotics (amikacin, gentamicin, kanamycin, neomycin, streptomycin), polymyxin antibiotics (polymyxin B sulfate, colistin), local anesthetics: potentiated neuromuscular blockade, leading to increased skeletal muscle relaxation and possible respiratory paralysis. Use cautiously during surgical and postoperative periods.

Quinidine: prolonged neuromuscular blockade. Use together with caution. Monitor closely.

Thiazide diuretics, furosemide, ethacrynic acid, amphotericin B, propranolol, methotrimeprazine, narcotic analgesics: potentiated neuromuscular blockade, leading to increased respiratory paralysis. Use with extreme caution during surgical and postoperative periods. Certain inhalation anesthetics exert curare-like activity and may elicit more pronounced blockade.

Clinical considerations

• Drug is contraindicated in asthmatics and other patients for whom histamine release is a hazard. Use cautiously in elderly or debilitated patients and in patients with hepatic or pulmonary impairment, respiratory depression, myasthenia gravis, myasthenic syndrome of lung cancer, dehydration, thyroid disorders, collagen diseases, porphyria, electrolyte disturbances, fractures, muscle spasms, and, in large doses, cesarean section.

• Small safety margin separates therapeutic dose from dose causing respiratory paralysis.

• Allow succinylcholine effects to subside before giving tubocurarine.

• Monitor baseline electrolyte levels (electrolyte imbalance can potentiate neuromuscular effects).

• Watch closely for early signs of paralysis—inability to keep eyelids open, changes in respirations (such as depth rate), unfocused eyes, and swallowing and speaking difficulty. Notify doctor immediately.

• Check vital signs every 15 minutes. Notify doctor of any changes at once.

• Measure intake and output (renal dysfunction prolongs duration of action, because much of drug is unchanged before excretion).

• Keep airway clear. Have emergency respiratory support (such as endotracheal equipment, ventilator, oxygen, atropine, edrophonium, epinephrine, and neostigmine) on hand.

• Decrease dose if inhalation anesthetics are used.

• Do not mix with barbiturates (such as methohexital or thiopental). Use only fresh solutions and discard if discolored.

• Give I.V. slowly (over 60 to 90 seconds); give deep I.M. in deltoid muscle.

• Do not give without doctor's direct supervision.

• Neostigmine or edrophonium may be used to reverse drug effects.

vecuronium bromide
Norcuron

Mechanism of action
Nondepolarizing agent; prevents acetylcholine from binding to muscle end plate receptors, thus blocking depolarization.

Respiratory indications and dosage
• Adjunct to general anesthesia, to facilitate endotracheal intubation and to provide skeletal muscle relaxation during surgery or mechanical ventilation (dose depends on anesthetic used, individual needs, and response; doses are representative and must be adjusted)— *Adults and children over age 9:* Initially, 0.08 to 0.10 mg/kg I.V. bolus. Administer maintenance doses of 0.010 to 0.015 mg/kg within 25 to 40 minutes of initial dose during prolonged surgical procedures. Maintenance doses may be given q 12 to 15 minutes in patients receiving a balanced anesthetic.

Children under age 10 may require a slightly higher initial dose and slightly more frequent supplementation than adults.

Adverse reactions
Respiratory: prolonged dose-related apnea.

Interactions
Aminoglycoside antibiotics (amikacin, gentamicin, kanamycin, neomycin, streptomycin), polymyxin antibiotics (polymyxin B sulfate, colistin), clindamycin, quinidine, local anesthetics: potentiated neuromuscular blockade, leading to increased skeletal muscle relaxation and possible respiratory paralysis. Use cautiously during surgical and postoperative periods.
Narcotic analgesics: potentiated neuromuscular blockade, leading to increased skeletal muscle relaxation and possible respiratory paralysis. Use with extreme caution, and reduce vecuronium dose.

Clinical considerations
• Drug is contraindicated in patients with hypersensitivity to bromides. Use cautiously in patients with altered circulation time caused by cardiovascular disease, advanced age, and edematous states; hepatic disease; severe obesity; and neuromuscular disease.
• Unlike other nondepolarizing neuromuscular blockers, vecuronium has no effect on the cardiovascular system. Also, the drug causes no histamine release and therefore no histamine-related hypersensitivity reactions, such as bronchospasm, hypotension, or tachycardia.
• Drug is well tolerated in patients with renal failure.
• Prior administration of succinylcholine may enhance vecuronium's neuromuscular blocking effect and duration of action.
• Vecuronium provides conditions for intubation within 2½ to 3 minutes. Duration of effect is 25 to 40 minutes.
• Once spontaneous recovery starts, vecuronium-induced neuromuscular blockade may be reversed with an anticholinesterase agent, together with an anticholinergic drug.

• Have emergency respiratory support (such as endotracheal equipment, ventilator, oxygen, atropine, and neostigmine) on hand.
• Store reconstituted solution in refrigerator. Discard after 24 hours.

Miscellaneous respiratory drugs

Chromones
A difficult drug to classify therapeutically, cromolyn sodium is an antiallergenic prophylactic agent used to prevent an acute allergic attack (it is not useful once an attack has begun). Cromolyn sodium isn't a corticosteroid anti-inflammatory agent.

cromolyn sodium
Intal, Intal Inhaler, Intal p, Nasalcrom, Rynacrom

Mechanism of action
Inhibits the degranulation of sensitized mast cells that follows exposure to specific antigens. This, in turn, inhibits release of histamine and slow-reacting substance of anaphylaxis (SRS-A).

Respiratory indications and dosage
• Adjunct in treatment of severe perennial bronchial asthma—
Adults and children over age 5: Inhale contents of one 20-mg capsule q.i.d. at regular intervals, or administer two metered sprays using inhaler q.i.d. at regular intervals. Also available as an aqueous solution administered through a nebulizer.
• Prevention and treatment of allergic rhinitis—
Adults and children over 5: 1 spray in each nostril t.i.d. or q.i.d. May give up to six times daily.
• Prevention of exercise-induced bronchospasm—
Adults and children over age 5: Inhale contents of one 20-mg capsule or inhale two metered sprays no more than 1 hour before anticipated exercise.

Adverse reactions
CNS: dizziness, headache.
EENT: irritation of the throat and trachea, cough, bronchospasm following inhalation of dry powder, esophagitis, nasal congestion, pharyngeal irritation, wheezing.
GI: nausea.
GU: dysuria, urinary frequency.
Skin: rash, urticaria.
Other: joint swelling and pain, lacrimation, swollen parotid gland, angioedema, eosinophilic pneumonia.

Interactions
None significant.

Clinical considerations
• Drug is contraindicated in patients with acute asthma attacks and status asthmaticus.
• Use cautiously in patients with coronary artery disease or history of cardiac dyshythmias.
• Drug should be discontinued if patient develops eosinophilic pneumonia.
• Capsule should not be swallowed; insert capsule into inhaler provided. Follow manufacturer's directions.
• Watch for recurrence of asthma symptoms when dosage is decreased, especially if patient is also receiving corticosteroids.
• Use only when acute episode has been controlled, airway is clear, and patient can inhale.
• Patients considered for cromolyn therapy should undergo pulmonary function tests to show significant bronchodilator-reversible component to airway obstruction.
• Teach patient correct use of Spinhaler: insert capsule in device properly, exhale completely before placing mouthpiece between lips, then inhale deeply and rapidly with steady, even breath. Remove inhaler from mouth, hold breath a few seconds, and exhale. Repeat until all powder has been inhaled.
• Store capsules at room temperature in a tightly closed container; protect from moisture and temperatures higher than 104° F. (40° C.).

• Instruct patient to avoid excessive handling of capsule.
• Esophagitis may be relieved by antacids or a glass of milk.

Antitussives

Antitussives, or cough suppressants, constitute a therapeutic class of agents containing compounds with a wide variety of pharmacologic activity. Coughing is a complex reflex involving local receptors in the lungs and nasopharynx as well as central medullary reflex centers. Cough suppression, when desirable, can be obtained using agents with a local, peripheral, or CNS location of action. Antitussives with a CNS location of action are reviewed in this section.

Drugs that depress the medullary respiratory center also depress the medullary cough center. Although most narcotic analgesics possess this effect, codeine is the most widely used agent. Dextromethorphan, chemically related to the potent opiate levorphanol, can depress medullary cough reflexes, but lacks opiate analgesic and abuse potential.

codeine phosphate

codeine sulfate
(Controlled Substance Schedule II)

Mechanism of action
Binds with opiate receptors at many CNS sites (brain, brain stem, and spinal cord), altering perception of and emotional response to pain through an unknown mechanism. Also supresses the cough reflex by a direct central action in the medulla.

Respiratory indications and dosage
• Nonproductive cough—
Adults: 8 to 20 mg P.O. q 4 to 6 hours. Maximum dosage is 120 mg/day.
Children: 1 to 1.5 mg/kg P.O. daily in four divided doses. Maximum dosage is 60 mg/day.

Adverse reactions
CNS: sedation, clouded sensorium, euphoria, convulsions (with large doses), dizziness.
CV: hypotension, bradycardia.
GI: nausea, vomiting, constipation, dry mouth, ileus.
GU: urinary retention.
Skin: pruritus, flushing.
Other: respiratory depression, physical dependence.

Interactions
Alcohol, CNS depressants: additive effects. Use together cautiously.

Clinical considerations
• Use with extreme caution in patients with head injury, increased intracranial pressure, increased cerebrospinal fluid pressure, hepatic or renal disease, hypothyroidism, Addison's disease, acute alcoholism, seizures, severe CNS depression, bronchial asthma, chronic obstructive pulmonary disease, respiratory depression, and shock; and in elderly or debilitated patients.
• Warn ambulatory patients to avoid activities that require alertness.
• Monitor respiratory and circulatory status.
• Monitor cough type and frequency.
• Don't use when cough is beneficial (as after thoracic surgery), or serves as a valuable diagnostic sign.
• Drug causes increased CNS depression if used with general anesthetics, other narcotic analgesics, tranquilizers, sedatives, hypnotics, alcohol, tricyclic antidepressants, or monoamine oxidase (MAO) inhibitors. Use together with extreme caution.

benzonatate
Tessalon

Mechanism of action
Suppresses the cough reflex by direct action on the medullary cough center. Also has local anesthetic action.

Respiratory indications and dosage
• Nonproductive cough—
Adults and children over age 10: 100 mg P.O. t.i.d., up to 600 mg/day.
Children under age 10: 8 mg/kg P.O. in three to six divided doses.

Adverse reactions
CNS: dizziness, drowsiness, headache.
EENT: nasal congestion, burning sensation in eyes.
GI: nausea, constipation.
Skin: rash.
Other: chills.

Interactions
None significant.

Clinical considerations
• Instruct patient not to chew capsules or leave them in mouth to dissolve; local anesthesia will result. If capsules dissolve in mouth, CNS stimulation may cause restlessness, tremors, and, possibly, convulsions.
• Don't use when cough is beneficial (as after thoracic surgery) or serves as a valuable diagnostic sign.
• Monitor cough type and frequency.
• Use with chest percussion and vibration.
• Maintain fluid intake to help liquefy sputum.

dextromethorphan hydrobromide
Balminil DM, Broncho-Grippol-DM, Delsym, Pertussin 8-Hour, St. Joesph's Cough Syrup for Children, Silence Is Golden. More commonly available in such combination products as Benylin-DM, Coryban-D Cough Syrup, Dimacol, 2G-DM, Naldetuss, Novahistine DMX, Ornacol, Phenergan Expectorant with Dextromethorphan, Robitussin DM, , Rondec-DM, Triaminicol, Trind-DM, Tussi-Organidin-DM

Mechanism of action
Suppresses the cough reflex by direct action on the medullary cough center.

Respiratory indications and dosage
• Nonproductive cough—
Adults: 10 to 20 mg q 4 hours, or 30 mg q 6 to 8 hours. Or controlled-release liquid twice daily (60 mg b.i.d.). Maximum of 120 mg daily.
Children age 6 to 12: 5 to 10 mg q 4 hours, or 15 mg q 6 to 8 hours. Or 30 mg of controlled-release liquid b.i.d. Maximum of 60 mg/day.
Children age 2 to 6: 2.5 to 5 mg q 4 hours, or 7.5 mg q 6 to 8 hours. Maximum of 30 mg/day.

Adverse reactions
CNS: drowsiness, dizziness.
GI: nausea.

Interactions
MAO inhibitors: hypotension, coma, hyperpyrexia, and possibly death. Do not use together.

Clinical considerations
• Drug is contraindicated in patients currently taking or within 2 weeks of stopping MAO inhibitors.
• Drug produces no analgesia or addiction and little or no CNS depression.
• Don't use when cough is beneficial (as after thoracic surgery) or serves as a valuable diagnostic sign.
• Use with chest percussion and vibration.
• Monitor cough type and frequency.
• Drug is available in most over-the-counter cough medicines.
• As an antitussive, 15 to 30 mg dextromethorphan is equivalent to 8 to 15 mg codeine.

diphenhydramine hydrochloride
Allerdryl, Baramine, Bax, Benachlor, Benadryl, Benahist, Ben-Allergin, Bendylate, Bentrac, Bonyl, Compoz, Diphenacen, Fenylhist, Nordryl, Nytol with DPH, Rodryl, Rohydra, Sominex Formula 2, Span-Lanin, Valdrene, Wehdryl

Mechanism of action
Competes with histamine for H_1-receptor sites on effector cells. Prevents but doesn't reverse histamine-mediated responses, particularly histamine's effects on smooth muscle of the bronchial tubes, GI tract, uterus, and blood vessels. Structurally related to local anesthetics, diphenhydramine provides local anesthesia by preventing initiation and transmission of nerve impulses. Also suppresses the cough reflex by a direct effect in the medulla.

Respiratory indications and dosage
• Rhinitis, allergy symptoms, nighttime sedation, motion sickness, and antiparkinsonism—
Adults: 25 to 50 mg P.O. t.i.d. or q.i.d.; or 10 to 50 mg deep I.M. or I.V. Maximum dosage is 400 mg/day.
Children under age 12: 5 mg/kg/day P.O., deep I.M., or I.V. divided q.i.d. Maximum dosage is 300 mg/day.
• Nonproductive cough—
Adults: 25 mg P.O. q 4 hours (not to exceed 100 mg/day).
Children age 6 to 12: 12.5 mg P.O. q 4 hours (not to exceed 50 mg/day).
Children age 2 to 6: 6.25 mg P.O. q 4 hours (not to exceed 25 mg/day).

Adverse reactions
CNS: drowsiness, confusion, insomnia, headache, vertigo (especially in elderly patients).
CV: palpitations.
EENT: photosensitivity, diplopia, nasal stuffiness.
GI: nausea, vomiting, diarrhea, dry mouth, constipation.
GU: dysuria, urinary retention.
Skin: urticaria.

Interactions
CNS depressants: increased sedation. Use together cautiously.

Clinical considerations
• Drug is contraindicated in patients with acute asthmatic attack. Use cau-

tiously in narrow-angle glaucoma, prostatic hypertrophy, pyloroduodenal and bladder-neck obstruction, or stenosing peptic ulcers; in newborns; and in asthmatic, hypertensive, or cardiac patients.
• Alternate injection sites to prevent irritation. Administer deep I.M. into large muscle.
• Warn patient against drinking alcoholic beverages during therapy and against driving or other hazardous activities until CNS response to drug is determined.
• Reduce GI distress by giving with food or milk.
• Coffee or tea may reduce drowsiness. Sugarless gum, sour hard candy, or ice chips may relieve dry mouth.
• If tolerance develops, another antihistamine may be substituted.
• Warn patient to stop taking drug 4 days before allergy skin tests to ensure test accuracy.
• Drug is used with epinephrine in patients with anaphylaxis.
• Drug is among the most sedating antihistamines; it is used commonly as a hypnotic.

Expectorants

Expectorants are used to enhance the output of respiratory tract secretions by decreasing the viscosity of nasopharyngeal mucus. Although clinical data have not yet proven their effectiveness, expectorants are used widely and included in many over-the-counter preparations.

ammonium chloride
Mechanism of action
Acts as an expectorant by causing reflex stimulation of bronchial mucous glands.

Respiratory indications and dosage
• Expectorant—
Adults: 250 to 500 mg P.O. q 2 to 4 hours.

Adverse reactions
(Adverse reactions usually result from ammonia toxicity.)
CNS: headache, confusion, progressive drowsiness, excitement alternating with coma, hyperventilation, calcium-deficient tetany, twitching, hyperreflexia, EEG abnormalities.
CV: bradycardia.
GI: with oral dose—gastric irritation, nausea, vomiting, thirst, anorexia, retching.
GU: glycosuria.
Metabolic: acidosis, hyperchloremia, hypokalemia, hyperglycemia.
Skin: rash, pallor.
Other: irregular respirations with apneic periods.

Interactions
Spironolactone: systemic acidosis. Use together cautiously.

Clinical considerations
• Drug is contraindicated in patients with severe hepatic or renal dysfunction. Use cautiously in patients with pulmonary insufficiency or cardiac edema and in infants.
• Give after meals to decrease adverse GI reactions. Enteric-coated tablets also minimize GI symptoms; however, they're absorbed erratically.
• Do not administer drug with milk or other alkaline solutions, because they are not compatible.
• Determine CO_2 combining power and serum electrolyte levels before and during therapy.
• Monitor rate and depth of respirations frequently.
• When using as an expectorant, give with full glass of water.

guaifenesin (formerly glyceryl guaiacolate)
Anti-Tuss, Balminil, Bowtussin, Breonesin, Colrex, Cosin-GG, Dilyn, 2/G, G-100, GG-CEN, Glycotuss, Gly-O-

Tussin, Glytuss, G-Tussin, Guaiatus-sin, Hytuss, Malotuss, Nortussin, Proco, Recsei-Tuss, Resyl, Robitussin, Tursen, Wal-Tussin DM

Mechanism of action
Increases production of respiratory tract fluids to help liquefy and reduce the viscosity of thick, tenacious secretions.

Respiratory indications and dosage
• Expectorant—
Adults: 100 to 200 mg P.O. q 2 to 4 hours. Maximum dosage is 800 mg/day.
Children: 12 mg/kg P.O. daily in six divided doses.

Adverse reactions
CNS: drowsiness.
GI: vomiting, nausea with large doses.

Interactions
None significant.

Clinical considerations
• Drug may interfere with certain laboratory tests for 5-hydroxyindole-acetic acid and vanillylmandelic acid.
• Watch for bleeding gums, hematuria, and bruising when administering to patients on heparin. Discontinue guaifenesin, as ordered, if these signs occur.
• Drug liquefies thick, tenacious sputum. Maintain fluid intake and advise patient to take drug with a glass of water whenever possible.
• Monitor cough type and frequency.
• Encourage deep-breathing exercises.
• Although guaifenesin is a popular expectorant, its efficacy has not been established.

iodinated glycerol
Organidin

Mechanism of action
Increases production of respiratory tract fluids to help liquefy and reduce viscosity of thick, tenacious secretions.

Respiratory indications and dosage
• Bronchial asthma, bronchitis, emphysema (adjunct)—
Adults: 60 mg (tablets) P.O. q.i.d., 20 drops (solution) P.O. q.i.d. with fluids, or 5 ml (elixir) P.O. q.i.d.
Children: Up to ½ adult dose based on child's weight.

Adverse reactions
After long-term use:
GI: nausea, distress.
Skin: eruptions.
Other: acute parotitis, thryroid enlargement, hypothyroidism.

Interactions
None significant.

Clinical considerations
• Drug is contraindicated in patients with hypothyroidism and iodine sensitivity.
• Skin rash or other hypersensitivity reaction may warrant stopping drug.
• Drug may liquefy thick, tenacious sputum. Maintain fluid intake.
• Monitor cough type and frequency.
• Encourage deep-breathing exercises.

potassium iodide (SSKI)
Mechanism of action
Increases production of respiratory tract fluids to help liquefy and reduce viscosity of thick secretions.

Respiratory indications and dosage
• As expectorant for chronic bronchitis, chronic pulmonary emphysema, bronchial asthma—
Adults: 0.3 to 0.6 ml P.O. q 4 to 6 hours.
Children: 0.25 to 0.5 ml of saturated solution (1 g/ml) b.i.d. to q.i.d.

Adverse reactions
GI: nausea, vomiting, epigastric pain, metallic taste.

Metabolic: goiter, hyperthyroid adenoma, hypothyroidism (with excessive use), collagen disease-like syndrome.
Skin: rash.
Other: drug fever; with prolonged use, chronic iodine poisoning, mouth soreness, coryza, sneezing, swelling of eyelids.

Interactions
Lithium carbonate: may cause hypothyroidism. Don't use together.

Clinical considerations
• Drug is contraindicated in patients with iodine hypersensitivity, tuberculosis, hyperkalemia, acute bronchitis, and hyperthyroidism.
• Maintain fluid intake.
• Drug has strong salty, metallic taste. Dilute with milk, fruit juice, or broth to reduce GI distress and disguise taste.
• Sudden withdrawal may precipitate thyroid storm.
• If rash appears, discontinue use and contact doctor.

terpin hydrate
Mechanism of action
Increases production of respiratory tract fluids to help liquefy and reduce viscosity of thick secretions.

Respiratory indications and dosage
• Excessive bronchial secretions—
Adults: 5 to 10 ml P.O. of elixir q 4 to 6 hours.

Adverse reactions
GI: nausea, vomiting.

Interactions
None significant.

Clinical considerations
• Drug is contraindicated in patients with peptic ulcer or severe diabetes mellitus.
• Don't give in large doses; elixir has high alcoholic content (86 proof).
• Monitor cough type and frequency.

Mucolytics
Acetylcysteine is the prototype mucolytic now available. Although it has questionable clinical efficacy, it is used to increase production of respiratory tract fluids to help liquefy and reduce the viscosity of thick, tenacious secretions. It is also used to restore liver stores of glutathione in the treatment of acetaminophen toxicity.

acetylcysteine
Airbron, Mucomyst

Mechanism of action
Splits disulfide linkages between mucopolysaccharide polymers in mucus, resulting in decreased fluid viscosity.

Respiratory indications and dosage
• Pneumonia, bronchitis, tuberculosis, cystic fibrosis, emphysema, atelectasis (adjunct), complications of thoracic and cardiovascular surgery—
Adults and children: 1 to 2 ml 10% to 20% solution by direct instillation into trachea as often as every hour; or 3 to 5 ml 20% solution, or 6 to 10 ml 10% solution, by mouthpiece t.i.d. or q.i.d.

Adverse reactions
EENT: rhinorrhea, hemoptysis.
GI: stomatitis, nausea.
Other: bronchospasm (especially in asthmatics).

Interactions
Activated charcoal: don't use together in treating acetaminophen toxicity; activated charcoal limits acetylcysteine's effectiveness.

Clinical considerations
• Use cautiously in patients with asthma or severe respiratory insufficiency and in elderly or debilitated patients.
• Use plastic, glass, stainless steel, or another nonreactive metal when ad-

ministering by nebulization. Hand bulb nebulizers are not recommended because output is too small and particle size is too large.

• After opening, store in refrigerator; use within 96 hours.

• Drug is incompatible with oxytetracycline, tetracycline, erythromycin lactobionate, amphotericin B, ampicillin, iodized oil, chymotrypsin, trypsin, and hydrogen peroxide. Administer separately.

• Monitor cough type and frequency. For maximum effect, instruct patient to clear his airway by coughing before aerosol administration.

Respiratory stimulants

Except for aromatic spirits of ammonia, used for its local effect to irritate nasal mucous membranes, respiratory stimulants have been used in the past allegedly to stimulate central respiratory centers that moderate ventilatory function. Although they may be somewhat beneficial and remain in use as respiratory stimulants, they should not be used in place of more direct supportive therapy, such as mechanical ventilation, because their effectiveness is still questioned.

ammonia, aromatic spirits
Mechanism of action
Irritates sensory receptors in the nasal membranes, producing reflex stimulation of the respiratory centers.

Respiratory indications and dosage
• Fainting—
Adults and children: Inhale as needed.

Adverse reactions
None reported.

Interactions
None significant.

Clinical considerations
• Drug stimulates mucous membranes of upper respiratory tract.

doxapram hydrochloride
Dopram

Mechanism of action
Acts either directly on the medullary respiratory centers or indirectly on chemoreceptors in the carotid body.

Respiratory indications and dosage
• Postanesthesia respiratory stimulation, drug-induced CNS depression, and chronic pulmonary disease associated with acute hypercapnia—
Adults: 0.5 to 1 mg/kg of body weight (up to 2 mg/kg in CNS depression) I.V. injection or infusion. Maximum dosage is 4 mg/kg, up to 3 g/day. Infusion rate is 1 to 3 mg/minute (initially 5 mg/minute for postanesthesia).
• Chronic obstructive pulmonary disease—
Adults: For infusion, 1 to 2 mg/minute. Maximum dosage is 3 mg/minute for a maximum duration of 2 hours.

Adverse reactions
CNS: seizures, headache, dizziness, apprehension, disorientation, pupillary dilation, bilateral Babinski's reflex, flushing, sweating, paresthesias.
CV: chest pain and tightness, variations in heart rate, hypertension, lowered T waves.
GI: nausea, vomiting, diarrhea.
GU: urinary retention, bladder stimulation with incontinence.
Other: sneezing, coughing, laryngospasm, bronchospasm, hiccups, rebound hypoventilation, pruritus.

Interactions
Monoamine oxidase inhibitors: potentiate adverse cardiovascular effects. Use together cautiously.

Clinical considerations
• Drug is contraindicated in patients with convulsive disorders; head injury; cardiovascular disorders; frank

uncompensated heart failure; severe hypertension; cerebrovascular accidents; respiratory failure or incompetence secondary to neuromuscular disorders, muscle paresis, flail chest, obstructed airway, pulmonary embolism, pneumothorax, restrictive respiratory disease, acute bronchial asthma, or extreme dyspnea; and hypoxia not associated with hypercapnia. Use with caution in patients with bronchial asthma, severe tachycardia, cardiac dysrhythmias, cerebral edema, increased cerebrospinal fluid pressure, hyperthyroidism, pheochromocytoma, or metabolic disorders.

• Most doctors strongly discourage doxapram's use as an analeptic.

• Establish adequate airway before administering drug. Prevent patient from aspirating vomitus by placing him on his side.

• Assess blood pressure, heart rate, deep tendon reflexes, and arterial blood gas measurements before giving drug and every 30 minutes afterward.

• Stay alert for signs of overdose: hypertension, tachycardia, dysrhythmias, skeletal muscle hyperactivity, and dyspnea. Discontinue if patient shows signs of increased arterial carbon dioxide or oxygen tension, or if mechanical ventilation is initiated. As necessary, give I.V. injection of anticonvulsant.

• Use only in surgical or emergency department situations.

• Do not combine with alkaline solutions, such as thiopental sodium; doxapram is acidic.

• Respiratory stimulation lasts only 2 to 5 minutes.

nikethamide
Coramine

Mechanism of action
Acts either directly on medullary respiratory centers or indirectly on chemoreceptors of the carotid body.

Respiratory indications and dosage
• Carbon monoxide poisoning—
Adults: 1.25 to 2.5 g I.V. initially, then 1.25 g q 5 minutes for first hour, depending on response.
• Cardiac arrest associated with anesthetic overdose—
Adults: 125 to 250 mg intracardially.
• Respiratory paralysis—
Adults: 3.75 g I.V.; repeat as required.
• Respiratory depression—
Adults: 1.25 to 2.5 g I.V.
• Shock—
Adults: 2.5 to 3.75 g I.V. or I.M. initially; repeat as indicated.
• Shortened narcosis—
Adults: 1 g I.V. or I.M.
Adjunct in neonatal asphyxia—
Neonates: 375 mg injected into umbilical vein.

Adverse reactions
CNS: seizures, restlessness, muscle twitching or fasciculations, fear.
CV: increased heart rate and blood pressure.
EENT: unpleasant burning or itching at back of nose, sneezing, coughing.
GI: nausea, vomiting.
Other: increased respiratory rate, flushing, feeling of warmth, sweating.

Interactions
None significant.

Clinical considerations
• Monitor patient's respiratory rate and volume frequently during therapy.
• Mechanical ventilatory support is preferred over nikethamide administration.
• Check for signs of overdose: muscle tremors or spasm, retching, tachycardia, dysrhythmias, hyperpyrexia, hyperpnea, convulsions, psychotic reactions, and postictal depression.
• Respiratory stimulation lasts only 2 to 5 minutes.

Selected References

American Hospital Formulary Service. Bethesda, Md.: American Society of Hospital Pharmacists Staff, 1988.

American Medical Association Department of Drugs Staff. *Drug Evaluations,* 6th ed. Philadelphia: W.B. Saunders Co., 1987.

Gilman, A.G., et al., eds. *Goodman and Gilman's The Pharmacological Basis of Therapeutics,* 7th ed. New York: Macmillan Publishing Co., 1980.

Kastrup, E.K., and Olan, B., eds. *Drug Facts and Comparisons 1987.* Philadelphia: J.B. Lippincott Co., 1987.

Nursing88 Drug Handbook. Springhouse, Pa.: Springhouse Corp., 1988.

Petty, T.A. "Drug Strategies for Airflow Obstruction," *American Journal of Nursing* 87(2):180-84, February 1987.

Physician's Desk Reference, 41st ed. Oradell, N.J.: Medical Economics Co., 1987.

Respiratory Problems. NurseReview Series. Springhouse, Pa.: Springhouse Corp., 1986.

United States Pharmacopeia Dispensing Information (USPDI). Rockville, Md.: United States Pharmacopeia Convention, Inc., 1987.

APPENDICES

Basic Life Support

Basic life support (BLS) aims to achieve one of the following goals:
• prevent respiratory or circulatory arrest (for example, by clearing an obstructed airway)
• support respiration and circulation with cardiopulmonary resuscitation (CPR) after an arrest.

The BLS guidelines presented here reflect the latest American Heart Association (AHA) standards. Always follow the *ABC* sequence: open the victim's *airway* and restore his *breathing* and *circulation*, as necessary. Note that CPR procedures for adults and children are the same, with these exceptions: for most children, seal both the nose and mouth, use only one hand for chest compressions, and compress only 1″ to 1½″ (compared to 1½″ to 2″ for adults).

C.P.R. AND DISEASE TRANSMISSION

Some health care workers who perform CPR frequently worry about the risk of contracting such diseases as hepatitis B and acquired immunodeficiency syndrome (AIDS). To safeguard against this infection risk, the AHA suggests using disposable airway equipment or resuscitation bags and wearing gloves when you anticipate contact with blood or other body fluids. Clear plastic face masks with one-way valves, which direct the victim's exhalations away from the rescuer, may provide added protection.

Similar concerns have been raised about mannequin use during CPR training. However, the AHA points out that the hepatitis B and AIDS viruses succumb to chemical disinfectants when outside a living organism.

The following precautions help minimize the risk of disease transmission:
• Students with AIDS, hepatitis, upper respiratory tract infection, or hand or mouth lesions shouldn't participate in CPR training.
• Students should work in pairs, with each pair using only one mannequin. Each student should practice good hygiene—for example, hand washing before mannequin contact.
• Change individual face shields (if used) between contacts by different students. Vigorously wipe the mannequin's face and airway with dry gauze between contacts (including finger sweeps), then wet with either sodium hypochloride or a 70% alcohol solution. Allow surfaces to remain wet for at least 30 seconds, then dry them with clean gauze.
• During two-person CPR training, when the mannequin can't be disinfected between students, the second student should simulate ventilation rather than blow into the mannequin airway.
• After training sessions, scrub and disinfect mannequins with sodium hypochloride according to manufacturer's specifications. Inspect mannequins routinely for cracks, which harbor microbes.

OPENING THE AIRWAY

Currently recommended for opening an airway under most circumstances, the head-tilt/chin-lift maneuver works more effectively than the previously recommended head-tilt/neck-lift maneuver.

To use the head-tilt/chin-lift maneuver, place one hand on the victim's

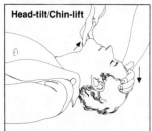

Head-tilt/Chin-lift

Basic Life Support (continued)

Jaw thrust without head tilt

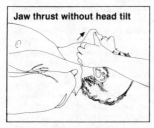

forehead and tilt his head back by applying firm backward pressure with your palm. Then put the fingers of your opposite hand under the lower jaw's bony portion (near the chin), and bring the chin forward. Don't close the victim's mouth completely (unless you're performing mouth-to-nose respiration). Remove his dentures if they interfere with positioning.

If you suspect cervical spine injury, use the jaw-thrust without head-tilt manuever. Begin by resting your elbows on the surface supporting the victim's head, and place a hand on each side of his lower jaw, at its angles. Lift with both hands to displace the mandible forward. Support his head so that it doesn't tilt backward or turn to the side. If his lips close, retract them with your thumb. After opening the victim's airway, check to see if his breathing has been restored.

MOUTH-TO-MOUTH RESUSCITATION
For adults and children
If the victim is not breathing even after you've opened his airway, begin artificial respiration immediately.
1. Keep the victim's neck hyperextended (unless you're using the jaw-thrust without head-tilt maneuver).
2. With your hand on the victim's forehead, pinch his nostrils closed. Maintain pressure on his forehead. (If you're using the jaw-thrust without head-tilt maneuver, seal his nostrils by pressing your cheek against them.)

3. Take a deep breath, then place your mouth around the victim's mouth, creating a tight seal.
4. Give two full breaths (each lasting 1 to 1½ seconds), pausing in between so that you can take a breath. The breaths you give should have sufficient volume to make the victim's chest rise.
5. If you can't observe the chest rise and fall and can't hear or feel air escaping during exhalation, reposition the victim's head and administer two more full breaths.
6. If ventilation is still unsuccessful, perform all procedures for clearing an obstructed airway.
7. If ventilation proves successful, check the victim's carotid pulse.
8. If you feel a pulse but the victim is still not breathing, give him one breath every 5 seconds. Until he begins to breathe again, check for a carotid pulse after every 12 ventilations.
9. If you can't feel a pulse, initiate CPR immediately.

Mouth-to-mouth resuscitation

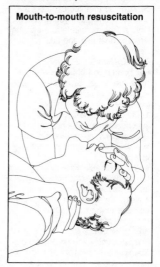

(continued)

Basic Life Support *(continued)*

Mouth-to-mouth-and-nose resuscitation

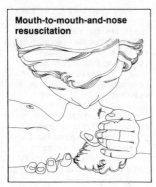

For infants
Modify the resuscitation procedure slightly, as follows:
1. Tilt the infant's head back only *slightly*, to prevent tracheal collapse.
2. Place your mouth over his mouth *and* nose.
3. Give two *slow* breaths (each lasting 1 to 1½ seconds), pausing in between so that you can take a breath. The breaths you give should have sufficient volume to make the infant's chest rise and fall.

PERFORMING C.P.R.
For adults and children
After you've determined that the victim has no pulse, take the following steps:
1. Position yourself for administering chest compressions. Before beginning chest compressions, position your hands at the correct location:
• With the middle and index fingers of the hand closer to the victim's legs, locate the rib cage's lower margin.
• Next, run these two fingers up the rib cage to the notch where the ribs meet the sternum.
• Put your middle finger on this notch, and place your index finger next to it. Then place the heel of your opposite hand next to the index finger, on the long axis of the sternum.

• Now place your first hand on top of the other, so that both hands are parallel and the fingers point away from you. Extend or interlace your fingers.
2. Compress the victim's sternum 1½″ to 2″. During the upstroke, keep your hands in position on the sternum and allow the chest to relax. Deliver four cycles of 15 compressions (compressing and relaxing evenly) and 2 ventilations. (Use a compression rate of 80 to 100/minute and a ventilation duration of 1 to 1½ seconds each).
3. Check for a pulse and spontaneous breathing. If these haven't returned, deliver 15 compressions and 2 ventilations; deliver four cycles of compressions and ventilations.

Positioning for chest compressions

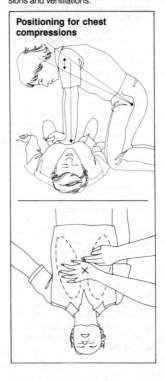

Basic Life Support *(continued)*

4. Pause for 5 seconds at the end of the first minute, and every few minutes thereafter, to determine whether spontaneous breathing and circulation have returned.

5. If a second rescuer arrives, the rescuer should announce that he knows CPR and get into position to deliver chest compressions. Complete the ventilation/compression cycle and check for a pulse and breathing. If you don't detect a pulse or breathing, say, "No pulse. Continue CPR."

6. Resume the head-tilt/chin-lift maneuver to open the airway. Deliver one ventilation; the second rescuer then delivers five compressions within 3 to 4 seconds (using a compression rate of 80 to 100/minute). Continue ventilating the victim once for every 5 compressions. To maintain rhythm, the second rescuer should say, "One-and-two-and-three-and-four-and-five, pause, vent."

7. Between ventilations, check the victim's pulse to determine if compression is effective. Deliver at least 10 compression/ventilation cycles.

8. When the second rescuer tires, he should say, "Change one-and-two-and-three-and-four-and-five." Immediately after the ventilation, both rescuers should change positions simultaneously.

9. The second rescuer now opens the airway; he also performs a 5-second pulse check. If he fails to detect a pulse, he should say, "No pulse. Continue CPR" and then deliver one ventilation. Resume compression/ventilation cycles.

For infants

1. Determine absence of pulse by feeling for a brachial pulse.

2. Position your fingers for chest compressions by drawing an imaginary horizontal line between the infant's nipples. Then place two or three fingers on his sternum, one finger's width below the imaginary line.

3. Compress vertically ½" to 1", keeping your fingers on the sternum during the upstroke. Keep compression and relaxation times equal; maintain a compression rate of at least 100/minute (5 compressions in 3 seconds or less).

4. Perform 10 cycles of 5 compressions and 1 ventilation. To remember this, use this mnemonic: one-two-three-four-five-pause-head tilt-chin lift-ventilate-continue compressions. After 10 cycles, check the brachial pulse to determine pulselessness.

CLEARING AN OBSTRUCTED AIRWAY

For adults and children

1. To help a person who appears to be choking, first determine if he can speak by asking, "Are you choking?" If he can speak, cough, or breathe, stand by but don't intervene.

2. If he *can't* speak, cough, or breathe, perform abdominal thrusts (the Heimlich maneuver). To do this, stand behind him, wrap your arms around his waist, and place the thumb side of one fist against his abdomen at midline (slightly above

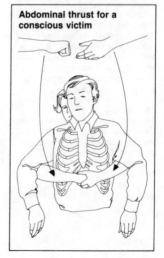

Abdominal thrust for a conscious victim

(continued)

Basic Life Support *(continued)*

the navel and well below the xyphoid tip). Grasp the fist with your other hand and make quick upward thrusts. Repeat until you're successful (the object is dislodged and the victim resumes breathing) or the victim loses consciousness.

3. If the victim loses consciousness, place him in the supine position, call for help, and activate the emergency medical services system. Open his mouth with a tongue-jaw lift, and sweep deeply into his mouth with your finger (finger sweep). *Caution*: If the victim is a child, do the finger sweep maneuver *only* if you can see a foreign object.

4. Open his airway with the head-tilt/chin-lift maneuver, and attempt to ventilate.

5. If you're unsuccessful, straddle the victim's thighs and position the heel of one hand against his abdomen at the midline point described in Step 2. Place your other hand on top of it, as shown here, and deliver 6 to 10 abdominal thrusts. *Note:* Use chest thrusts for obese victims and women in the late stages of pregnancy.

6. Open the victim's mouth and perform a finger sweep. (Again, if the victim is a child, do this step only if you can see the object.) Then open his airway with the head-tilt/chin-lift maneuver, and attempt to ventilate. If you're unsuccessful, repeat the procedure as necessary.

For infants

If a conscious infant appears to be choking, assess his condition by looking, listening, and feeling for breathing. Observe for blue lips, which indicate a lack of oxygen. To clear an obstruction:

1. Support the infant's head and neck by holding his jaw with one hand. Position him face down over your arm with his head lower than his trunk. Use your thigh to support your forearm.

2. With the heel of your hand, deliver four forceful back blows between the shoulder blades.

3. Next, sandwich the infant between your hands and turn him on his back, with his head lower than his trunk. Continue to support his head throughout.

4. Deliver four chest thrusts in the midsternal region. Use the same technique you would use to deliver chest compressions (see "Performing CPR for Infants," page 397), but deliver the thrusts at a slower rate. Repeat back blows and chest thrusts until you dislodge the foreign object or the infant loses consciousness.

5. If the infant becomes unconscious, call for help and activate the emergency medical services system. Then open the airway with a tongue-jaw lift and look for the foreign body. Attempt to remove it only if you can see it.

6. Open the infant's airway with a head-tilt/chin-lift maneuver, and attempt to ventilate.

7. If you can't ventilate the infant, position him head-down and deliver four back blows.

8. Then turn the infant on his back and deliver four chest thrusts.

9. Open the airway with a tongue-jaw lift, and look for the foreign body. Attempt to remove it only if you can see it. Then open the airway with a head-tilt/chin-lift maneuver and attempt to ventilate.

10. Repeat the sequence until it is effective.

Equations

The equations presented here are special condensed formulas that can be used conveniently at the bedside. While not appropriate for highly sophisticated research, the results can be used for patient monitoring. For complete formulas, refer to respiratory physiology texts.

ALVEOLAR AIR EQUATION
Explanation

With this equation, you can determine the partial pressure of oxygen in the alveoli (PAO_2), expressed in millimeters of mercury (mm Hg). Once you've determined the PAO_2, you can use it to find the ratio of the partial pressure of oxygen in arterial blood (PaO_2) to the PAO_2. This is known as the a/A ratio (see below).

Equation

$$PAO_2 = (PB - 47)\,(FIO_2) - PaCO_2$$

Where:
- PAO_2 = partial pressure of alveolar oxygen in (mm Hg)
- PB = barometric pressure (mm Hg)
- 47 = pressure taken up by water vapor in the alveoli (mm Hg)
- FIO_2 = fraction of inspired oxygen, expressed in decimals
- $PaCO_2$ = partial pressure of carbon dioxide in arterial blood, used as an estimation of partial pressure of alveolar carbon dioxide (mm Hg)

Example A: Mr. Jones has an FIO_2 of 0.40 and a $PaCO_2$ of 50 mm Hg. Barometric pressure at sea level is approximately 760 mm Hg. (Adjust accordingly for high altitudes.)

$$
\begin{aligned}
PAO_2 &= (760 - 47) \times (0.40) - 50 \\
&= (713 \times 0.40) - 50 \\
&= 285 - 50 \\
&= 235 \text{ mm Hg}
\end{aligned}
$$

a/A RATIO
Explanation

You can use the a/A ratio to assess a patient's oxygenation status. This equation uses the $PCAO_2$ value.

Equation

$$\text{a/A ratio} = \frac{PaO_2}{PAO_2}$$

(The normal a/A ratio is approximately 0.80 to 0.85)

Example B: To find Mr. Jones' a/A ratio from Example A, assume he had a PaO_2 level of 70 mm Hg.

$$
\begin{aligned}
\text{a/A ratio} &= \frac{70 \text{ mm Hg}}{235 \text{ mm Hg}} \\
&= 0.3
\end{aligned}
$$

Example C: To understand fully the value of the a/A ratio, you must compare the a/A ratio from Example B to this example. Returning to Mr. Jones in Example A, assume that after viewing arterial blood gas (ABG) measurements, the doctor decided to increase the FIO_2 to 0.50.

Repeat ABG measurements (taken after the FIO_2 change) showed a PaO_2 level of 80 mm Hg and a $PaCO_2$ level of 50 mm Hg. These results suggest that the patient's oxygenation status has improved. To confirm this, check it with the a/A ratio, as follows.

First, calculate PAO_2 based on the increased FIO_2.

$$
\begin{aligned}
PAO_2 &= (713 \times 0.50) - 50 \\
&= 356 - 50 \\
&= 306 \text{ mm Hg}
\end{aligned}
$$

In Example B, the a/A ratio is $70/235 = 0.3$. This means that almost one-third of the oxygen available in the alveoli is reaching the arterial blood.

In Example C, the a/A ratio is $80/306 = 0.26$. As you can see, even less available oxygen is getting into the arterial blood.

Thus, even though the PaO_2 level has improved, the patient's oxygenation has deteriorated. The a/A ratio can be recalculated with changing FIO_2, giving you an objective reference to assess your patient's oxygenation status.

(continued)

Equations *(continued)*

ESTIMATING VENTILATION
Explanation

You can use the following equation to calculate new ventilator settings to manipulate a patient's $Paco_2$ level.

Equation

$$\frac{\text{Present } Paco_2 \times}{\text{present } \dot{V}E} = \frac{\text{desired } Paco_2 \times}{\text{desired } \dot{V}E}$$

The minute volume (respiratory rate times tidal volume, $\dot{V}E$) is inversely related to $Paco_2$. That is, if minute volume increases, $Paco_2$ decreases and vice versa.

Example D: Mr. Smith is on a mechanical ventilator with a tidal volume of 800 ml at a rate of 10. His $Paco_2$ level is 60 mm Hg. The doctor wants to decrease his $Paco_2$ level to 48 mm Hg. Using the equation given:

$$\frac{\text{Present } Paco_2 \times}{\text{present } \dot{V}E} = \frac{\text{Desired } Paco_2 \times}{\text{Desired } \dot{V}E}$$

$$60 \times (800 \times 10) = 48 \times$$

$$60 \times 8,000 = 48 \times$$
$$480,000 = 48 \times$$
$$10,000ml = \times = \text{desired } \dot{V}E$$

You now have a choice: you can leave the rate at 10 and increase the tidal volume to 1,000 ml, or you can leave the tidal volume at 800 ml and increase the rate to 12. (*Note:* This equation is effective only if the patient's condition remains stable without complicating pulmonary factors, such as intrapulmonary shunting.)

ESTIMATING COMPLIANCE
Explanation

Compliance reflects lung stiffness, indirectly showing how easily the lungs can be ventilated. In a mechanically ventilated patient, you can estimate compliance from inspiratory pressure (shown on the manometer on a volume-cycled ventilator) and the tidal volume.

Dynamic compliance refers to lung elasticity during airflow—while the breath is delivered. It's measured using the peak inspiratory pressure appearing on the manometer. (In mea-suring compliance, consider the pressure change from baseline most important; therefore, subtract positive end-expiratory pressure (PEEP) from the pressure registered.)

Equation

$$\text{Compliance} = \frac{\text{volume}}{\text{pressure}}$$

Volume here refers to tidal volume; you can use the tidal volume set on the ventilator when using this equation.

One compliance value provides less information than serial values indicating a trend. Increasing compliance signals greater lung elasticity resulting in easier ventilation. Decreasing compliance indicates that lungs are becoming stiffer, usually from fluid accumulation, as in pulmonary edema or interstitial changes occurring in adult respiratory distress syndrome. Normal compliance values vary from one patient to the next; for best results, compare your patient's values over time rather than comparing them to a normal value.

Example E: Mr. Baker was admitted after a myocardial infarction and cardiac arrest. He's on a mechanical ventilator with a tidal volume of 1,000 ml, a peak inspiratory pressure of 30 cm H_2O, and PEEP of 5 cm H_2O.

To calculate compliance (C):

$$C = \frac{1,000}{30\text{-}5}$$
$$= \frac{1,000}{25}$$
$$= 40 \text{ ml/cm } H_2O$$

Four hours later, Mr. Baker's tidal volume remains at 1,000, and his PEEP remains at 5. However, his peak inspiratory pressure has increased to 45.

To calculate compliance:

$$C = \frac{1,000}{45\text{-}5}$$
$$= \frac{1,000}{40}$$
$$= 25 \text{ ml/cm } H_2O$$

Equations *(continued)*

Thus, his compliance has decreased—a change accompanied by falling blood pressure and increased pulmonary capillary wedge pressure. Pulmonary edema from pump failure has made his lungs more difficult to ventilate.

DURATION OF FLOW FROM AN OXYGEN TANK
Explanation
This simple formula allows you to calculate how long a small or large oxygen tank will last, giving you ample time to prepare a replacement tank in advance.

Equation
Duration (D) of flow (minutes) $= \dfrac{\text{gauge psi} \times \text{factor}}{\text{LPM}}$

Here's the value of the factor for each type of tank:
• E oxygen cylinder (a small cylinder)—0.28
• H & K oxygen cylinder (large cylinders)—3.14.

LPM value is the number of liters of oxygen the patient is receiving per minute. The gauge psi is the pounds per square inch which is shown on the gauge on the oxygen tank. This is 2,200 psi on a full tank of oxygen.

Example F: Mr. Ingram is using a nasal cannula continuously at 2 LPM. To calculate how long (D) a large oxygen cylinder would last with a gauge psi of 2,200, use this formula:

$$D = \frac{(2{,}200 \text{ [psi]} \times 3.14)}{2}$$
$$= \frac{6{,}908}{2}$$
$$= 3{,}454 \text{ minutes}$$

To calculate D in days (24 hours = 1,440 minutes), use this formula:

$$D = \frac{3{,}454 \text{ minutes}}{1{,}440 \text{ minutes}}$$
$$= 2.4 \text{ days}$$

For a small tank:

$$D = \frac{2{,}200 \text{ (psi)} \times 0.28}{2}$$
$$= \frac{616}{2}$$
$$= 313 \text{ minutes; or } 5 \text{ hours, } 13 \text{ minutes}$$

Pulmonary Rehabilitation Program

The progressively debilitating effects of a chronic pulmonary disease can limit a patient's work capacity, daily activities, and psychosocial outlook. These effects may also require recurrent hospitalization. To minimize these consequences, the doctor may recommend a pulmonary rehabilitation program designed to improve the patient's activity level and to teach him about measures to prevent disease exacerbation. However, the effectiveness of such a rehabilitation program in reversing the disease process hasn't been established. The following information serves as a general review of the definition, goals, and components of a typical pulmonary rehabilitation program.

DEFINITION

A pulmonary rehabilitation program is an individually tailored multidisciplinary program involving therapy, emotional support, and education to stabilize or reverse the physiologic and psychopathologic effects of pulmonary disease. Such a program also attempts to restore the patient to the maximal functional capacity that his pulmonary handicap and overall life-style will allow.

GOALS

The general goals described below may be accompanied by individualized patient goals—for example, gardening or walking around the block without becoming short of breath.

• Reduce the frequency of hospitalizations by promoting improved health and providing comprehensive outpatient support in the most cost-effective manner.

• Shorten hospital length of stay for patients whose medical, nursing, and other needs can be met at home or through an outpatient program.

• Increase exercise tolerance, functional level, and work capacity through a comprehensive, progressively graded exercise program, thereby appropriately encouraging a return to activities of daily living and vocational endeavors.

• Create a positive patient attitude toward accepting responsibility for personal health and thereby attaining and maintaining optimal physical and psychological functioning.

• Teach the patient and family about pulmonary disease, including its causes, effects, risk factors, and management. Involve the family in the patient's recovery or in maintaining optimal patient functions.

• Prevent and promptly recognize exacerbations secondary to infection or cardiac and respiratory failure and, through proper health maintenance, avoid future hospitalization.

STAGES OF A REHABILITATION PROGRAM

Stage 1 (inpatient)

This stage begins when the patient is first referred to the program. The initial goal is to provide pulmonary hygiene when needed and to teach symptom recognition and self-management. The beginning concepts of exercise tolerance and pulmonary rehabilitation are explained. During this stage, the patient is seen at least once a day, or more often if indicated.

Stage 2 (outpatient)

This stage starts when the patient is medically stable and ready to commit himself to the program. It's designed to improve exercise tolerance and to provide the education and psychological support that will enable the patient to attain his optimal level of health and functioning. The patient participates in hour-long sessions twice a week for 14 weeks.

ADMISSION CRITERIA

• Referral by the attending doctor
• For stage 1, a clinical diagnosis of symptomatic chronic obstructive

Pulmonary Rehabilitation Program *(continued)*

or restrictive pulmonary disease
• For stage 2, chronic obstructive or restrictive pulmonary disease and medical stability

CONTRAINDICATIONS FOR ADMITTANCE TO STAGE 2
• Significant pulmonary disease, such as active tuberculosis, neoplasm, pulmonary embolus, or acute pulmonary infection
• Any other disabling medical problem, such as uncontrolled diabetes mellitus, renal insufficiency, or hepatic insufficiency
• Significant cardiac impairment, such as uncontrolled dysrhythmia
• Disorientation or psychological instability
• Refusal to stop smoking during the exercise program or teaching sessions
• Acute illness, such as fever, gastrointestinal bleeding, or influenza
• Failure to sign an informed consent form

PROGRAM COMPONENTS
• Chest physiotherapy and respiratory therapy
• Individualized, monitored exercise program
• Educational program that includes information about:
—the purpose of pulmonary rehabilitation
—exercise principles
—the anatomy and physiology of respiratory disease
—the pathophysiology of pulmonary disease
—risk factors and life-style modifications
—work simplification and energy conservation methods related to activities of daily living
—diet and nutrition
—medications, indications, and contraindications
—symptom management and breathing retraining
—stress management and relaxation exercises
—sexuality issues
—vocational outlook
—oxygen therapy
—equipment management
• Professional social services
• Psychological counseling, as indicated
• Occupational and physical therapy, as required

Abbreviations and symbols

ABG Arterial blood gas

A/C MODE Assist/control mode

ARDS Adult respiratory distress syndrome

ARF Acute respiratory failure

BPD Bronchopulmonary dysplasia

CF Cystic fibrosis

CO Carbon monoxide

CO_2 Carbon dioxide

COLD Chronic obstructive lung disease

COPD Chronic obstructive pulmonary disease

CPAP Continuous positive-airway pressure

DLco Diffusing capacity for carbon monoxide

EGTA Esophageal gastric tube airway

EOA Esophageal obdurator airway

ERV Expiratory reserve volume

FEF Forced expiratory flow

FEV Forced expiratory volume

FEV_1 Forced expiratory volume in the 1st second

FIo_2 Fraction of inspired oxygen

H^+ Hydrogen ion

HbO_2 Oxyhemoglobin

HCO_3^- Bicarbonate ion

H_2CO_3 Carbonic acid

HFJV High-frequency jet ventilation

HFV High-frequency ventilation

IC Inspiratory capacity

IMV Intermittent mandatory ventilation

IPPB Intermittent positive-pressure breathing

IRDS Infant respiratory distress syndrome

IRV Inspiratory reserve volume

MBC Maximum breathing capacity

MDI Metered-dose inhaler

MLT Minimal leak technique

MMEF Maximal midexpiratory flow

MOV Minimal occlusive volume

MVV Maximal voluntary ventilation

NIF Negative inspiratory force

O_2 Oxygen

O_2Sat Oxygen saturation

$Paco_2$ Partial pressure of carbon dioxide in arterial blood

PAo_2 Partial pressure of oxygen in the alveolar air

Pao_2 Partial pressure of oxygen in arterial blood

PAP Pulmonary artery pressure

PAWP Pulmonary artery wedge pressure

PB Barometric pressure

Pco_2 Partial pressure of carbon dioxide

PCWP Pulmonary capillary wedge pressure

PE Pulmonary embolism

PEEP Positive end-expiratory pressure

PEFR Peak expiratory flow rate

PFT Pulmonary function test

Po_2 Partial pressure of oxygen

RV Residual volume

SIMV Synchronized intermittent mandatory ventilation

Svo_2 Mixed venous oxygen saturation

TGV Thoracic gas volume

TLC Total lung capacity

TV Tidal volume

VC Vital capacity

$\dot{V}E$ Minute volume or minute ventilation

$\dot{V}/\dot{Q}$ Ventilation/perfusion ratio

Pulmonary Toxicity: Causative Drugs

Anaphylaxis

- Cephalosporins
- Immune globulins, vaccines, and toxoids
- Insulin
- Iodinated drugs and contrast media
- Lidocaine
- Penicillins
- Procaine
- Streptokinase
- Streptomycin

Bronchospasm or airway obstruction

- Beta-blocking agents
- Cephalosporins
- Cholinergic agonists
- Nonsteroidal anti-inflammatory agents
- Penicillins
- Pentazocine
- Streptomycin
- Drugs containing tartrazine (FD&C Yellow No. 5—a coloring agent used in some tablets)

Respiratory depression or arrest

- Aminoglycosides
- Barbiturates
- Benzodiazepines
- Opiates (narcotic analgesics)
- Polymyxin B
- Streptomycin
- Trimethaphan

Pulmonary infiltrates, edema, or fibrosis

- Amiodarone
- Amphotericin B
- Bleomycin
- Busulfan
- Carbamazepine
- Carmustine (BCNU)
- Colchicine
- Cyclophosphamide
- Gold salts
- Hydrochlorothiazide
- Iodinated drugs and contrast media
- Melphalan
- Nonsteroidal anti-inflammatory agents
- Opiates
- Penicillins
- Phenytoin

INDEX

i refers to an illustration, t to a table

C

i refers to an illustration, t to a table

J

K

L

I

i refers to an illustration, t to a table

M

N

i refers to an illustration, t to a table

i refers to an illustration, t to a table

W

i refers to an illustration, t to a table

Notes

Notes